Clinical Manual of Gerontological Nursing

Clinical Manual of Gerontological Nursing

Mildred O. Hogstel, Ph.D., R.N., C.

Editor
Abell-Hanger Professor of Gerontological Nursing
Harris College of Nursing
Texas Christian University
Fort Worth, Texas

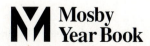
Mosby
Year Book

St. Louis   Baltimore   Boston   Chicago   London   Philadelphia   Sydney   Toronto

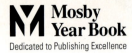
Mosby
Year Book
Dedicated to Publishing Excellence

Editor: Linda L. Duncan
Developmental Editor: Kathy Sartori
Project Manager: Barbara Merritt
Editing and Production: University Graphics
Designer: Jeanne Wolfgeher

Mosby–Year Book, Inc.
11830 Westline Industrial Drive
St. Louis, Missouri 63146

The following pages may be duplicated for use in clinical practice: 34, 44, 56, 64, 76, 80, 85, 89, 100, 104, 109, 113, 119, 130, 135, 138, 149, 155, 156, 164, 165, 169, 172, 178, 185, 191, 193, 195, 198, 209, 214, 216, 221, 229, 236, 242, 243, 249, 250, 251

International Standard Book Number 0-8016-2814-8

92 93 94 95 96 GW/VH 9 8 7 6 5 4 3 2 1

To my father,
who at age 95
is my inspiration

PREFACE

The purpose of this *Manual* is to provide a clear, concise, practical guide to the specialized nursing care of older adults. The nursing implications presented are based on theories, facts, and principles that nurses must know to provide quality care to older adults in a variety of clinical settings. Older adults have many unique needs and problems. Those who have an acute illness often show symptoms and responses to treatment that are different from those shown by younger adults. Many older adults have one or more chronic health problems that interfere with their quality and quantity of life. Some have minor symptoms and health problems that can lead to acute illness and disability if not recognized and treated early. Prompt attention to these problems is essential to avoid the need for long-term care.

Nurses have a professional responsibility and obligation to become aware of the special needs and problems of older adults. This *Manual* focuses on the unique, special, and often covert health problems of older adults, presenting them in a way that will enable the nurse to establish priorities and concentrate on providing the most effective nursing care possible. The content is primarily organized around the most common medical problems older adults have in each of the various body systems. For each medical condition, basic definitions are followed by a discussion of the pathophysiology, signs and symptoms, common diagnostic procedures, medical management including pharmacology, prognosis (if appropriate), and nursing management based on the nursing process with special emphasis on discharge planning and teaching older adults. Essential information is presented in short paragraph, outline, table, figure, and box format for easy access and quick reference by the busy nurse. Sample nursing care plans, with practical nursing interventions, are included for many of the most common medical diagnoses. These care plans will be helpful to nurses in hospitals, nursing homes, outpatient clinics, physician's offices, outpatient surgery centers, and agencies providing hospice and home health care.

Chapter 1 presents an introduction to some of the demographics and definitions important in gerontological nursing. Nursing implications related to the common physical, psychological, and sociocultural aspects of aging are also presented. In Chapter 2, two certified ger-

ontological nurse practitioners who work with older adults in several settings give a thorough overview of the assessment of older adults. Chapter 3 summarizes the basic information nurses need to know about the administration, absorption, distribution, biotransformation, and excretion of medications in older adults. Chapters 4 through 12 cover the medical and nursing management of the most common medical problems of older adults. Chapter 13 summarizes components of discharge planning for older adults and suggests important guidelines and techniques for use in teaching this age group. Throughout the *Manual,* guides for discharge planning and teaching are presented in large print. Nurses may make copies of these guides for distribution to older patients and their families during the process of discharge planning and teaching.

The appendixes include the American Nurses' Association Standards of Gerontological Nursing Practice, sample assessment tools, and a list of organizations and journals helpful to nurses caring for older adults. Because this *Manual* is primarily a concise, quick reference to essential facts, the reader should refer to the general bibliography at the back of the book for a list of books that will provide greater depth and breadth on specific topics as needed.

Some of the information in this *Manual* may be new to graduate nurses and students who have not had a specific course in gerontological nursing or have had limited exposure to this topic in their nursing curriculums. Also, new information is being discovered every day through research and is made available through publication, workshops, seminars, and symposiums. It is important for nurses to recognize that older patients do have special and unique needs. Doing so will help nurses provide the quality nursing care these patients deserve.

Appreciation is expressed to all of the authors who contributed their knowledge and expertise to this manual, to Peggy Mayfield for reviewing and making valuable suggestions on several chapters, to Susan Moore, Esther Ochoa, Melissa McInnis, and Martha Thomas for their excellent typing assistance, and to Tim Kuchta for some of the sketches.

Mildred O. Hogstel

CONTRIBUTORS

Marta A. Browning, M.S.N., R.N.
Assistant Professor
Department of Nursing
Temple University College of Allied Health
Philadelphia, Pennsylvania

Lisa L. Havens, M.S.N., R.N., C.C.R.N.
Cardiovascular Clinical Nurse Specialist
Formerly Methodist Medical Center
Dallas, Texas

Mildred O. Hogstel, Ph.D., R.N., C.
Abell-Hanger Professor of Gerontological Nursing
Harris College of Nursing
Texas Christian University
Fort Worth, Texas

Peggy Mayfield, M.S.N., R.N.
Adult Nurse Practitioner
Associate Professor Emeritus
Harris College of Nursing
Texas Christian University
Fort Worth, Texas

Pamela F. Millsap, M.S.N., R.N., C.
Gerontological Nurse Practitioner
Gerontological Assessment and Planning Program
Department of Medicine
Division of Geriatrics
Texas College of Osteopathic Medicine
Fort Worth, Texas

Ann S. Reban, M.S.N., R.N., C.
Gerontological Nurse Practitioner
Gerontological Assessment and Planning Program
Research Associate
Center for Studies in Aging
University of North Texas
Denton, Texas

Clinical Instructor
Department of Medicine
Texas College of Osteopathic Medicine
Fort Worth, Texas

Carol A. Stephenson, Ed.D., R.N.
Associate Professor of Nursing
Harris College of Nursing
Texas Christian University
Fort Worth, Texas

Danna Strength, D.N.Sc., R.N.
Assistant Professor of Nursing
Harris College of Nursing
Texas Christian University
Fort Worth, Texas

Laura Talbot, Ph.D., R.N., C.
Assistant Professor of Nursing
Harris College of Nursing
Texas Christian University
Fort Worth, Texas

Joycelyn W. Weaver, M.S.N., R.N., C.C.R.N.
Critical Care Clinical Nurse Specialist
Methodist Medical Center
Dallas, Texas

CONTENTS

Clinical Manual of
Gerontological Nursing

CHAPTER 1

Introduction

Mildred O. Hogstel

DEMOGRAPHICS

The number of older adults in our society is increasing tremendously (Table 1-1). More than 12% of the U.S. population is over age 65, and older adults are increasing not only in numbers but also in longevity. It is estimated that about 235 people reach age 100 every day (Special report on health, 1989, p. 45).

Chronic health problems increase as age increases (Table 1-2). Between 50% and 60% of the patients in general medical-surgical hospitals are estimated to be age

Table 1-1. Major demographic statistics related to the older population

Population	Number	Percentage
Persons >65 (1900)	3.1 million	4.1
Persons >65 (1989)	31 million	12.5
Older women	18.3 million	
Older men	12.6 million	
65-74 age group	18.2 million	
75-84 age group	9.8 million	
>85 age group	3.0 million	
Persons reaching age 65 in 1989 (5960/day)	2.2 million	
Married men >65		77
Married women >65		42
Racial/ethnic composition		
White >65		90
Black >65		8
Other >65		2
Institutionalized >65		5
Institutionalized >85		22
Predictions of >65 by 2000		13
Predictions of >65 by 2030		21.8

From American Association of Retired Persons and Administration on Aging (1990). A profile of older Americans, Washington, DC, US Department of Health and Human Services.

Table 1-2. Most frequently occurring health problems of older adults

Problem	Percentage
Arthritis	49
Hypertension	37
Heart disease	30
Hearing impairment	32
Orthopedic impairments	16
Cataracts	17
Sinusitis	17
Diabetes	9
Tinnitus	8

From American Association of Retired Persons and Administration on Aging (1990). A profile of older Americans, Washington, DC, US Department of Health and Human Services.
Note: Many older people have multiple chronic health problems.

65 or older. This age group "accounted for 33% of all hospital stays and 44% of all days of care in hospitals in 1988," and their hospital stays averaged 8.9 days whereas those of people below age 65 averaged only 5.4 days (American Association of Retired Persons and Administration on Aging, 1990, p. 14).

DEFINITIONS

gerontological nursing Comprehensive assessment and management of the physical, mental, psychological, socioeconomic, and cultural aspects of the nursing care of older adults in a variety of settings

geriatrics Study and treatment of the diseases of older adults by physicians

gerontology A multidisciplinary approach to the study of factors affecting older people

geriatric nursing The care of older patients with medical problems

gerontic nursing A term preferred by some to refer to the nursing care of older adults

ageism A negative stereotyped view of old age (for example, use of the word *senile*)

life expectancy The number of years an individual can be expected to live based on the year of birth

life span The total number of years that a human being is capable of living (probably 110 to 120)

longevity Long duration of individual life (e.g., reaching 90s and 100s)

senescence Biological aging

young-old Ages 55 to 65

old Ages 65 to 85

old-old Over age 85

COMMON PHYSICAL CHANGES

The process of aging begins at conception and continues until death. Each individual ages at a different rate, and each organ system within an individual may age at a different rate. Biological age is more important than chronological age. Some individuals age faster than others, possibly because of genetic makeup, lifestyle, and environment.

Aging is not a disease, although many diseases increase as a person ages. One of the major problems in gerontology is determining what is normal aging and what is disease. Perhaps it is better to describe aging changes as *common* rather than *normal* because it is not

known what is normal. The major biological theories of aging are categorized in Table 1-3, and Table 1-4 lists the most common, not necessarily pathological, aging changes that occur in each major organ system along with some of the most important nursing implications related to each change where appropriate. Assessment for these changes is presented in Chapter 2. Problems and nursing management related to each system are given in Chapters 4 through 12.

Table 1-3. Biological theories of aging

Category	Theory
Wear and tear theories	Free radical—Free radicals disrupt normal chemical bonds
	Lipofuscin accumulation—Insoluble lipid pigments increase
	Cross-linkage—Molecules are linked and DNA is damaged
Genetic programming theories	Finite doubling potential—Cells can divide just so many times
	Immunological—Decreased immune system produces autoimmune problems
	Neuroendocrine—All changes are due to losses in neurologic and endocrine systems

Data compiled from Graves (1988, pp. 63-64).

Table 1-4. Common physical changes of aging and related nursing implications

System	Changes	Nursing implications
Integumentary		
Skin	Thin	Keep intact, clean, free of injury.
	Fragile	
	Dry	Use emollient lotions.
	Decreased elasticity	Check turgor on forehead, chest, abdomen.
	Increased wrinkles	Use lotions, massage, cosmetics (female), beard (male).
	Less perspiration	No deodorants are needed.
Hair	Gray	Color if desired.
	Fine	Prevent damage from tight braids, hair curlers.
	Thin	
	Alopecia	Use wig, medication (men).
	Decreased body hair	
	Increased facial hair	
	Lips, chin—women	Remove hair.
	Ears, eyebrows—men	Trim excess hair.
Nails	Hard	Keep clean. Dry well between toes. Use manicure stick instead of nail file because of less trauma.
	Thick	
	Hypertrophied	
	Brittle	
	Friable	
	Scaly	

Table 1-4. Common physical changes of aging and related nursing implications—cont'd

System	Changes	Nursing implications
	Opaque	Refer to podiatrist for cutting.
	Split	Teach to wear clean hose (socks) and shoes at all times.
	Onychomycosis (fungus)	Observe for infection. Refer for treatment if severe.
Sensory		
Eyes	Decreased acuity	Provide large-print reading materials and labels in home (e.g., stove dials and telephone dial).
	Decreased pupil size	
	Greater sensitivity to glare	Use well-diffused light.
	Lens become yellow, thick, stiff; crack	Use yellows, reds, and oranges instead of purples, pinks, or blues.
	Arcus senilis (lipid deposits around iris)	Does not affect vision.
	Impaired accommodation	Have well-lit stairs, steps, rooms.
	Poorer night vision	Teach care while walking and driving at night.
	Poorer peripheral vision	
	Dark, puffy or sunken tissue under eyes	Decrease or increase fluids Use appropriate cosmetics.
	Less tearing	Use artificial tears.
Ears	Increase in hard, thick cerumen	Soften and wash out with care. Refer to otologist if needed.
	Impaired balance	Teach to rise and move slowly.
Taste	Decreased sensitivity of taste buds, especially to bitterness and salt	Make foods look attractive. Add seasonings other than salt (e.g., lemon, other spices if tolerated).
	Decreased saliva production	Encourage frequent oral hygiene.
Smell	Decreased sensation	Warn about possibility of fires, smoke, spoiled food.
Tactile	Decreased perception to touch	Prevent injuries from extreme heat or cold.
Cardiovascular		
	Heart increased in size	Have physical exam yearly and before beginning any exercise program.
	Cardiac muscle atrophies	
	Decreased density of collagen fibers	
	Decreased elastic fibers	
	Endocardium thickens	
	Decreased contractile force	
	Aortic and mitral valves stiffen	
	Pacemaker cells decrease	Take pulse monthly.
	Cardiac output decreases 40% by age 65	If allowed, exercise (e.g., walking) 20 min a day three times a week.
	Sluggish blood flow	
	Ventricular and atrial premature contractions increase	Limit fat, salt, calories, cholesterol in diet.
	Increased collagen and stiffness	Stop smoking.
	Decreased elasticity of all vessels	Reduce stress. Follow medication regimen exactly.
	Increased pulse pressure	Take blood pressure monthly.
	Decreased diastolic pressure (e.g., 140/40)	

Continued.

Table 1-4. Common physical changes of aging and related nursing implications—cont'd

System	Changes	Nursing implications
Respiratory		
	Decreased vital capacity and diffusing capacity	Avoid large crowds to prevent upper respiratory infections.
	Increased collagen in lung	Encourage influenza and pneumonia vaccines.
	Decreased lung elasticity	
	Increased lung size	Exercise as for cardiovascular system.
	Thoracic cage stiffens due to decreased bone and respiratory muscle mass and kyphoscoliosis	Avoid oversedation.
	Abdominal and diaphragmatic respiration decrease	Prevent aspiration.
	Loss of lung elastic recoil	Provide adequate hydration.
	Decreased ability to cough	Give frequent oral hygiene.
	High risk for aspiration because of dysphagia, less ciliary activity	
Musculoskeletal		
Muscles	Decreased muscle mass, size, strength; increased fat, collagen, interstitial fluid	Maintain physical activity through regular mild exercise (walking is best for all older age groups).
	Muscle atrophy	
	Increased flexion contractures	
	Leg cramps	Assess diet.
	Restless legs	Prevent falls.
Bones	Decreased bone mass and density	Maintain good posture and safe exercise.
	More porous bones	
	Decrease in height of 1-4 inches between ages 20 and 90	Assure adequate nutrition, especially calcium.
	Increased kyphosis	
	Less flexible rib cage	
	Joints less mobile	Take hormones if appropriate.
	Decreased bone marrow function	
Endocrine		
	Decreased glucose intolerance	Check blood glucose and thyroid hormone level yearly and compare to norms for age group.
	Higher blood glucose levels; increase 1-2 mg/dl (fasting) per decade	
	Decreased thyroid hormone	
	Absence of fever when infection present	Report oral temperature of 99° F or more.
Hematological		
	No change in hemoglobin hematocrit, white blood cells (WBC), or platelets	Anemias are due to causes other than chronological age (e.g., bleeding or inadequate diet).
	Decreased bone marrow function	White blood cells may not increase with infection.
Gastrointestinal		
Mouth	Teeth worn down, transparent, dark	Provide nutritious foods able to be chewed.
	Gum recedes	Provide frequent mouth care.
		Prevent periodontal disease and eventual loss of teeth.
	Lips turn in and nose down	
Esophagus	Dilated	Keep in semi-Fowler's position for 30 min to 1 hr after eating.
	Thin	

Table 1-4. Common physical changes of aging and related nursing implications—cont'd

System	Changes	Nursing implications
	Dysphagia	Observe for choking and aspiration while eating and drinking.
Stomach	Gastric mucosa thins	Eat five small meals a day instead of three large ones.
	Decreased secretion of acids and digestive enzymes	
	Decreased hunger contractions	Restrict caffeine, fats, chocolate, spices.
	Decreased gastric emptying	
Intestines	Atrophy of muscle layer and mucosa	Provide high-bulk nutritious diet with adequate fruits and vegetables.
	Decreased tone of smooth muscle	
	Decreased peristalsis	
	Decreased sensation for defecation	
	Decreased absorption of calcium and vitamins	
Genitourinary		
Kidney	Loss of one third to one half of nephrons by age 80	
	Loss of 50% of glomerular filtration by age 70-80	
	Decreased creatinine production	
	Decreased excretion of drugs	Observe for medication overdose and toxicity.
	Decreased thirst	Maintain at least 2000 ml fluid intake/24 hr.
Bladder	Decreases in size and becomes funnel shaped	Assist to void, if needed, as soon as possible.
	Decreased muscle tone	
	Decreased control	Keep clean and dry.
	Increased frequency	Provide bladder training and Kegel exercises if needed.
Uterus	Decreased size	
Ovaries	Decreased hormone production	Estrogen replacement therapy may be helpful.
Fallopian tubes	Decreased length	
Vagina	Shortens; muscles and mucosa thin	Suggest artificial lubrication if intercourse is painful.
	Decreased vaginal secretions	
	Loss of labia firmness	
Testes	Decreased sperm production	
Seminal fluid	Decreased volume and viscosity	
Prostate	Hypertrophies	Assess for benign prostatic hypertrophy and nodules, urinary output, and infection.
Nervous		
	Loss of neurons	Keep active mentally.
	Brain loses water, weight, and size	
	Cells degenerate	Assess mental status yearly for noninstitutionalized and monthly for institutionalized patients.
	Increased senile plaques	
	Decreased cerebral blood flow	
	Decreased nerve conduction velocity	
	Decreased functioning of hypothalamus	Maintain comfortable temperature of environment (72°-78° F).
		Assess and treat low-grade fever (99° F) promptly.
	Decreased quality (not quantity) of sleep	Encourage exercise.
		Reduce stress.

Data compiled from Burggraf and Stanley (1989), Graves (1988), and Jones (1988).

COMMON PSYCHOLOGICAL CHANGES

Nurses and others who work with and care for older people also need to be aware of the common psychological changes that occur in the aging process as well as those characteristics that do not change. The major psychological changes of aging together with samples of related nursing implications are summarized in Table 1-5.

Table 1-5. Common psychological changes of aging and related nursing implications

Characteristic	Changes	Nursing implications
Stress	Increased if multiple physical problems	Assess and help with problems early.
Reaction time	Slowed response to sensory stimuli	Wait for verbal response.
		Validate cues.
		Assure effective communication.
		Teach safety while driving.
	Slower pace	Do not rush with nursing care or mobility.
		Be patient.
Intelligence	No decline until a few years before death	Treat with respect as intelligent adult human beings.
	Affected by decreased attention span and hearing and seeing problems	Check ears and eyes.
		Clean glasses.
	Decreased motivation to do well on standardized intelligence tests	Look for new ways to test intelligence in old age.
Learning	No major change until late 80s or 90s	Older people *can* learn.
	More cautious and hesitant; afraid to make errors for fear of being called "senile"	Decrease stress.
		Provide a quiet environment.
		Speak slower.
	Will learn useful information—what they need and want to know	Present needed information slower in small sections at a time.
		Goals should be clear.
	Vocabulary increases; learning new motor skills declines.	Provide for repetition when learning new motor skills (e.g., testing blood for glucose level).
Problem-solving	Use previous experiences for solutions	Relate new problems to old experiences.
	More cautious	Do not push.
		Give choices.
		Be supportive
Memory		
Immediate (seconds)	Rarely impaired	Assess (e.g., ask nurse's name seconds after introduction).
Recent (24 hr to 1 week)	May be impaired	Assess (e.g., ask what the patient had for breakfast).
		Practice memory of recent events.
		Stimulate recall of recent events to help person remember.
		Do not embarrass because of decreased memory—decreases self-esteem.
Remote (many years earlier)	Usually not impaired	Assess (e.g., ask about year of marriage).
		Use reminiscence to talk about happy events in the past (anyone can do); life review (evaluation of life) should be used only by a skilled therapist.
Attitudes	No major changes throughout life	Respect different sociocultural and economic attitudes and values.
Values		
Interests	Changes in physical condition, family, environment, and economic status may change interests	Help substitute new interests more appropriate for current status.
Self-concept	Feelings of self-esteem often decrease	Help with general hygiene and appearance.
	Sense of belonging is lost (home and work)	Encourage to keep personal belongings (pictures, furniture).
	Fewer successes	Reward and compliment when appropriate.
	Many losses (friends, family, income) decrease self-concept	Encourage to meet new friends.

Table 1-5. Common psychological changes of aging and related nursing implications—cont'd

Characteristic	Changes	Nursing implications
Personality	No basic change May become exaggerated (more of the same) Some withdraw and become severely depressed Some become more aggressive and paranoid (especially if multiple health problems)	Refer for a specific diagnosis and treatment if a sudden change in behavior occurs. Refer for treatment. Be calm, accepting, and patient.
Emotions	May become more labile	Assess for possible problems needing diagnosis and treatment.

Data compiled from Hogstel (1990) and Lancaster and Simpson (1988).

Table 1-6. Sociological theories of aging and related nursing implications

Theory	Explanation	Nursing implications
Disengagement	Proposed in early 1960s Mutual withdrawal of older person from society and society from older person Older person is free to "sit in a rocking chair" Society needs to make room for the younger age group	This theory is not accepted by most gerontologists.
Activity	Developed in opposition to disengagement theory and widely accepted Successful aging implies keeping as physically and mentally active as possible Life satisfaction increases when activity increases The more activities, the more role supports	Help older people to develop new roles to replace old roles and new friends to replace lost friends (e.g., volunteer instead of employee).
Continuity	Maintaining the same patterns of living through life If active in young adulthood, active in old age If inactive in young adulthood, inactive in old age	Assess types of activities preferred. Do not push older people to participate in activities they do not care for.

Data compiled from Jones (1988, pp. 53-54).

SOCIOLOGICAL THEORIES OF AGING

The three major sociological theories of aging are presented in Table 1-6. Older people might naturally fit into one of these theories, depending on their personal and individual situations, interests, and environments. Although the activity theory is the one considered to be most related to successful aging, some older people prefer to be less active physically and socially because that has been their lifestyle all of their lives. They should not, therefore, be forced to participate in physical and social activities when they seem to be happy, content, and relaxed in the lifestyle they have chosen. For example, a nursing home resident who prefers to be alone, read, or watch television and is doing well should be allowed to

do so rather than be continually asked to participate in group exercises or other social activities.

SUMMARY

Many physiological, psychological, and sociocultural changes occur in the aging process. However, older people are not homogeneous. In fact, they probably differ more than any other age group because of their differing backgrounds, lifelong experiences, and interests. They do not feel the need to "keep up with the Joneses" or be like everyone else. Many reach a point where they feel secure and satisfied with their lives.

Nurses need to be aware of the unique differences and needs of older people, incorporating the knowledge of these differences and needs into the nursing process in all clinical settings.

REFERENCES

American Association of Retired Persons and Administration on Aging (1990). A profile of older Americans, Washington, DC, US Department of Health and Human Services.

Burggraf V and Stanley M, editors (1989). Nursing the elderly: A care plan approach, Philadelphia, JB Lippincott Co.

Graves M (1988). Physiologic changes. In Hogstel MO, editor: Nursing care of the older adult, ed 2, New York, John Wiley & Sons, Inc, pp 63-90.

Hogstel MO (1990). Geropsychiatric nursing, St Louis, Mosby–Year Book, Inc.

Jones A (1988). Developmental changes. In Hogstel MO, editor: Nursing care of the older adult, ed 2, New York, John Wiley & Sons, Inc, pp 42-47, 53-54.

Lancaster J and Simpson KR (1988). Psychologic changes. In Hogstel MO, editor: Nursing care of the older adult, New York, John Wiley & Sons, Inc, pp 91-115.

Special report on health (1989). Knoxville, Tenn, Whittle Communications LP.

CHAPTER 2

Assessment of Older Adults

Ann S. Reban
Pamela F. Millsap

The nurse can look and not see, can listen and not hear. Being perceptive is an important key to assessing the health of older individuals, given the frequent biopsychosocial complexity of their situations. In *Webster's Ninth New Collegiate Dictionary, perceptive* is defined as "responsive to sensory stimulus: DISCERNING . . . capable of or exhibiting keen perception: OBSERVANT . . . characterized by sympathetic understanding or insight." In some instances, perceptual powers can be heightened. It is important when approaching health assessment with the older adult to purposely put one's "antennae" out. Realizing that older people defy generalization and that they are more heterogeneous than younger populations can stimulate one's interest in perceptively gathering data on each older individual presenting for health assessment.

Assessment is that important first step in the nursing process. Assessing the older individual requires a holistic approach that takes into account many elements. Perceptive data collection allows interventions in even seemingly small areas of concern that can make a difference to the older adult's overall functioning.

The health history and physical exam are different for the older adult than for other clients. The nurse's basic skills in history taking and physical examination require special refinements because the health history and physical examination become unique when applied to an older adult. The biological changes that occur in normal aging must be taken into account and differentiated from changes caused by disease. For example, a soft systolic heart murmur can be a normal finding in the healthy older adult.

HEALTH HISTORY

Setting the Stage

More time and patience tend to be required for taking the health history of an older adult (Burggraf and Donlon, 1985). The nurse should allow a minimum of 30 minutes and may need to gather the health history in several sessions if fatigue is a factor. Questions may have to be repeated and extra time given to respond. Establishing rapport and communication is vital to obtaining a valid health history.

Showing respect by addressing the older client as Mr., Mrs., Ms., or Miss Brown (unless an individual requests otherwise) helps to establish rapport. Above all, the nurse must avoid a patronizing manner, even when faced with obvious functional and cognitive deficits (Stokes, Rauckhorst, and Mezey, 1980). The nurse should seat the older person in a straight-back chair, not in a low-slung lounge chair that makes rising a struggle, and should sit facing the client to facilitate eye contact and lip reading (if applicable). Small amplified listening devices with small earphones are available at nominal cost from electronics stores and should be a part of the gerontological nurse's tool kit. Such a device may be particularly effective when an older adult with hearing loss does not have a working hearing aid or will not wear one.

Other interviewing tips include eliminating background noise, lowering voice pitch, talking slowly, avoiding shouting (which obscures consonants), using commonly accepted vocabulary and simple, direct questions, and resorting to writing if necessary. A visual deficit calls for frequent verbal cues and the use of touch to establish rapport. Touch is also useful in redirecting older clients who get off track when providing their personal health history.

Focused Data Collection

Taking a functional approach to the assessment process means determining where the older person fits on a continuum between dependency and independence. The first step in this process is to discover what brings the older adult to the health assessment encounter. This involves asking older clients how they view their health in general and trying to gather information on their use of the health care system. Who is their primary care physician? Are specialists, nurses, or therapists involved? Client satisfaction with current medical care may influence compliance with the physician's recommendations and affect care planning.

Chief concerns or complaints should be explored. Are these long-standing or of recent origin? What changes have taken place? When? How have these changes affected everyday functioning? How is the individual coping?

Because of the frequently encountered problems of sensory loss and cognitive deficit, these same exploratory questions need to be asked of the frail older client's family or significant other. In this case, gathering the health history is very much a family affair from start to finish.

Vague symptoms mentioned by the older person or a family member deserve attention. Loss of interest, fatigue, confusion, weight loss, or a change in behavior such as grooming are examples. Infections, malignancies, stroke, heart failure, myocardial infarction, and dehydration are among the conditions that may present atypically (Andresen, 1989; Santo-Novak, 1988). More obvious problems such as falling, bladder or bowel incontinence, or memory loss may surface.

It is important to ask follow-up questions and to use previous records in an effort to uncover information that may link vague symptomatology with events in the individual's life and later with physical examination findings. For example, visual loss might turn out to be linked to frequent falling or frequent falling may be connected to the untoward effect of an antihypertensive. Or recent widowhood might be connected to recent weight loss. Only through careful attention to detail and nuance can the nurse decide if a client is providing consistent answers, confabulating, or having difficulty with both reception and perception.

The usual list of previous hospitalizations, surgeries, illnesses, and accidents may be extensive. It should include nursing home stays.

Medication Review

Since many health problems for older adults stem from adverse reactions to medications, a medication history is critical to the assessment process. Asking the older client to bring in all medications, including over-the-counter, vitamins, supplements, and "home remedies" such as herbal preparations is the best way to obtain an accurate listing. During such a "brown bag autopsy," the nurse can ask various questions about the medications: which ones are actually taken, in what pattern, and for how long? What are their effects? Are there any adverse reactions? Are several doctors prescribing medications? Are the cost of the medications and the ease of obtaining them factors in compliance? In addition, any difficulties in medication administration can be discussed. Older clients' knowledge of the reason they are taking a specific drug and its side effects can be determined. For a comprehensive discussion of medication history as a part of the nursing assessment of older clients, see Carnevali and Enloe (1986).

Nutritional Status Screen

As normal aging proceeds, the basal metabolic rate decreases, calcium and iron absorption declines, and fat digestion is less efficient. There are declines in cell mass and lean body mass whereas total body fat increases (Spence, 1989). As a result of a number of contributing factors such as living alone, inadequate income, functional disabilities, alcoholism, and lack of knowledge about nutrition, older people are frequently deficient in total calories, calcium, iron, folate, zinc, vitamin A, ascorbic acid, thiamine, and riboflavin (Reber, 1988). Low or deficient blood levels of serum albumin, protein, and hematocrit may be present.

A 24-hour diet recall can be used to screen for lack of one or more of the basic four food groups and to learn how foods are prepared. The older client and family member should be asked whether this pattern is typical. Fluid intake, which according to Spence (1989) should be 1 liter per day with a balanced diet, needs to be assessed because older persons tend to drink less and may become dehydrated. Questions should be asked to determine whether the older client is on any special diet, such as salt restriction; whether there has been a change in appetite or weight in the past 6 months; and whether there are any problems with choking, swallowing, or chewing.

If indicated, requesting that a diet diary be kept for 1 to 3 weeks will provide additional data that can be used to verify initial impressions and to plan interventions and possible referral for nutritional counseling. Nutritional indicators such as height, weight, protein, albumin, hemoglobin, hematocrit, and white cell count are usually available to nurses assessing clients who are at nutritional risk or are nutritionally depleted (Collinsworth and Boyle, 1989).

Functional Deficits and Strengths

It is often a family member who reports deficits in the older person's ability to perform the activities of daily living (ADL), including eating, ambulation, dressing and grooming, transferring, toileting, and maintaining continence. In addition, a family member or friend must frequently step in to perform the instrumental activities of daily living (IADL)—telephoning, shopping, preparing food, doing housekeeping chores and laundry, providing transportation, and managing financial affairs. Changes tend to occur slowly, and older clients may not be aware of the gradual reduction in their ability to perform ADL and IADL independently.

Inquiry into performance of ADL and IADL leads naturally to questions about bath routine, whether or not bathroom aids and other equipment or supplies are being used.

Asking the older client and family member to describe a typical day may uncover such problems as sleep or eating disorders, depression, constipation, the occurrence of symptoms, financial hardship, or elder abuse.

Social Support Network

The nurse should assess the degree to which the formal network of service providers is involved. Is the older client visiting the local senior center, receiving home health care, or using chore service or Meals on Wheels?

The extent and effectiveness of the older client's informal support network are also evaluated. Are family members, friends, or neighbors providing assistance? What kinds? Is there caregiver strain—perhaps to the burnout stage? A home visit, if possible, provides data on the condition and layout of the older client's home, the presence or absence of environmental barriers, and safety issues, as well as further information about strengths and weaknesses in the support system.

Health Maintenance Activities

Questions related to self-care habits include frequency and kinds of health maintenance activities such as routine health checkups or regular exercise that provide information relative to the older client's health perception–health maintenance pattern. This information should include detrimental habits such as smoking, the use of chewing tobacco or snuff, and the consumption of alcohol or high levels of caffeine.

A sample of a comprehensive nursing health assessment form for use with older adults that includes space for or questions related to the list in Box 2-1 can be found in Eliopoulos (1987). This form is adaptable for use in a variety of settings. The sample form also covers identifying information, family profile, and other social data, and incorporates physical and mental status assessment. The reader is referred to Nelson and Mayfield (1988) for additional explanations of the components of the health history as applied to older persons.

Box 2-1.

Important primary components of the health history for the older client

Focused data collection
Subjective view of current health
Current use of health care system
Chief concern or complaint
Other symptomatology
Past illnesses, accidents, and use of health care system
Medication review
Nutritional status screen
Functional deficits and strengths
Social support network
Health maintenance activities

Note: Review of systems is a part of the standard health history but is covered later in this chapter under the system-by-system physical assessment.

PHYSICAL EXAMINATION
Preparation of the Client and the Environment

Preparation of older clients does not differ in the need for the examiner to offer explanations of the procedures, protection of privacy, and a chance to have questions answered. If anything, the examiner should be even more cognizant of these areas (Nelson and Mayfield, 1988). Sensory losses make it incumbent on the nurse to explain each step fully before it happens. The minimum time allowed for the physical examination of an older client should be 1 to 1½ hours. It may be necessary for the comprehensive examination to occur over two or three visits.

Again, setting the stage to allow for the changes that accompany aging is important. The examination room should be well lighted to compensate for visual deficits. Ideally, the examination room is equipped with a well-padded high-low examination table with slight elevation on the edges. These specifications help to compensate for loss of subcutaneous fat tissue, the frequently encountered limitations in mobility or cognition, and the presence of dizziness, balance, and proprioceptive problems. Leaving the older individual alone on a high examination table is very risky and should be avoided.

In the ideal room setup, two straight, sturdy arm chairs are available, one for the caregiver and one for the family member who may be in the room for parts of the health assessment process. One of the chairs provides a safe and comfortable seat while the older client undresses. The ideal gown is specially constructed of heavier cotton material, has overlapped openings in both the front and back, and is longer than most hospital gowns. A cotton flannel sheet helps to compensate for the older client's reduced skin vascularity, which leads to complaints of feeling cold.

Keeping the room temperature between 68° and 75° F also prevents chilling.

Ideally, there is a safe surface on which to carefully place removed glasses, dentures, and hearing aids and a spare corner where the quad cane or walker can be stowed temporarily. The head of the examination table can be raised to provide back support or to facilitate breathing, and the stirrups have soft, cotton terry footlets over the foot pieces to provide warmth and cushioning.

Finally, the ideal examination room contains a step stool with a hand rail, a sit-down scale to measure weight, a knee-high caliper to measure the height of a client unable to stand, and a lighted Snellen chart.

It is possible for the creative nurse to modify some existing equipment to approximate the ideal examination room, for example, through the use of padding and pillows on the examination table. A nonclinical look to the room and a slower pace will do much to forestall fatigue and ensure a more relaxed and cooperative client.

The order in which the various systems are examined may have to be adjusted so that the older client's energy is conserved. For example, a combination of gait, equilibrium, and range of motion of the legs may be evaluated at the beginning or end of the examination while the client is standing. Be prepared to assist the older client to change positions frequently in an attempt to increase comfort. System-related physical examination tips appear in the sections that follow.

Overview

Mental status assessment, general survey, and vital signs are important aspects of the health history and physical examination process. These aspects of the assessment process may occur at individualized times during the collection of data.

The mental status is assessed in an interview format during the health history. Factors that can affect the results are hearing, visual, and communication deficits. Components of a mental status examination include speech, mood and attitude, symptoms of anxiety, and cognitive tests (Eliopoulos, 1984; Bates, 1987). Cognitive tests assess orientation, level of consciousness, long- and short-term memory, and simple calculation and language skills. Many reliable instruments are available for use in testing cognition; the Mini Mental Status (Folstein, Folstein, and McHugh, 1975) is an example of such a tool.

A general survey of the client includes observation of level of consciousness, posture, gait, grooming and hygiene, manner and affect, facial expression, and speech. The general survey begins at first contact with the client and continues throughout the assessment.

Vital signs include height, weight, pulse, temperature, blood pressure, and respiratory rate. The blood pressure is always taken in both arms, first supine and then sitting and standing. Blood pressure readings taken in this manner allow assessment of postural changes that are common in older adults. Use of the proper cuff size will ensure accurate blood pressure readings.

The physical exam incorporates the skills of inspection, auscultation, percussion, and palpation in a systematic examination of each body part and system. The physical exam is presented in a system-by-system format in the boxes and tables that follow. The systems are addressed in terms of technique tips, health history questions, and physical exam/normal aging changes specific to the older client.

Integumentary System

See Boxes 2-2 and 2-3 and Table 2-1.

Box 2-2.

Health history questions—integumentary system

Does a functional problem such as impaired mobility or mental status deficit create a problem with carrying out grooming or hygiene needs?

Does the client have external supports to complete grooming or hygiene needs?

How often does the client bathe?

Does the client avoid use of drying soaps, rubbing alcohol?

Does the client use any medications or over-the-counter creams or lotions on the skin?

Does the client lead a lifestyle that involves extended sun exposure?

Has the client noticed a skin lesion that bleeds, fails to heal, or has changed in size or appearance?

Does the client have a history of diabetes, anemia, or previous skin lesions?

Box 2-3.

Technique tips—integumentary system

The pinch test is best done on the abdomen in determining dehydration.

Look for sagging skinfolds or pronounced bony prominences that may indicate cachexia.

If the skin is very fragile, place the palms of your hands under joints when moving or repositioning the client to prevent trauma to the skin.

A skinfold exam may reveal hygienic problems.

Multiple bruises and welts may indicate elder abuse.

Fungal infection of the nails starts at the tip and invades toward the nail base.

Normal age-related changes can be confused with cancerous lesions. Look for new growths and recent changes in moles, such as increased size, bleeding, or pain. Lesions that are dark or hyperpigmented, have variegated color, or exhibit surface scaliness, erosion, oozing, crusting, or ulceration need further evaluation.

Table 2-1. Physical exam—integumentary system

Physical exam	Changes of normal aging	Physical exam	Changes of normal aging
Inspection/palpation			
Skin			
Color	Paleness of skin in white clients	Lesions—cont'd	Senile purpura—well-defined purplish-colored bruises usually found on dorsum of forearm and hands (fade after several weeks)
	Hypopigmentation (local or generalized)		
Moisture	Increased drying and flaking of the skin		
	Decreased perspiration		Sebaceous hyperplasia—yellow papular or flat thickening with central depression found on face, forehead, and nose*
Temperature	Slightly cooler to touch		
Texture	Facial and sun-exposed areas wrinkle		
Mobility and turgor	Generalized loss of turgor	*Nails*	
	Thinner, translucent skin over dorsal areas and bony prominences of extremities	Color	Yellowing may occur; translucent
		Shape	Toenails may be thickened, distorted with previous fungal infections
	Fat deposits thicker over abdomen and torso		
Lesions†—note color, size, texture, borders, distribution pattern or arrangement	Skin tags—pink to light tan in color, often multiple and pedunculated, found on face, axillae, and neck	Texture	Fingernails may be brittle or have ridges; a downward curve may occur
		Hair and scalp	
		Distribution	Alopecia with visible scalp; symmetrical hair loss and decreased facial hair in men
	Seborrheic keratosis—appear as "stuck on," greasy, yellow-brown, thickened, scaly, irregular or round lesions on trunk or back		Less axillary, pubic, and body hair
			Increased facial hair in white women
	Cherry angiomas—smooth, purplish or red, soft papules found on trunk	Color	Graying or whitening of hair
		Texture	Eyebrow, ear, and nose hairs may be coarse and grow more rapidly in men
	Senile lentigo—"age spots," yellow-brown pigmented maculae or areas found on the dorsum of hands, forearms	Quality	
			Hair on head may become more fine

Data compiled from Bates (1987), Burggraf and Donlon (1985), DeWitt (1990), Eliopoulos (1984), Stokes, Rauckhorst, and Mezley (1980), and Thompson and Bowers (1980).

*Further evaluation is needed.

†Abnormal skin findings often seen in the older client are actinic keratosis and the skin cancers: basal cell carcinoma, squamous cell carcinoma, and melanoma. (Refer to Chapter 4 for a detailed discussion of the diagnosis and treatment of skin lesions.)

Head and Neck

See Boxes 2-4 and 2-5 and Table 2-2.

Box 2-4.

Health history questions—head and neck

Symptom review of headaches, neck tremor, head injury, dizziness, syncope, enlarged lymph nodes or thyroid, and any history of previous thyroid problems.

Does the client have any limitations of neck range of motion? How does this affect daily living (driving, ability to look at stairs while walking down them, cooking, bathing, socialization)?

Box 2-5.

Technique tips—head and neck

View face from the side as well as from the front.

Check for temporomandibular joint degeneration as a factor in mastication.

Place one hand over the back of neck to feel crepitation of cervical arthritis.

Cardiac murmurs may be referred to neck vessels.

Although mild tremors of the head are thought by some clinicians to be normal, the beginner should seek further evaluation.

Range of motion of the neck should be done carefully and slowly in the older client. Pain, limitations, crepitation, muscle tension, and dizziness should be assessed in range of motion.

Table 2-2. Physical exam—head and neck

Physical exam	Changes of normal aging
Physical exam	
Hair (see Table 2-1)	
Skull—note contour and size	
Face—note symmetry of expression, any involuntary movement	Dentures or missing teeth may alter facial symmetry
Neck—note range of motion of neck and head, muscle development	Shortening of neck Clients with cervical arthritis will not be able to place chin to chest
Faciocervical lymph nodes	Lymph nodes are not usually palpable; small, shotty, nontender nodules may be remnants of a past infection
Trachea	
Thyroid	Thyroid not usually palpated; if felt, should be small, smooth, nontender
Auscultation	
Carotid artery	
Thyroid (bruits are abnormal)	

Data compiled from Bates (1987), Burggraf and Donlon (1985), Matteson and McConnell (1988), and Thompson and Bowers (1980).

Nose, Sinuses, Mouth, and Pharynx

See Boxes 2-6 and 2-7 and Table 2-3.

Box 2-6.

Health history questions—nose, sinuses, mouth, and pharynx

Symptom review of any soreness or bleeding of gums, lips, tongue, or throat; salivation problems, hoarseness, missing teeth, or chewing difficulty.

Symptom review of any sinus drainage, nasal drainage, loss of smell, allergies, mouth breathing, sneezing, or epistaxis.

Medication review: Does the client use any oral or nasal medications, over-the-counter drugs, or home remedies?

Does a functional problem impede the client's ability to perform oral hygiene or care for dentures?

If client wears dentures, how well do they fit, how old are they, and are they in good repair?

What is the routine pattern of dental care? Last exam?

Does the client smoke?

Box 2-7.

Technique tips—nose, sinuses, mouth, and pharynx

Look for ill-fitting dentures or edentulousness.

Look for evidence of denture rub. Look for presence of cracks or fissures. Ask client to bite down with dentures in place; overclosure of mouth (folding of skin at angle of mouth) indicates poorly fitting dentures.

Remove any dentures before examining the mouth.

Using a glove, palpate cheeks and lips between thumb and first two fingers.

Palpate alveolar ridges in edentulous clients for signs of tenderness.

The tongue should be grasped with a gauze pad to examine the lateral borders, base, and floor of mouth.

Most malignancies develop on the floor of mouth and on the tongue (Bates, 1987). The incidence of mouth cancer increases in males over age 50 who have a smoke or alcohol intake history.

Having the client tightly compress lips will assist in visualizing masses.

Voice qualities may be concurrently assessed when mental status exam is administered during the overview.

Table 2-3. Physical exam—nose, sinuses, mouth, and pharynx

Physical exam	Changes of normal aging
Inspection/palpation	
Nose	
External	Increased number and coarseness of nasal hairs
Nasal mucosa	Drier
Sense of smell (cranial nerve I)	Decreased sense of smell but should be able to smell strong odors
Lips	May be drier
Color	
Presence of ulcers, cracks, or masses	
Teeth	May be darker, yellow in color
	May appear elongated because of increased tooth exposure with supporting bone resorption
Buccal mucosa	Thinner, less vascularity
Color	Fordyce granules (yellow papules) may be seen on oral mucosa
Gums	Pale in color
Tongue	Varicosities (caviar spots) on under surface of tongue.
Color	
Papillae	Papillae may be smoother and shiny
Cranial nerve XII (hypoglossal)	
Pharynx	
Uvula	
Cranial nerve X (vagus)	Slower gag reflex*
Tonsils, hard and soft palate, posterior pharynx	Drier mucosa
	Midline exostosis (torus palatinus) may be noted
	Tonsils may be too small (cryptic) to be seen
Palpation	
Frontal and maxillary sinuses	
Temporomandibular joint (tenderness, crepitation, and decreased mobility are abnormal)	
Alveolar ridges	
Crepitation	

Data compiled from Bates (1987), Burggraf and Donlon (1985), Eliopoulos (1984, 1987), Matteson and McConnell (1988), and Thompson and Bowers (1980).
*Further evaluation may be needed.

Eyes

See Boxes 2-8 and 2-9 and Table 2-4.

Box 2-8.

Health history questions—eyes

Symptom review of decreased vision, acute eye pain, halos around lights, clouding of vision, increased eye tearing, double vision, tunnel vision, headaches, eye fatigue, or transient blindness.

Does the client wear glasses? For what problem?

Does the client wear contact lenses?

Does the client use aids or environmental adaptations to improve sight, function?

What impact does a visual problem have on the lifestyle of the client?

Does client have a history of glaucoma, diabetes, or cataracts?

Box 2-9.

Technique tips—eyes

Explain every activity before it happens; use touch to communicate when needed.

For vision testing, use a lighted Snellen chart or a light behind the client. Newspaper print is an alternative to vision testing if Snellen or Jaeger chart is not available.

Vision test with corrective lenses and without if possible. Test each eye separately.

Note behaviors accompanying the attempt to read that indicate difficulty—squinting or adjusting distance of reading material from eyes.

Fundoscopy may be limited by small pupil size and lens opacity.

Table 2-4. Physical exam—eyes

Physical exam	Changes of normal aging
Inspection	
External eye—lids, lacrimal ducts	Xanthelasma (cutaneous fat deposits in medial aspects of eye) may be present
	Skin around eyes may be darker with pouching
	Eyeballs may be deeper into sockets
	Eyelids may droop slightly
Conjunctiva	Yellow tinge to conjunctiva*
Sclera	
Cornea	Arcus senilis (a thin white-blue ring) may be seen around the cornea
	Decreased tear production and excessive dryness of eyes may cause corneal irritation
Pupils—size, shape, equality	Bilaterally smaller, irregular, but equal
	Slowed pupillary response to light
	Decreased light accommodation response
Fundoscopy	Crystalline lens opacity
Optic disc	
Fundus	Pale fundus
Vision	Presbyopia (farsightedness)
Snellen chart	
Jaeger chart	Slowed accommodation to darkness, glare
Newspaper print	
Peripheral vision	Peripheral vision diminishes
Glare	
Light/dark accommodation	Depth perception declines
Color	May not be able to distinguish blue from green

Data compiled from Bates (1987), Blair (1990), Matteson and McConnell (1988), and Thompson and Bowers (1980).
*Further evaluation is needed.

Ears

See Boxes 2-10 and 2-11 and Table 2-5.

Box 2-10.

Health history questions—ears

Symptom review of earache, dizziness, vertigo, infections, ringing in ears, and excessive ear cerumen.

Has family member or caregiver noticed that the client cannot understand shouted voice?

Has inability to hear sounds been accompanied by suspiciousness, depression, isolation, or confusion?

If hearing aid is used, how, why, when, and where was it obtained?

When was last audiometric examination?

Does client have a history of long-term exposure to loud noise?

Box 2-11.

Technique tips—ears

Speak clearly; avoid shouting and reduce background noise.

Establish eye contact.

Check for irritation of external canal by ill-fitting earmolds of hearing aids.

Inspect for ceruminous plugs before assessing hearing.

Deep insertion of ear speculum elicits normal tenderness.

Audiometry is the best assessment tool for hearing.

Test each ear separately at 40 decibels (dB) at frequencies of 500, 1000, 2000, and 4000 hertz (Hz) (Collinsworth and Boyle, 1989). Keep your face out of direct view, so the client cannot lip read. Repeat the test facing the client to assess for lip reading. An alternative is the whisper test.

Table 2-5. Physical exam—ear

Physical exam	Changes of normal aging
Inspection	
External ear	Pinna is without lesion; it may continue to grow
Ear canal	Impacted cerumen
	Tympanic membrane may appear dull and retracted bilaterally, with diminished light reflex
Hearing	If atrophic or sclerotic changes occur, the
Weber test	tympanic membrane landmarks may
Rinne test	appear more pronounced
Audiometry	

Data compiled from Bates (1987), Blair (1990), Matteson and McConnell (1988), Scura (1988), and Thompson and Bowers (1980).

Thorax and Lungs

See Boxes 2-12 and 2-13 and Table 2-6.

Box 2-12.

Health history questions—thorax and lungs

Symptom review of cough (acute or chronic), sputum production, dyspnea on exertion or rest, breathlessness (any associated heart symptoms?), chest pain, low-grade fever, night sweats, and weight loss or gain.

Does the client have a history of respiratory disease?

Do respiratory problems prevent the client from carrying out activities of daily living?

Is there a history of smoking?

Are there seasonal effects on respiratory pattern?

Does client have a history of past exposure to environmental pollutants (coal, pollution, asbestos)?

When was last chest x-ray? Last tuberculin skin test?

Box 2-13.

Technique tips—thorax and lungs

It will be very difficult for many clients to breathe deeply or hold their breath on command during the exam.

Many of the respiratory changes take place slowly; the client adjusts to these changes, and symptoms occur only with exertion beyond ADL.

Table 2-6. Physical exam—thorax and lungs

Physical exam	Changes of normal aging
Inspection	
Posture	Kyphosis may be present
Symmetry of chest expansion	Increased anteroposterior diameter—senile emphysema*
	A barrel chest is not normal
	General chest expansion decreases with calcification at rib articulation points and decreased vital capacity
	With decrease in subcutaneous fat, increase in bony prominences of rib cage
Respiratory pattern—rate, rhythm, depth, length	
Cough reflex (strong is normal)	
Sputum production	
Skin color	
Nailbed color	
Palpation	
Temperature of skin	
Areas of tenderness	Rib fractures are common in older adults even with mild trauma
Percussion	
Normal—equal resonance	Normal hyperresonance with decreased distensibility of lungs*
Auscultation	
Breath sounds—vesicular throughout; abnormal sounds are rales, wheezes, or rhonchi	Equal breath sounds; breath sounds may be distant in areas of kyphosis or with decreased respiratory effort

Data compiled from Bates (1987), Blair (1990), Matteson and McConnell (1988), and Thompson and Bowers (1980).
*Further evaluation is needed.

Breast and Axillae

See Boxes 2-14 and 2-15 and Table 2-7.

Box 2-14.

Health history questions—breast and axillae

Symptom review of changes in nipples, discharge, lumps, tenderness, dimpling in breasts or axillae.

Is there a history of breast cancer in self or family?

Is there a history of mastectomy and any past or present use of prostheses?

Does client perform breast self-examination? When was the last time?

When was last mammogram?

Box 2-15.

Technique tips—breast and axillae

This is a good opportunity to teach breast self-examination.

Elongation of breast tissue makes careful assessment difficult; "pancaking" breast tissue between two hands may improve assessment of large pendulous breasts.

To assess contour, have client (1) lean forward, (2) place hands on hips and press, (3) hold arms over the head.

Masses that tend to suggest breast cancer are those that are nontender, form a single mass, cause asymmetry of breasts with unilateral changes, dimpling of skin, nipple retraction, nipple bleeding, or axillae mass.

Table 2-7. Physical exam—breasts and axillae

Physical exam	Changes of normal aging
Inspection	
Size	Decrease of subcutaneous fat
Symmetry	means an increase in the bony prominences
Contour	Ligaments relax—breasts may appear elongated/ pendulous
	Breast tissue atrophies
	Inspect under breasts for rash/irritation
Scars	
Palpation	
Breast	"Stringy" breast tissue
Nipple	Increased evidence of cystic changes common after menopause
Axillae—lateral, central, pectoral, and subscapular areas	
Lumps—all are significant; note location, size, shape, consistency, tenderness, "fixed" or "non-fixed," and mobility of lump	

Data compiled from Bates (1987), Eliopoulos (1984), Nelson and Mayfield (1988), and Thompson and Bowers (1980).

Cardiovascular System

See Boxes 2-16 and 2-17 and Table 2-8.

Box 2-16.

Health history questions—cardiovascular system

Symptom review of any mental status changes, orthopnea, dyspnea, syncope, edema, palpitations, cough, paroxysmal nocturnal dyspnea, hemoptysis, resting leg pain, cool extremity, nighttime awakening, exercise intolerance, and chest pain.

Review of medications, with particular attention to potassium, antihypertensives, and digoxin.

Review of diet, with particular attention to sodium-containing foods.

Lifestyle review: life stressors, ability to carry out ADL/IADL, energy levels for social activities. Comparison of present to 5 years and 10 years ago.

Does client have a history of cardiovascular problems?

Is there a family history of cardiovascular diseases?

Box 2-17.

Technique tips—cardiovascular system

Mental confusion may present as a decrease in cardiac output in the older adult.

Chest pain in the older adult may present as a "tightness" and may be associated with dyspnea or palpitations.

Perform the heart exam in two positions, lying and sitting.

Table 2-8. Physical exam—cardiovascular system

Physical exam	Changes of normal aging	Physical exam	Changes of normal aging
Inspection/palpation			May be difficult to assess because of increased anteroposterior diameter
Neck vein distension—examine client at 45 degree angle to elicit distension	Kinking of right common carotid artery is seen as a pulsation above the right clavicle	Extremities—assess presence of edema (abnormal); document edema as pitting or nonpitting; note location and degree of pitting	
Extremities—color, warmth, evidence of vascular insufficiency			
Elicit Homan's sign		**Auscultation**	
Chest wall—apical pulse; any thrill, heave	Kyphosis may distort normal symmetrical contour of chest wall	Bruits (abnormal finding)—carotid, femoral, abdominal	
Palpation		Heart sounds	
Carotid, radial, femoral, popliteal, dorsalis pedis, and posterior tibial pulses		Rate	Rate slower with age
		Rhythm	Arrhythmias may be present as a result of the increase in connective tissue in sinoatrial/atrioventricular nodes and decrease in number of pacemaker cells
		S_1	
		S_2	
		S_3, S_4	
		Murmurs	
Apical pulse—supine and in left lateral position	Located in fourth to fifth intercostal space, 5-7 cm from midclavicular line		Early, soft systolic murmur in aortic area heard in half of the population over age 85 (Bates, 1987) as a result of changes in aorta*
	Rate 60-90; heart rate slows with aging		S_4 may be heard as a result of decrease in left ventricle compliance*

Data compiled from Bates (1987), Blair (1990), Eliopoulos (1984), Matteson and McConnell (1988), Nelson and Mayfield (1988), and Thompson and Bowers (1980).

*Further evaluation is needed.

Abdomen

See Boxes 2-18 and 2-19 and Table 2-9.

Box 2-18.

Health history questions—abdomen

Symptom review of appetite changes, nausea, vomiting, pain (and its relationship to eating patterns), weight loss, burning in throat, premature fullness when eating, change in bowel habits, hemorrhoids, change in appearance of stool, tarry or bloody stools, constipation or diarrhea.

Medication review.

Nutritional assessment (see earlier discussion in section on health history).

Are there any functional problems that prevent client from preparing or shopping for meals?

Is external support for meal preparation available?

Is lifestyle sedentary or active?

What is elimination pattern? Are aids or laxatives used?

When was last gastrointestinal examination, last formal assessment for blood in stool?

Box 2-19.

Technique tips—abdomen

The older client experiences less pain and less rigidity of the abdomen with acute or chronic conditions.

Deeper, firmer palpation may be required to elicit pain or rebound tenderness.

The client should always void before the abdominal exam.

Table 2-9. Physical exam—abdomen

Physical exam	Changes of normal aging
Inspection	
Symmetry	Deposition of fat in lower abdomen
Contour	and hips along with a decrease
Masses	in abdominal muscle strength
Presence of hernias	may give "potbelly" appearance
Striae	
Scars	
Auscultation	
Bowel sounds	
Bruits (abnormal)	
Percussion	
Liver size	Decreased liver size
Ascites (abnormal)	
Tympany normal (dullness may indicate mass or full bladder)	
Palpation	
Liver span	Decrease in liver size
Kidneys	Liver may be palpated 1-2 cm below right costal margin
Spleen (abnormal if felt)	
Organ tenderness	
Masses (abnormal)	

Data compiled from Bates (1987), Blair (1990), Eliopoulos (1984), Matteson and McConnell (1988), Nelson and Mayfield (1988), and Thompson and Bowers (1980).

Musculoskeletal System

See Boxes 2-20 and 2-21 and Table 2-10.

Box 2-20.

Health history questions—musculoskeletal system

Symptom review of loss of range of motion, painful joint, change in size or shape of joint, stiffness, muscle weakness, muscle cramps, or back pain.

Medication review for use of pain relievers.

Does client use assistive devices: cane, walker, crutch, wheelchair, prosthesis, grab bars in bathroom, or elevated toilet seat?

Is there a history of spontaneous fractures, falls, stumbling, loss of balance, or unsteady gait?

When are the client's peak activity times, morning or afternoon?

Does the client exercise? Discover type, frequency, intensity, need for special equipment to perform the activity.

Is the client able to carry out ADL/IADL? Who assists if unable?

Box 2-21.

Technique tips—musculoskeletal system

Observe client sitting, standing, and walking.

Use active range of motion (ROM) to assess for movement limitations; use passive ROM to test resistance to flexor and extensor muscle groups.

Omit resistance to hip flexion, which increases pressure on lumbar vertebrae; rely instead on active hip flexion.

Any decrease in muscle strength should correlate with muscle size decrease.

Note onset and duration of tremors, whether resting or intention.

Test for mild residual "drift" (hemiparesis) during ambulation.

Weak or unsteady clients will watch their feet as they walk.

Observe for misuse of walking aids.

Check shoes for fit; ill fit may cause unsteady gait.

Demonstrate moves; if necessary, hold both hands and walk backward facing client to provide support.

Make note of client's ability to flex spine, finger and hand dexterity, shoulder rotation, arm strength, wrist flexion, finger-thumb opposition.

Table 2-10. Physical exam—musculoskeletal system

Physical exam	Changes of normal aging
Inspection	
General appearance	Slightly flexed posture
Gait—note symmetry	Wider-based stance
	Narrowed shoulders
	Slightly increased difficulty in tandem walking
	Smaller steps, wider-based gait
	Gait should remain normal: arm swing is symmetrical, heel strikes floor, weight shift is stable, length of stride is normal, legs swing freely to new position
Inspection/palpation	
Note muscle symmetry, range of motion, and muscle strength; look at the joint and the skin and muscles around the joint, and "feel" the joint through range of motion	Upper and lower extremity symmetry
	Joints able to pass through full range of motion
Spine	Decreased endurance
Head and neck	*
Hands and wrists	Hand grip stays strong
Elbows	Diminished ability to perform sudden, intense exercise
Shoulders	
Arm muscles	
Feet and ankles	
Knees	
Hips and pelvis	
Leg/hip/pelvis muscles	
Upper and lower extremity symmetry	
Performance of ADL: able to rise from lying to sitting position, able to rise from chair to standing position, able to climb and descend a step, able to retrieve an item from the floor, able to tie shoes in sitting position, and able to dress, comb hair, and button buttons.	

Data compiled from Bates (1987), Burggraf and Donlon (1985), Kane, Ouslander, and Abrass (1984), Matteson and McConnell, (1988), and Thompson and Bowers (1980).
*See previous table (2-2).

Nervous System

See Boxes 2-22 and 2-23 and Table 2-11.

Box 2-22.

Health history questions—nervous system

Symptom review of dizziness, syncope, headache, falls, loss of balance or coordination, speech changes, mental status changes, weakness, numbness or loss of sensation, memory changes, and loss of consciousness.

How do nervous system changes affect client's ability to carry out ADL and general well-being?

Does the client have a history of nervous system problems? A seizure history?

Does the client have diabetes, hypertension, cardiovascular disease, or family history of these?

Box 2-23.

Technique tips—nervous system

Client response to exam may be slower.

Be alert to facial asymmetry, weakness of extremities, gait disturbances, tremors, and alteration in mental ability as clues to problems during the exam.

A decrease in deep sleep and REM time is normal; the client may experience an increase in light sleep and sleep fewer hours.

Table 2-11. Physical exam—nervous system

Physical exam	Changes of normal aging
Inspection/palpation	
Mental status interview (see overview earlier in this section)	
Speech	Receptive language does not alter; process is slowed
Gait—have client walk, stop, turn, and start; note any tremor, gait disturbance	Decreased postural balance and muscle tone
Romberg sign	
Upper extremity coordination	Decreased coordination of fine motor movements, worsened by demand for rapid response
	Decreased motor readiness
Cranial nerves I-XII	Decreased sense of smell, but should smell strong odors
	Decreased sense of taste
	Decreased visual acuity, decreased peripheral vision
	Conductive hearing loss
	Slower gag reflex*
	Pupils smaller but should constrict with light stimulus
Sensory Touch Pain Vibration	Decreased vibratory sense in feet and ankles; should be normal at calf level
Lower body coordination	As for upper extremities
Reflexes Triceps Biceps Brachioradialis Knee Ankle Babinski's reflex	Decreased reflexes in ankle, knee

Data compiled from Bates (1987), Blair (1990), Matteson and McConnell (1988), Nelson and Mayfield (1988), and Thompson and Bowers (1980).
*Further evaluation is needed.

Male Genitourinary System

See Boxes 2-24 and 2-25 and Table 2-12.

Box 2-24.

Health history questions—male genitourinary system

Carefully question about sexuality. Needs met? Problems in function? These needs, functions remain throughout the life cycle.

Symptom review of urinary frequency, nocturia, urgency, urinary hesitancy, abnormal flow of urine (start/stop? dribbling after termination of stream?), incontinence, urethral discharge, scrotal masses, impotence, pain with erection, perineal pain, flank pain, abdominal pain.

How do problems affect the client as a whole?

Does client have a history of prostate, testicular, venereal disease?

What is client's fluid intake? Pattern of fluid intake?

Does client perform testicular self-examination?

Does client have a history of diabetes, hypertension, cardiovascular disease?

Box 2-25.

Technique tips—male genitourinary system

Cancer of prostate is often asymptomatic.

Bates (1987) reported that half of all colorectal cancer is detected on a simple digital exam.

Genitourinary pain is often vague and ill defined by the client; careful assessment is needed.

Patient should stand and lie for hernia exam.

Look at the undersurface of scrotum; elongation of the scrotal sac leaves the skin susceptible to irritation.

Table 2-12. Physical exam—male genitourinary system

Physical exam	Changes of normal aging
Inspection	
Penis	
Skin	
Scrotum	Scrotal sac is elongated
Testes	
Hernias—natural posture and with strain	
Sacrococcygeal and perianal area	
Palpation	
Abdomen for bladder fullness	
Check for costovertebral angle tenderness	
Penis	
Scrotal sac	
Testicles	Decrease in testicular size; testicles less firm
Hernias	
Anus—note nodules, fissures, sphincter tone	
Rectum—note nodules, irregular features	
Prostate—note size, texture	May feel larger*

Data compiled from Bates (1987), Matteson and McConnell (1988), Nelson and Mayfield (1988), and Thompson and Bowers (1980).
*Further evaluation is needed.

Female Genitourinary System

See Boxes 2-26 and 2-27 and Table 2-13.

Box 2-26.

Health history questions—female genitourinary system

Question client carefully about sexuality, and problems that she may be having. Active? Painful intercourse? Satisfied with current status?

Symptom review of frequency, urgency, nocturia, incontinence, hesitancy, abnormal flow of stream, urethral discharge, pelvic heaviness, pain, and bleeding.

Establish usual voiding pattern.

If incontinent, does the client use devices to keep dry? What, how many per day, and when? How does the incontinence affect the client? Does she isolate herself? Do functional or mental status problems affect her ability to be continent?

Obtain a full history as to number of children, types of deliveries, and any complications; date of menopause and any difficulties during menopause; use of estrogen, now or in the past, and any history of problems while using estrogen (bleeding, fluid retention, breast enlargement); past gynecological surgeries

---

Box 2-27.

Technique tips—female genitourinary system

Help client to maintain lithotomy position by supporting her legs with pillows. Client will tire easily; hips cannot remain abducted for an extended period of time.

If client is disabled, has changes of arthritis, or has other mobility impairments, the left lateral prone position may be the best position for examination.

Perform test of urinary incontinence: With client standing, pad in place, have her cough several times and observe any leakage of urine; with client in the lithotomy position, have her cough and evaluate urine leakage.

Table 2-13. Physical exam—female genitourinary system

Physical exam	Changes of normal aging
Inspection/palpation	
Abdomen—assess for fullness and for costovertebral angle tenderness	Decreased bladder capacity, increased urine residual (>100 ml is abnormal)
External structures—pad stress test: natural and strained postures to check for urethral leakage	Atrophy of vulva, decreased subcutaneous fat
	Decreased pubic hair
	Shiny, drier appearance
Vagina—note cystocele, rectocele	Thinner epithelium, decreased vascularity, paler, decreased rugae with smoother surface and drier environment
Cervix—Pap smear, bimanual exam	May not palpate cervix/uterus because of decreased size
	Ovaries should not be palpated
Anus	
Rectum	

Data compiled from Bates (1987), Matteson and McConnell (1988), Nelson and Mayfield (1988), and Thompson and Bowers (1980).

GERIATRIC LABORATORY VALUES

Assessment of laboratory values can play an important role in obtaining a comprehensive data base for the older client. Because there are normal aging differences in the healthy older adult, studies are indicating that there are "normal laboratory values" for the older adult. The term "normal value" has been replaced with "standard," and the term "reference interval" has been designated to represent those laboratory values that are more closely associated with a given population (Carnevali and Enloe, 1986). Determining a reference interval for the older population is limited by differences in factors such as use of prescription medications, diet, sex, community living ver-

---

Box 2-28.

Laboratory values that remain constant with increasing age

Platelet count
Bilirubin
Chloride
Sodium
Magnesium
Lactic dehydrogenase (LDH)
Bicarb
Aspartate aminotransferase (AST) (formerly
  SGOT—serum glutamic-oxalacetic transaminase)

Date compiled from Andresen (1989) and Jeppesen (1986).

Table 2-14. Laboratory values that change with increasing age

Test	General trend from standards	Range
Hematology		
Hemoglobin	Decreases to lower limits of normal	M—12.4-14.9 g/100 ml F—11.7-13.8 g/100 ml Lower standard ranges
Hematocrit	Decreases to lower limits of normal	M—42%-54% F—38%-46% Lower limits of standard range
Sedimentation rate	Mild increase	0-20 units
Chemistry		
Albumin	Decreases	3.3-4.9 g/100 ml
Creatinine	Increases	0.6-1.8 mg/100 ml*
BUN	Increases	M—8-35 mg/100 ml F—6-30 mg/100 ml
Potassium	Increases	Runs higher to upper limits of standard
Glucose	Increases somewhat	150 mg/100 ml proposed upper limit†
Calcium	Changes occur	Stay within standard ranges
Uric acid	Increases somewhat	7.7 mg/100 ml upper limit of standard
Enzymes		
Alkaline phosphatase	Increases	M—80 units average F—79 units average
Urine chemistry		
Creatinine clearance	Must be calculated for age-related changes‡	
Specific gravity	Decreases maximum value	1.028-1.024
Blood gases		
P_{CO_2}	Increases	
P_{O_2}	Decreases	
Hormones		
Thyroid stimulation hormone (TSH)	Increases§	

Data compiled from Andresen (1989) and Jeppesen (1986).
*Age and creatinine must be taken into account; may have normal values even in renal failure.
†Common to have higher values but reflects carbohydrate intolerance.
‡Creatinine clearance calculated as: $\dfrac{(140 - age) \times body\ weight\ (kg)}{serum\ creatinine \times 72\ kg}$ ($\times 0.85$ for women)
§Common but related to abnormal thyroid function.

sus institutional living arrangements, use of alcohol or tobacco, and ethnicity.

Box 2-28 lists laboratory values that are not thought to alter with the aging process, and Table 2-14 gives reference intervals for the older adult identified in the literature. In evaluating laboratory values for the older client it is important to remember that the laboratory value is a tool; it can be used in adding a piece to the data base. All laboratory values must be compared with the clinical picture the client presents and the client's established baseline laboratory values.

SUMMARY

Assessment is the important first step in the nursing process. A comprehensive assessment identifies positive and negative factors affecting the older client's quality of life. Perceptive assessment skills promote nursing diagnoses that reflect deficits as well as strengths and resources. The health care provider must be knowledgeable about normal physiological changes of aging and their influence on functional status as reflected in the health assessment.

REFERENCES

Andresen GP (1989). A fresh look at assessing the elderly, RN 52(6):28-40.

Bates B (1987). A guide to physical examinations and history taking, ed 4, Philadelphia, JB Lippincott Co.

Blair KA (1990). Aging: Physiological aspects and clinical implications, Nurse Pract 15(2):14-28.

Burggraf V and Donlon B (1985). Assessing the elderly, part one of two parts, system by system, Am J Nurs 85(9):974-984.

Carnevali D and Enloe C (1986). Assessment in the elderly. In Carnevali DL and Patrick M, editors: Nursing management for the elderly, ed 2, Philadelphia, JB Lippincott Co, pp 26-38.

Collinsworth R and Boyle K (1989). Nutritional assessment of the elderly, J Gerontol Nurs 15(12):17-21.

DeWitt S (1990). Nursing assessment of the skin and dermatologic lesions, Nurs Clin North Am 25(1):235-245.

Eliopoulos C (1984). Assessment of the feet. In Eliopoulos C, editor: Health assessment of the older adult, Menlo Park, Calif, Addison-Wesley, pp 219-228.

Eliopoulos C, editor (1984). Health assessment of the older adult, Menlo Park, Calif, Addison-Wesley.

Eliopoulos C (1987). Gerontological nursing, ed 2, Philadelphia, JB Lippincott Co.

Folstein MF, Folstein SD, and McHugh PR (1975). Mini mental state, a practical method for grading the cognitive state of patients for the clinician, J Psychiatr Res 12:189-198.

Jeppesen ME (1986). Laboratory values for the elderly. In Carnevali DL and Patrick M, editors: Nursing management for the elderly, ed 2, Philadelphia, JB Lippincott Co.

Kane RL, Ouslander JG, and Abrass IB (1984). Essentials of clinical geriatrics, New York, McGraw-Hill.

Matteson MA and McConnell ES (1988). Gerontological nursing, Philadelphia, WB Saunders Co.

Nelson MD and Mayfield P (1988). Health assessment. In Hogstel M, editor: Nursing care of the older adult, ed 2, New York, John Wiley & Sons, Inc.

Reber A (1988). Nutrition and aging, ed 2, Denton, University of North Texas, Center for Studies in Aging.

Santo-Novak DA (1988). Seven keys to assessing the elderly, Nursing 1988 18(8):60-63.

Scura KW (1988). Audiological assessment program, J Gerontol Nurs 4(10):19-25.

Spence AP (1989). Biology of human aging, Englewood Cliffs, NJ, Prentice-Hall.

Stokes SA, Rauckhorst LM, and Mezey MD (1980). Health assessment—considerations for the older individual, J Gerontol Nurs 6(6):328-337.

Thompson JM and Bowers AC (1980). Clinical manual of health assessment, St Louis, The CV Mosby Co.

CHAPTER 3

Medications

Mildred O. Hogstel

It is estimated that people aged 60 and over make up about 16% of the population in the United States and take almost 40% of the prescription medications. Nursing home residents take an average of four to seven different medications several times a day. Some take many more. Because of comorbidity, or the presence of several chronic, long-term disease processes, older people are prescribed a number of medications for the relief of various symptoms. When medications are prescribed by a variety of physicians for different problems, patients may not inform each physician of their total medication regimen.

Although older adults do have more chronic diseases than those who are younger and therefore may need more drugs than younger people, there is mounting evidence that many of our older citizens are getting prescription drugs which are entirely unnecessary (the wrong diagnosis has been made or nondrug therapy would work), or they are getting a more dangerous drug when a much less dangerous one would work, or a lower dose of the same drug would give the same benefits with lower risks (Wolfe et al, 1988, p. 7).

Table 3-1. Most common prescription and over-the-counter types of medications taken by older adults

Prescription	Over-the-counter
Cardiovascular drugs	Laxatives
Antihypertensive agents	Vitamins
Diuretics	Antacids
Analgesics	Analgesics
Hypnotics	Antihistamines
Sedatives	Medications for colds/flu
Tranquilizers	
Antidepressants	
Antianxiety agents	

POLYPHARMACY

The problem of multiple medications in older adults is a major one. Polypharmacy has been defined as one more medication than that which is clinically indicated for a specific diagnosis or condition. The more medications taken, the greater the chance there is for adverse effects, toxicity, and harmful drug–drug interactions.

A very serious problem concerning the use of drugs by older adults is that many of the "illnesses" for which they seek and are given drug treatment are problems which are, in fact, adverse drug reactions to drugs already being used which were not recognized by either patient or doctor as such (Wolfe et al, 1988, p. 7).

The category of medication most overused with older adults is psychotropic medication, particularly antidepressants, antipsychotics such as neuroleptics and major tranquilizers, and antianxiety agents. In one study reported by Wolfe et al (1988), 61% of 65- to 84-year-old residents in nursing homes were given mind-affecting drugs. The Federal Omnibus Budget Reconciliation Act (OBRA) of 1987, implemented in full on October 1, 1990, has started to have a positive effect on this problem. Psychotropic medications that had often been used as chemical restraints may not now be used without a specific medical reason (diagnosis or condition). Such medications are being discontinued or reduced in dosage whenever possible.

Some geriatricians recommend that older adults should not be taking any more than three different medications at one time. When assessing a new patient with multiple problems, the physician may stop all medications and then start specific ones as symptoms reappear. However, some symptoms often fail to reappear because they were due to the interaction of multiple medications. Guidelines used in prescribing medications for older adults are listed in Box 3-1.

After an extensive review of the research and literature on medications and older adults, and evaluation and comments by a wide variety of medical specialists, Wolfe et al (1988) provided a classic reference, *Worst Pills, Best Pills.* Although primarily written for lay readers (it is in large print), the 532-page book is an excellent reference for all health care professionals who work with older adults. The book discusses the problem of medication overuse by older adults and includes recommendations about specific medications that should and should not be used by older people (see Table 3-2 and reference list). The book can be purchased in most local book stores or by writing to:

PILLS
2000 P Street, NW, Suite 700
Washington, DC 20036

Table 3-2. Medications that should and should not be used by older adults

Category	Do not use	Limited use	Okay
Cardiovascular	Aldomet	Capoten	Inderal
	Catapres	Dyazide	Lopressor
	Serpasil	Minipress	Tenormin
	Persantine	Lasix	Lanoxin
	Cyclospasmol		Nitrobid
	Pavabid		Coumadin
	Trental		K-Lor
Tranquilizers and hypnotics	Ativan	Serax	
	Dalmane		
	Halcion		
	Librium		
	Nembutal		
	Restoril		
	Valium		
	Xanax		
Antidepressants	Elavil	Desyrel	Norpramine
	Triavil	Sinequan	Aventyl
		Tofranil	Pamelor
Antipsychotics		Haldol	Lithium
		Mellaril	
		Navane	
		Prolixin	
		Stelazine	
		Thorazine	
Medications for pain and arthritis	Bufferin	Clinoril	Advil
	Feldene		Aspirin
	Darvocet		Ecotrin
	Darvon		Empirin
	Talwin		Tylenol
	Wygesic		Demerol
			Dilaudid
			Percodan
			Vicodin
Gastrointestinal	Mylanta	Antivert	Tagamet
	Tigan	Compazine	Zantac
	Colace	Phenergan	Maalox
	Dialose Plus	Reglan	Metamucil
	Doxidan	Milk of Magnesia	
	Surfak		
	Donnatal		

Continued.

Table 3-2. Medications that should and should not be used by older adults—cont'd

Category	Do not use	Limited use	Okay
Antiinfectives	Furadantin	Achromycin	Bactrim
			Gantrisin
			Keflex
			Penicillin
			Septra
			Vibramycin
Neurological	Artane	Hydergine	Sinemet
	Cogentin		Dilantin
			Tegretol
Nutritional supplements	Vitamin E		Calcium
			Feosol
			Fergon
			Niacin
			Vitamins
Others	Norflex	Premarin	Synthroid

Data compiled from Wolfe SM et al (1988).

PHARMACOKINETICS AND PHARMACODYNAMICS

The absorption, action, duration of action, distribution, and excretion of medicines in older adults differ significantly from those in other adults. For these reasons, the choice of medications and dosages should be made carefully and monitored closely.

Absorption of oral medications can be delayed by the following conditions and factors common in older adults:

Decreased amount of hydrochloric acid in the stomach

Delayed emptying of food in the stomach

Use of antacids

Multiple oral medications taken at one time, especially those that prevent absorption of other medications (e.g., cholestyramine [Questran], a cholesterol-lowering medication, prevents the absorption of fat-soluble vitamins)

Decreased motility of the gastrointestinal tract

Decreased blood flow to the gastrointestinal tract

Decreased enzyme production

After absorption, the distribution of medications may be decreased because of the following conditions and factors common in older adults (Medicating the elderly, 1987):

Decreased cardiac output

Decreased total body water (TBW) due to

Decreased thirst

Dehydrating drugs

Increased fat and decreased muscle mass (where most of the water is); some medications accumulate in fatty tissue

Blood-brain barrier less effective (increased permeability due to central nervous system effects)

Altered protein binding (the increased number of drugs compete for the proteins in the blood stream thus delaying distribution)

Metabolism of medications is also slowed in older adults. The majority of medications are metabolized in the liver. Older people often have decreased metabolism (see Chapter 1), decreased liver mass, decreased blood flow to the liver, decreased enzyme activity, and lack of protein in the diet. Therefore medications stay in the body longer, and substances with a long half-life should be used cautiously with older adults. When the half-life increases, there is a greater chance for side effects. Examples of medications with long half-lives that generally are not recommended for older adults are given in Table 3-3. It is obvious that if a hypnotic with a long half-life is administered to an older adult at 9 PM each night for one week, the accumulative effect of that medication over a period of 1 week could cause confusion, decreased cognition, and poor balance with a high risk for falling during waking hours. A medication such as oxazepam (Serax)

Table 3-3. Examples of medications with long half-lives

Medication	Half-life (hr)
Flurazepam (Dalmane)	30-200
Diazepam (Valium)	36-200
Amitriptyline (Elavil)	10-50
Chlordiazepoxide (Librium)	36-200
Fluoxetine (Prozac)	>300 (in older adults)

Data compiled from Deglin, Vallerand, and Russin (1991), Kushnir (1990), and Luke (1990).

would be much better because it would be excreted from the body in 4 to 6 hours (Allen, 1983).

Excretion of medications also is slowed in older adults as a result of decreased blood supply to the kidneys, decreased kidney function, and decreased glomerular filtration rate. Urinary excretion also may be slowed because of inadequate fluid intake or dehydration due to other factors such as fever.

DOSAGE

Although the dosage of many medicines for older adults is generally recommended to be one third to one half of the dose used for younger adults, there has been little research to determine the most effective dose for the older age group. Most randomized clinical research trials on medicines have been tested on healthy adult males weighing about 150 pounds (Medicating the elderly, 1987). Therefore the most effective dose of medicines for older adults has not been scientifically determined. The reason for the lack of such research on older adults is not clear, but it may be because of the prevalence of comorbidity and polypharmacy among this age group (Generic drugs. Myths vs. facts, 1987). Few medicine references (books and manuals) include recommended geriatric doses, whereas they do include pediatric doses.

ADVERSE EFFECTS

The most common side effects of many medicines in older adults are sedation and lethargy, which can lead to other complications such as falling. The behaviors may be mistakenly considered a normal part of the aging process instead of adverse medicine reactions. The action of some medicines in older adults also may have a paradoxical effect, or an effect opposite to that intended. For example, some hypnotics (especially the barbiturates) may produce increased activity and restlessness instead of sleep and relaxation.

Sometimes the side effects are worse than the illness for which the person is taking medication and may cause severe long-term problems. The following are examples:

Dry mouth that decreases the appetite in a person who already has a poor appetite

Symptoms of tardive dyskinesia that will last a lifetime and inhibit eating and social activities

Urinary retention when an antidepressant is given to a patient with benign prostate hyperplasia

Need for a permanent urinary catheter following long-term use of an antidepressant

Many older people are admitted to the hospital for a medicine-related illness as a result of severe adverse reactions. The most common medicines that cause the need for hospital admission are the following:

Digitalis

Diuretics

Antihypertensive agents

Tranquilizers

Antidepressants

Hypoglycemic agents

Over-the-counter medications such as laxatives, that result in increased sodium intake, and aspirin, which causes gastrointestinal bleeding

NONCOMPLIANCE

One of the major problems in prescribing medications for older people is noncompliance. The most common problem is not taking the medication exactly as prescribed. Some of the reasons for noncompliance are listed in Box 3-2. Nurses in all settings—hospitals, clinics,

---

Box 3-2.

Reasons for medication noncompliance in older adults

Do not understand the purpose/benefit of the medication

Do not understand the exact instructions for taking the medicine (e.g., 3 times a day, before meals, every 4 hours)

Do not have enough money to buy the medicine (many prescriptions are never filled because patients spend their limited financial resources on food instead of medicine)

Try to save on the amount of money spent on medications by cutting a pill in two or four, skipping a dose, or taking a regularly scheduled medication only when they feel bad

Cannot remove the cap on a bottle of medicine (the pharmacist should be instructed not to use a child-proof cap)

Cannot read the instructions on the label of a medication bottle (the pharmacist should be requested to use a large-print label)

Fear that asking the physician or nurse questions about the medication regimen will result in being labeled "senile"

Do not remember whether a medication has been taken as a result of confusion or drowsiness that may be caused by the medication and omit or double a dose

Do not believe the medicine is needed

Do not trust the physician, nurse, or caregiver

Take more than the prescribed dose when they feel like they need it or take none at all when they feel well

Take over-the-counter medications they see advertised on television instead of medications prescribed by their physician

nursing homes, home health care—should carefully assess the older patient's knowledge of the medication regimen and ensure that, when possible, the patient understands the medications. This process is especially important in the discharge planning process when the older person is being discharged from the hospital. See Chapter 13 for more details on discharge planning and teaching the older adult.

It may be difficult for some older people to understand or remember a complex medication regimen. Sometimes they do not remember that they took a certain medication and then repeat the medication, doubling the dose. Specific, clear, written instructions are essential and can be supplemented by one of the many devices available to help older people organize and remember their medication schedule. Among these devices are the following:

Empty egg carton with medicines in each compartment and date/times printed clearly on the top of each compartment

Small clear bottles with medicines for certain days or times and labels on the top of each one

Small plastic containers with compartments labeled by day or time (also in braille for blind persons), which can be purchased at a minimal cost in most pharmacies

Battery-operated containers similar to the above that beep at appropriate times to alert the person to take a medicine

Elaborate electronic devices that hold a 30-day supply of medicines compartmentalized by day and time

Even with devices such as these, however, the older person with mobility, vision, or finger manipulation problems will usually need to have another person check and perhaps fill the device on a weekly or monthly basis.

GENERIC MEDICINES

Generic medicines are drug products that are not protected by a patent awarded to a specific pharmaceutical company for a brand-name medication. A patent gives the company that discovered the medicine the sole right to sell it for as long as the patent is in effect, usually about 17 years after the medicine has been approved for use. This period allows the pharmaceutical company to recover its investment in the discovery of the medicine. After the patent expires, other companies may produce and sell the medicine, usually at a lower price because they did not have the expense of research, experimentation, or advertising.

Generic medicines "contain exactly the same active ingredients as the brand-name drug and must be just as safe and effective" (Generic drugs. Myths vs. facts, 1987). They must also be "identical in strength, dosage form (tablet, solution, etc.), and route of administration" (Ge-

neric drugs. Myths vs. facts, 1987). However, some believe that certain generic medicines—for example, the loop diuretics and phenothiazines—are not exactly equivalent to brand-name preparations and therefore should be used carefully, especially with older adults (Lamy, 1985). Another example is generic calcium, often taken by older women, which may not be absorbed as well as a brand-name preparation. Calcium that is not absorbed, of course, is of no value in maintaining bone density.

Generic medications are important to older people because they are less expensive. They may cost 50% less than a similar brand-name medicine. Nurses should explain the benefits (less cost) and availability (e.g., by mail from the American Association of Retired Persons' Pharmacy) of generic medicines to their older patients and tell them to ask their physicians for generic prescriptions if there are no individual or medicine contraindications to their use.

NURSING IMPLICATIONS

Many medications can be very dangerous to older adults, and the nurse has an important responsibility to observe for early or covert adverse effects and complications. Because most older adults experience specific physical changes in many organ systems and often do not have typical presentation of an illness (see Chapters 1 and 2), the nurse must be alert to changes in behavior. For example, sudden confusion or memory loss, poor balance that may cause falls, or a minor temperature elevation may be early signs of medication overdose or toxicity.

Because absorption of medications takes longer in older adults, the nurse should recognize that onset and peak of action may be delayed so that relief of symptoms, such as pain, takes longer. Therefore, a second dose should not be given until the initial dose has had an opportunity to take full effect. Analgesics for pain should not be routinely given every 4 hours.

Both absorption and excretion can be hastened by ensuring that the patient takes an adequate amount of fluid. Older adults should take a minimum of 2000 ml of fluids every 24 hours, unless contraindicated by another condition (e.g., congestive heart failure or kidney failure). Because the sense of thirst is diminished in many older people, the nurse will need to encourage them to drink more by offering fluids frequently and by assisting persons with diminished mobility to obtain the needed fluids.

Nurses should always remember that they have a responsibility to confirm any medication order by a physician that is perceived to be questionable. Some physicians, for example, may not be aware of recent trends in geriatric pharmacology. Nurses should question a medication or dose not recommended for older people. A few excellent references on geriatric pharmacology are listed at the end of this chapter. Box 3-3 lists specific responsibilities of nurses administering medications to older people.

The Medicines I Take box below and boxes 3-4, 3-5, and 3-6 are examples of types of handouts that can be given to older patients as a part of the discharge planning and teaching process.

Box 3-3.

Nursing responsibilities in administering medications to older people

Take a complete medication history, including
   Past medications
   Present medications (prescription and over-the-counter)
   Allergies of all kinds
   Patient's understanding of medications being taken (name, purpose, dosage, method, times)
Space oral medications so that not more than one or two are taken at one time.
Have the patient drink a little fluid *before* taking oral medications (to ease swallowing).
Encourage the patient to drink at least 5 to 6 ounces of fluid *after* taking the medication (to assure that the medications have left the esophagus and are in the stomach and to speed absorption of the medications).
Do not routinely give analgesics for pain every 4 hours. Because of delayed absorption and distribution and the half-life of the medicine, there may be an adverse cumulative effect.
If the patient has difficulty swallowing a large capsule or tablet, ask the physician to substitute a liquid medication if at all possible. (Cutting the tablet in half or crushing it and placing it in applesauce or fruit juice may distort the action of some medications, reduce the dose, or cause choking or aspiration of particles of medication or applesauce).
Teach alternatives to medications, such as the following:
   Proper diet instead of vitamins
   Exercise instead of laxatives
   Bedtime snacks instead of hypnotics
   Decrease in weight, salt, fat, stress, and smoking, and increased exercise, instead of hypertensive agents (if approved by physician)

Medicines I Take

Name of Drug & What It's For	Color/Shape	Directions & Cautions	Times

Source: Using your medicines wisely: A guide for the elderly, U.S. Department of Health, Education, and Welfare Public Health Service. Alcohol, Drug Abuse, and Mental Health Administration, PF1436(1185), D317, p. 16.

Box 3-4.

Patient Education

How to Take Medicines at Home

Ask the physician or nurse the following:
   Name of medicine
   Amount to take
   Best time to take it
   How often to take it
   How to take it
   How long to take it
   Reason for taking it
   Most common side effects
   Whether any foods or other drugs
      should not be taken with it

Take all of the medicine prescribed unless the physician states otherwise.

Stop taking the medicine and report any new or unusual problems to the physician immediately, such as the following:
   Shortness of breath
   Nausea, vomiting, or diarrhea
   Sleepiness
   Dizziness
   Weakness
   Skin rash
   Fever

Never take a medicine prescribed for another person.

Do not take any medicine more than 1 year old or past the expiration date on the container.

Store medicines in a safe place, preferably the kitchen rather than the bathroom where moisture from bathing, especially showers, may affect the medicine.

Do not keep medicines, especially sedatives or hypnotics, on the bedside stand because when you are sleepy, you may forget that you have already taken the medicine earlier.

Do not place different medicines in the same container.

Take a sufficient supply of all medicines in their individual containers when traveling away from home.

Use a chart to keep track of medications to be taken. Cross through time after taken. See sample below.

NAME OF DRUG/ DIRECTIONS	SUN	MON	TUE	WED	THU	FRI	SAT
DRUG A — 3 Times a day	8 12 8	8 12 8	8 12 5	8 12 5	8 12 5	8 12 5	8 12 5
DRUG B — once a day in A.M.	8	8	8	8	8	8	8
DRUG C — 3 Times a day	8 12 6	8 12 6	8 12 5	8 12 5	8 12 5	8 12 5	8 12 5

Source: Using your medicines wisely: A guide for the elderly, US Department of Health, Education, and Welfare, Public Health Service, Alcohol, Drug Abuse, and Mental Health Administration, PF1436(1185), D317, p. 18.

Box 3-5.

Safe use of medicines by older people

Most people, and especially the elderly, use medicines at some point during their lifetime. When used correctly, medicines can be of great value. They can help heal wounds, stop the spread of infections, bring on sleep, and ease pain, both physical and mental. But when used incorrectly, drugs have the ability to injure the patient or change the effects of other medicines being taken at the same time.

Drugs can be divided into two major groups; over-the-counter drugs (also called patent medicines), which can be bought without a doctor's precription; and prescription drugs, which can be ordered only by a doctor and sold only by a pharmacist (druggist). Prescription drugs are usually more powerful and have more side effects than over-the-counter medicines.

People over 65 make up 11% of the American population, yet they take 25% of all prescription drugs sold in this country. One reason for this more frequent use of drugs by older people is that, as a group, they tend to have more long-term illnesses than they did when they were younger. Also, advancing age sometimes brings with it changes in physical abilities, eating habits, and social contacts. The result of these changes— whether it is aching muscles, constipation from lack of certain foods, or depression after the loss of a relative or friend—may often lead an older person to seek medical help. Drug treatment may be suggested to help overcome many of these physical and emotional problems.

Safe drug use requires both a well-informed doctor and a well-informed patient. New information about drugs and about how they affect the older user is coming to light daily. For this reason, those taking drugs should occasionally review with a doctor their need for each medicine.

In general, drugs given to older people act differently than they do when given to young or middle-aged people. This is probably the result of the normal changes in body makeup that occur with age. For example, as the body grows older, the percent of water and lean tissue (mainly muscle) decreases, while the percent of fat tissue increases. These changes can affect the length of time a drug stays in the body, how a drug will act in the body, and the amount of drug absorbed by body tissues.

The kidneys and the liver are two important organs responsible for breaking down and removing most drugs from the body. With age, the kidneys and the liver often begin to function less efficiently, and thus drugs leave the body more slowly. This may account for the fact that older people tend to have more undesirable reactions to drugs than do younger people.

Because older people can often have a number of physical problems at the same time, it is very common for them to be taking many different drugs. Two or more medicines taken at the same time can sometimes react with each other and produce harmful effects. For this reason, it is important to tell each doctor you go to about other drugs you are taking. This will allow the doctor to prescribe the safest medicines for your situation.

By taking an active part in learning about the drugs you take and their possible side effects, you can help bring about safer and faster treatment results. Some basic rules for safe drug use are as follows:

1. Take exactly the amount of drug prescribed by your doctor and follow the dosage schedule as closely as possible.
2. Medicines do not produce the same effects in all people. For this reason, you should never take drugs prescribed for a friend or relative, even though your symptoms may be the same.
3. Always tell your doctor about past problems you had with drugs, and be sure to mention other drugs (including over-the-counter medicines) you are taking.
4. It may help to keep a daily record of the drugs you are taking, especially if your treatment schedule is complicated or you are taking more than one drug at a time.
5. If child-proof containers are hard for you to handle, ask your pharmacist for easy-to-open containers. Always be sure, however, that such containers are out of the reach of children.
6. Make sure that you understand the directions printed on the drug container and that the name of the medicine is clearly printed. This will help you to avoid taking the wrong medicine or following the wrong schedule. Ask your pharmacist to use large type on the label if you find the regular labels hard to read.
7. Throw out old medicines, since many drugs lose their effectiveness over time.
8. Ask your doctor about side effects that may occur, about special rules for storage, and about which foods or beverages, if any, to avoid.
9. Always call your doctor promptly if you notice unusual reactions.

A useful booklet, *Using Your Medicines Wisely: A Guide for the Elderly*, has been published by the National Institute on Drug Abuse. Free single copies are available by writing to Elder-Ed, PO Box 416, Kensington, MD 20795. Multiple copies (in lots of 100) may be purchased for $17.00 by writing to the Superintendent of Documents, U.S. Government Printing Office, Washington, DC 20402

From U.S. Department of Health and Human Services, Public Health Service, National Institutes of Health.

Box 3-6.

Safe use of tranquilizers

Everyone is worried, tense, or nervous at one time or another. Most people have concerns that can cause them to feel uneasy or anxious, and older people are no exception. Sometimes these feelings of anxiety are accompanied by physical symptoms such as a tightness in the chest, trembling, choking, or rapid heart beat. Since a wide range of problems can produce these feelings, it is very important to have a thorough checkup if your symptoms continue.

There are many ways such symptoms can be managed. Sometimes physical activities or support from family or friends can make a difference. Sometimes professional assistance (individual, group, or family counseling) can be considered. And, sometimes, medications are helpful. "Minor" tranquilizers, or antianxiety drugs, recommended by a therapist and prescribed by a doctor, might be used at these times.

Ideally, tranquilizers are used in combination with counseling. The goal is usually to limit the dosage and length of an individual's tranquilizer use. This is especially important for older people because age-related changes often cause the body to use medications differently in later life. As a result, older people should pay close attention to side effects and safety considerations when taking tranquilizers.

Effects of tranquilizers

Tranquilizers are central nervous system (CNS) depressants. That is, they slow down the nervous system and can cause drowsiness. Some individuals, particularly older people, may become sleepy, dizzy, unsteady on their feet, and confused when taking these drugs. If the medication is taken at night, these side effects may occur the next day. As a result, when taking tranquilizers you should not drive, operate machinery, or do jobs that require you to be alert.

The effects of tranquilizers are greatly increased if they are taken at the same time as other CNS depressants such as antihistamines (medicines for allergies or colds), sleeping pills, prescription pain relievers, or muscle relaxants. It is also important to avoid alcohol when taking tranquilizers because it too is a powerful CNS depressant. Mixing large amounts of drugs and alcohol can cause unconsciousness and even death.

Some drugs, such as the ulcer drug cimetidine, may affect the body's use of tranquilizers. A doctor or pharmacist can tell you which drugs are safe to take with tranquilizers. Always tell the doctor what prescription and over-the-counter medications you are taking whenever he or she is considering a new medication for you.

Once you begin taking a tranquilizer, do not stop taking it suddenly. This can cause withdrawal symptoms including convulsions, muscle cramps, sweating, and vomiting. When it is time to stop your medication, the doctor will probably reduce the dose slowly to prevent these symptoms.

Sometimes people taking tranquilizers are afraid they will not be able to handle their problems without the medication. They may insist that their doctors prescribe tranquilizers for a longer period of time than is recommended. Since people who take tranquilizers for a long period of time may become dependent on them, it is very important to take this medication only under the careful supervision of a doctor.

Taking tranquilizers safely

When taking a tranquilizer you should observe the following safety tips:

- Make sure the doctor knows about all your current medications (prescription and over-the-counter) before you begin taking tranquilizers.
- Ask the doctor to explain any possible side effects of the tranquilizer he or she has prescribed.
- Follow the doctor's instructions exactly.
- Take only the amount of tranquilizer the doctor specifies—no more, no less.
- Take the tranquilizer only as often as prescribed—not more or less frequently.
- If you forget one dose of the medicine, do not double the next dose.
- Let the doctor know if you experience excessive drowsiness or other side effects—sometimes a shorter acting tranquilizer can relieve those complaints.
- Let the doctor know if you feel unusually chilly while taking tranquilizers. Sometimes they can cause a change in body temperature.
- Try to avoid caffeine (found in coffee, tea, cola drinks, and chocolate) while taking tranquilizers—it can counteract the effects of the tranquilizer.
- If you think you may have taken too many tranquilizers, get emergency help right away.

For more information

Tranquilizers can help many people manage the symptoms of anxiety. However, for these medicines to work safely and effectively, they must be taken as directed. Learning more about the medications the doctor prescribes will increase your health, safety, and well-being. For more information on the safe use of medications contact the following organizations.

The Elder Health Program provides patient information and service programs in geriatrics and gerontology.
University of Maryland
School of Pharmacy
20 North Pine Street
Baltimore, MD 21201
(301) 328-3243

Box 3-6.

Safe use of tranquilizers—cont'd

The AARP Pharmacy Service provides prescription drug information for older persons.
  1 Prince Street
  Alexandria, VA 22314
  (703) 684-0244

The Food and Drug Administration provides information about drugs and their side effects.
  Center for Drug Evaluation and Research
  Consumer and Professional Affairs (HFD-365)
  5600 Fishers Lane
  Rockville, MD 20857
  (301) 295-8012

The National Institute on Aging provides information about health and aging.
  Information Office
  Federal Building, Room 6C12
  Bethesda, MD 20892
  (301) 496-1752

From U.S. Department of Health and Human Services, Public Health Service, National Institutes of Health.

REFERENCES

Allen M (1983). Geriatric psychopharmacology, Fort Worth, Texas College of Osteopathic Medicine.

Deglin JH, Vallerand AH, and Russin MM (1991). Davis' drug guide for nurses, ed 2, Philadelphia, FA Davis Co.

Generic drugs. Myths vs. facts (1987). PL3987 (987), Washington, DC, Public Policy Institute, American Association of Retired Persons.

Kushnir SL (1990). PROZAC, Newsweek, p 10, April 16.

Lamy PP (1985). Are generic drugs dangerous for the aged? J Gerontol Nurs 12(2):36-37.

Luke EA (1990). Psychotropic drugs. In Hogstel MO, editor: Geropsychiatric nursing, St Louis, Mosby–Year Book, Inc.

Medicating the elderly (1987). Videotape L7508, New York, American Journal of Nursing.

Wolfe SM, Fugate L, Hulstrand EP, and Kamimoto LE (1988). Worst pills best pills, Washington, DC, Public Citizen Health Research Group.

CHAPTER 4

Skin

Peggy Mayfield

The skin serves as a window for viewing the age, race, and health of an individual. The appearance of the skin plays a major role in maintaining a positive self-image and sense of worth. Therefore the many changes and diseases of the skin that occur with increasing age cause concern to many older people. This chapter focuses primarily on neoplasms of the skin, some of which may be life-threatening if not detected early and promptly treated.

AGING OF THE SKIN

Intrinsic Aging

Intrinsic changes that are associated with the aging process include structural and functional changes such as the following:

The capacity to produce new cells diminishes, resulting in fewer cells (Marks, 1989).

The amount of pigmentation decreases as a result of the loss of melanocytes. Marks (1989) reported a 10% to 20% decrease per decade, occurring primarily in the non–sun exposed areas of the body. According to Fenske, Grayson, and Newcomer (1989), after age 30 there is a 20% loss of melanocytes per decade. This results in a significantly increased risk from ultraviolet radiation with aging.

A decrease in immunological function occurs that is related to a decrease in the Langerhans cells (Fenske, Grayson, and Newcomer, 1989). The older person is therefore more prone to skin cancers.

Cutaneous innervation decreases, resulting in an increased risk of injury (Fenske, Grayson, and Newcomer, 1989).

Dermal and epidermal circulation diminish and vascular walls thin, resulting in bruises (Fenske, Grayson, and Newcomer, 1989).

Subcutaneous fat thins, resulting in diminished insulation capacity and increased risk of hypothermia (Fenske, Grayson, and Newcomer, 1989).

Overall skin function is reduced as a result of thinning, structural breakdown, and loss of vascularity. Fenske, Grayson, and Newcomer (1989) stated that there is a 15% to 20% reduction in skin function of people in their 80s.

Photoaging

Photoaging denotes changes in the skin as a result of solar radiation. Changes in the skin that are generally equated with aging are actually the result of chronic solar damage (Epstein, 1989a). Solar damage causes wrinkles, dryness, atrophy, pigmentation changes, and fragility that results in ecchymoses and telangiectasia of the skin (Epstein, 1989a). Kligman (1989) stated that "photophobes who avoid the sun can have smooth, unblemished skin even into the ninth decade of life" (p. 331).

Kligman and Balin (1989) stated that solar damage also causes inelastic, saggy, wrinkled, coarse, redundant, yellow skin; benign growths (solar lentigo and freckles); precancerous growths (actinic keratosis); and cancers (basal cell carcinoma and squamous cell carcinoma). According to Fenske, Grayson, and Newcomer (1989), photoaging is responsible for 90% of skin cancers. Neoplasms and pigment changes are rare in protected skin.

Solar damage is caused by ultraviolet radiation. Ultraviolet B (UVB) rays are responsible for the most sun damage and have a high potential for causing burning, tanning, aging, and carcinogenesis, whereas ultraviolet A (UVA) rays have a low potential for burning, a high potential for tanning, and intermediate effects on aging and carcinogenesis (Wolfe and Davison, 1989). UVB rays are the most carcinogenic; however, UVA rays accelerate the damage done by UVB. Damage from ultraviolet radiation is cumulative throughout life and has a lag period of 10 to 20 years or more. In addition to solar damage, the skin is also damaged by chemical, mechanical, and physical trauma such as wind, cold, and low humidity (Kligman and Balin, 1989).

Table 4-1. Skin types and recommended sunscreen protection factor (SPF)

Skin type	Sensitivity to ultraviolet radiation*	Sunburn and tanning history*	Recommended SPF†
I	Very sensitive, + + + +	Always burns easily; never tans	15 or more
II	Very sensitive, + + + +	Always burns easily, tans minimally	15 or more
III	Sensitive, + + +	Burns moderately; tans gradually and uniformly (light brown)	10 to 15
IV	Moderately sensitive, + +	Burns minimally; always tans well (moderate brown)	6 to 10
V	Minimally sensitive, + to ±	Rarely burns; tans profusely (dark brown)	4 to 6
VI	Insensitive	Never burns; deeply pigmented (black)	None indicated

From Pathak MA (1987). Sunscreens and their use in the preventive treatment of sunlight-induced skin damage, J Dermatol Surg Oncol 13(7):741. Reprinted by permission of the publisher. Copyright 1987 by Elsevier Science Publishing Co, Inc.
Note: Constitutive color of unexposed buttock skin is white for individuals of skin types I-III and is white or faintly brown for those of skin type IV. Individuals of skin type V have brown buttock skin and those of skin type VI have dark brown or black buttock skin.
*Based on first 45 to 60 minutes of sun exposure after winter season or no sun exposure.
†Based on outdoor field studies.

Skin Types

The susceptibility of an individual to sun-induced skin damage varies on the basis of skin type, for example, the amount of melanin in the skin. The six skin types are shown in Table 4-1. Individuals with the first three skin types are more susceptible to solar damage than those with the last three, who have more melanin in the skin. The skin type is determined by determining the minimal erythema dose (MED), which is based on the number of minutes of noonday sun needed to cause minimal redness of the skin. For example, a skin of type I would become minimally red after 10 to 20 minutes of exposure, whereas a skin of type IV would take 40 to 50 minutes.

BENIGN SKIN NEOPLASMS
Solar Lentigo

Solar lentigines are harmless tan to brown macules that appear on sun-exposed skin areas following significant solar damage. They are frequently referred to as liver spots, age spots, or senile lentigo (Friedman, Rigel, and Kopf, 1985). They usually begin in adulthood, from age 40 upward. Balin and Lin (1989) reported results of a study that revealed solar lentigo present in 90% of persons over 80 years of age. Application of sunscreens and use of protective clothing before going outdoors will help prevent further lentigines.

Acrochordons

Acrochordons are soft, flesh-colored skin tags that occur primarily in middle-aged and older adults. They develop before age 40 in women and after age 50 in men (Fenske, Grayson, and Newcomer, 1989). The most common sites are in areas of skin laxity and friction such as the axillae, eyelids, groin, neck, and area beneath breasts. The size varies from 1 to 10 mm in diameter. Recent studies indicate a correlation between skin tags and adenomatous polyps of the colon (Goldman, 1989). There have been no reports of malignancy from skin tags; therefore removal is for cosmetic reasons or to prevent continued trauma from rubbing of clothing. They may be removed by electrodesiccation, cryosurgery, or simple snip excision, or chemically with trichloroacetic acid (Goldman, 1989).

Seborrheic Keratosis

Seborrheic keratoses are thick-crusted, warty, waxlike or greasy papules or plaques that range in color from yellow-orange through tan, brown, or black (Herten, 1989). They often have a "stuck on" appearance. They are most frequently located on the trunk, neck, scalp, face, and extremities and range in size from several millimeters up to 5 cm in diameter. Most persons have only a few of these lesions, but some have hundreds. Little is known about the etiology of seborrheic keratoses, but they are hereditary in approximately 50% of persons who have them (Herten, 1989). They are more common in the older adult, generally appearing in the early 50s. Balin (1989) reported results of a study that revealed the presence of seborrheic keratosis in 80% of persons over 64 years of age. They are benign but may be removed for cosmetic reasons. Liquid nitrogen cryotherapy is the simplest method of removal. Curettage and electrodesiccation are also used (Herten, 1989).

PREMALIGNANT NEOPLASMS
Actinic Keratosis

Actinic keratoses are slightly elevated, rough lesions that range in color from tan to dark brown, with a mild to moderate degree of erythema, and are usually less than

1 cm in diameter (Weiss, 1989). Solar damage rather than age is responsible for these lesions; hence the term *senile keratosis* is a misnomer. They occur on sun-exposed areas: the face, "V" of the chest, and the backs of arms and hands in the middle-aged and older adult, especially the fair-skinned person with solar damage. Actinic keratosis is the most common premalignant skin lesion and affects nearly 100% of the elderly white population (Epstein, 1989a; Schwartz and Howard, 1987). The lesions must be removed since approximately 20% will develop into squamous cell carcinoma. For small lesions, cryotherapy with liquid nitrogen is used, but for widespread lesions, topical 5-fluorouracil (5FU), dermabrasion, or chemical peel may be used (Weiss, 1989). Use of sunscreens and protective clothing will help prevent further solar damage.

Leukoplakia

Leukoplakia is a white plaque that may form on the lip or mucous membrane and is caused by chronic irritation such as pipe smoking, ill-fitting dentures, or smokeless tobacco. All forms of smokeless tobacco contain carcinogens that contribute to irritation of the mucosa, but the practice of greatest concern to the American Cancer Society is the habit of dipping snuff. Oral cancer is several times more frequent in those who use snuff as compared with non–tobacco users, and the risk of cheek and gum cancer is nearly 50 times greater among long-term snuff users (American Cancer Society, 1989).

In the older adult the oral mucosa becomes thin, smooth, and dry and has an edematous appearance (Epstein, 1989b). When inspecting the lips and oral mucosa, the examiner should look for abnormalities such as a white patch that cannot be rubbed off or a velvety red plaque that might indicate erythroplasia (erythroplakia). Among oral precancerous lesions 95% begin as erythroplasia, with or without leukoplakia, and 2% begin primarily as leukoplakia (Schwartz and Howard, 1987).

Early treatment of leukoplakia consists of eliminating irritants such as tobacco and strong toothpastes or mouthwashes and correcting dental problems. These measures, along with good oral hygiene, should permit the tissue to return to normal (Berliner, 1986). If the leukoplakia continues, referral is necessary. Differentiating leukoplakia of the lip from squamous cell carcinoma requires a biopsy. A biopsy of the oral cavity is used for a differential diagnosis to determine whether the lesion is premalignant or malignant. Squamous cell carcinoma that develops from mucosal leukoplakia metastasizes more frequently than cutaneous squamous cell carcinoma (Schwartz and Howard, 1987).

Dysplastic Nevi

Dysplastic nevi are abnormal nevi (moles). They are acquired pigmented lesions that are frequently familial. Dysplastic nevi have the following characteristics:

They are larger than common nevi, ranging from 6 to 12 mm or more in diameter.

Borders are irregular and poorly defined.

Color is variegated, ranging from tan to dark brown, and they may have a pinkish white center.

They are numerous, often exceeding 100, whereas a typical adult has 10 to 40 common moles.

They frequently occur on non–sun-exposed areas such as scalp, breast, and buttocks, as well as on sun-exposed areas (as with common nevi). The back is the most common site.

They continue to develop throughout adult life, whereas common nevi usually do not develop past age 40 (Friedman, Rigel, and Kopf, 1985; Green et al, 1985).

The risk of developing a malignant melanoma is 6% to 18% for persons with dysplastic nevi, as compared to 1% for the general population. The risk is especially high if there is also a family history of dysplastic nevi or malignant melanoma. Individuals and families with dysplastic nevi need to be followed closely by a dermatologist throughout life because the nevi are difficult to differentiate from malignant melanoma. Diagnosis is made by biopsy of several nevi. Subsequent biopsies are done if malignant melanoma is suspected or if a new nevus appears. It is impractical to remove all the dysplastic nevi.

SKIN CANCER

American Cancer Society statistics show that there are over 500,000 cases of skin cancer a year, with most of them being basal cell carcinoma (BCC) or squamous cell carcinoma (SCC). Malignant melanoma, which is the most serious skin cancer, has an incidence of 27,000 cases each year and is increasing at the rate of 3.4% a year. There are about 8200 deaths a year from skin cancer, with 6000 deaths from malignant melanoma and 2200 deaths from other skin cancers. The death rate from malignant melanoma is increasing faster than from any other cancer except lung cancer in women. Malignant melanoma, depending on subtypes, peaks in the fifth to eighth decades of life (Gilchrest, 1986). Persons over 60 years of age are at a greater risk of developing BCC and SCC than younger persons given the same amount of sun exposure, but solar damage is a much greater risk than advancing age (Epstein, 1989a). Each year 2% to 3% of the older population develop new cases of BCC and SCC (Gilchrest, 1986). According to Fenske, Grayson, and Newcomer (1989) most of the cancerous skin lesions on older adults tend to be slower in developing and spreading than on younger persons.

Box 4-1 lists risk factors for skin cancer.

Basal Cell Carcinoma

BCC is a malignant tumor that develops from the basal cell layer of the epidermis and most commonly presents

---

Box 4-1.

Risk factors for skin cancer

Overexposure to frost, wind, and ultraviolet radiation from the sun

Occupational exposure to radiation (e.g., radioisotopes, x-rays)

Exposure to chemical carcinogens (e.g., coal tars, arsenic, creosote, pitch, petroleum, paraffin)

Genetic predisposition

Thermal burn scars

Chronic trauma and irritation to an area

X-ray therapy (e.g., for acne, birthmarks)

Skin that is fair, ruddy, freckled; light hair or eyes; skin that burns easily

Precancerous skin lesions (e.g., actinic keratosis, Bowen's disease, dysplastic nevi)

Age over 50

Indoor occupation with blasts of outdoor recreation

History of severe sunburn before age 18

From Cancer prevention and detection in the cancer screening clinic (1988). Houston, The University of Texas MD Anderson Cancer Center.

---

as a firm, translucent nodule with a rolled, pearly border, telangiectasia and an umbilicated center. BCC is the most common skin cancer; in fact, it is the most common of all cancers.

▶ **PATHOPHYSIOLOGY, SIGNS, AND SYMPTOMS**

Chronic solar damage is the major cause of BCC. The lesions occur on the sun-exposed areas of the skin, with 85% occurring on the head and neck (Epstein, 1989a). High-risk persons are those with fair, freckled or ruddy skin who have light eyes and light-colored hair and who sunburn easily (Epstein, 1989a).

The warning signs of BCC (Fenske, Grayson, and Newcomer, 1989) are as follows:

A sore that lasts for 3 weeks or more

An irritated, reddened area that may be itchy or painful

A smooth growth with an elevated, shiny border

A pearly or translucent nodule that resembles a mole

A white or yellow lesion that resembles scar tissue

BCC rarely metastasizes, but local destruction and disfigurement can be extensive (Strick, 1989).

▶ **MEDICAL MANAGEMENT**

A biopsy is necessary for histologic diagnosis. Skin biopsies include the following:

Shave biopsy—A scalpel is used to shave off tissue, or scissors are used to snip off tissue for evaluation.

Punch biopsy—A sharp, circular instrument is used to obtain a specimen of the dermal, epidermal, and subcutaneous tissue. The wound is closed with a suture.

Excisional biopsy—The total lesion is excised with a scalpel and the wound is closed with sutures.

Treatment for BCC includes the following:

Radiation therapy (BCC is very radiosensitive)

Surgical excision (Mohs' microscopically controlled surgery is widely used)

Topical cytotoxic agents (5FU)

Cryosurgery (application of cold liquid nitrogen)

Electrodesiccation (use of high-frequency current through a needle) and curettage (Fry, 1985; Roses et al, 1989)

Squamous Cell Carcinoma

SCC is a malignant tumor arising from the squamous epithelium. The appearance varies from a rough, scaly tumor, to a red nodular mass, to an ulcerated or fungating mass. The lesions are opaque, in contrast to BCC lesions, which are translucent. SCC is the second most common skin cancer in whites. In blacks SCC is more common than BCC (Strick, 1989).

▶ **PATHOPHYSIOLOGY, SIGNS, AND SYMPTOMS**

Contributing factors for SCC include chronic solar damage and chronic irritation or trauma. Lesions occur in areas of chronic irritation and on sun-exposed areas including the back of the hand, rim of the ear, forehead, and lower lip; 75% occur on the head (face, cheeks, ears, nose, lips), 15% on the hands, and 10% elsewhere (Roses et al, 1989). Actinic keratoses are considered to be the premalignant form of SCC because approximately 20% progress to SCC (Schleper, 1984). Since chronic irritation is one of the causes, the lesions also appear in dark-skinned persons (Epstein, 1989a). Exposure to chemical carcinogens such as coal, pitch, asphalt, tar, soot, and creosote contribute to SCC, with an estimated latent period of 20 to 50 years (Schleper, 1984). Strick (1989) stated that SCC may metastasize depending on the etiology of the tumor, with a 0.5% to 5% rate of metastasis if secondary to sun damage and a 15% to 35% rate if secondary to other causes. Lesions that most frequently metastasize are those located at the mucocutaneous junctions (e.g., lip, vulva, glans penis), in the "H" area of the face, or on the oral mucous membrane and those greater than 5 cm in size.

▶ **MEDICAL MANAGEMENT**

Punch or incisional biopsies are made to confirm the diagnosis. There are three approaches to cure of SCC:

Surgical excision—the treatment of choice; Mohs' surgery

Radiotherapy

Local destruction by curettage and electrodesiccation, diathermy, or cryotherapy (Fry, 1985)

The cure rates for BCC and SCC are 90% to 95% or greater (Stegman, 1986; Strick, 1989).

Malignant Melanoma

Malignant melanoma is a malignant neoplasm of melanocytes (pigmented cells), which can spread throughout the body via the blood stream and lymphatics. It is less common than BCC or SCC but has a higher mortality rate.

▶ **PATHOPHYSIOLOGY, SIGNS, AND SYMPTOMS**

The etiology of malignant melanoma is less clear than that of the other skin cancers. Solar radiation seems to be a factor, especially a blistering sunburn before the age of 18, which is thought to damage the Langerhans cells and thus affect the immune response of the skin. Two thirds of malignant melanomas occur in preexisting moles and one third in new moles; therefore any change in a current mole or the development of a new mole after age 40 should be carefully examined.

There are several types of cutaneous melanomas:

Superficial spreading—65% to 75% of melanomas; spreads horizontally with minimal dermal invasion, has a favorable prognosis, affects middle-aged persons, and occurs most frequently on the back and lower extremities

Nodular—20% to 25%; convex, nodular lesion that grows vertically and becomes invasive more quickly, thus has a poor prognosis

Acral lentiginous—10%; seen on palms, soles, nail beds, and mucous membranes of blacks and orientals

Lentigo maligna melanoma or Hutchinson's melanotic freckle—5% to 7%; commonly seen on the face in persons over 60 years of age; appear as tan, flat lesions and slowly change in size and color (Schleper, 1984)

The danger signs of malignant melanoma are as follows:

Change in color—darkening, variegated shades of tan, brown, black, red, white, blue

Change in shape—irregular or notched margins; blending of color into surrounding skin.

Change in texture—rough or scaly; oozing, bleeding, or ulcerated

Change in sensation—itching, tingling, or painful; feels "strange"

Change in height—elevation of a previously flat mole or a "fried egg" appearance

Change in size—especially a sudden increase; moles larger than 6 mm (size of a pencil eraser) are suspicious

Development of a new mole—especially after age 40 (Roses et al, 1989).

The American Cancer Society lists simple melanoma ABCD rules that are easy to remember (Box 4-2).

▶ **MEDICAL MANAGEMENT**

An incisional or excisional biopsy is done for histologic diagnosis. Treatment consists of the following:

Surgical excision of the tumor, with microscopic clearance of all margins—Tumors less than 0.76 mm in depth rarely metastasize; they can be locally excised with a 2-cm margin and the wound closed by primary closure. Deeper lesions require wide local excision and a skin graft.

Isolated limb perfusion with chemotherapy for melanoma of an extremity

Prophylactic excision of regional lymph nodes (controversial)

Immunotherapy (e.g., interleukins, interferons, monoclonal antibodies) (White and Polk, 1986; Hirsch, 1989)

Box 4-2.

The ABCD rules of melanoma

A. *Asymmetry:* One half does not match the other half.
B. *Border irregularity:* The edges are ragged, notched, or blurred.
C. *Color:* The pigment is not uniform in color—shades of tan, brown, or black, or a mottled appearance with red, white, or blue areas
D. *Diameter:* The diameter is greater than 6 mm (size of a pencil eraser) or an increase in size.

▶ **NURSING MANAGEMENT—NURSING CARE PLAN**
The Patient with a Suspicious Skin Neoplasm

Assessment

SUBJECTIVE DATA
Risk factors for skin cancer (see Box 4-1)
Recent change in a wart or mole
A sore that has persisted for more than 3 weeks
Use of snuff or other smokeless tobacco
Knowledge of preventive measures
OBJECTIVE DATA
Presence of a suspicious skin lesion

Presence of firm, red, shiny or pearly lesion on sun-exposed areas
Presence of scaly, rough, keratotic lesion on sun-exposed areas
Presence of red or white patch on lip or mucous membrane
Presence of pigmented lesion that is irregular in shape, color, or size

	Nursing diagnoses	Expected outcomes	Nursing interventions (rationale)
N U R S I N G C A R E P L A N	Impairment of skin integrity related to premalignant or malignant skin lesions	Suspicious skin lesions will be assessed and treated.	Assess the skin and mucous membranes of the oral cavity for abnormal skin lesions or neoplasms.
		Client will be free of skin cancer and precancerous lesions.	Refer to dermatologist for evaluation and treatment of abnormal lesions or neoplasms.
	Knowledge deficit regarding prognosis and treatment of skin cancer	New skin lesions will be promptly detected, reported, and treated.	Emphasize the need for physician follow-up and annual skin examination.
	Knowledge deficit regarding prevention and early detection of skin cancer	Client and/or significant other will be able to describe risk factors for skin cancer and methods of diminishing the risks.	Teach the risk factors that are pertinent for the individual.
			Teach client to limit sun exposure to 20 min a day, avoiding the sun if possbile between 10 AM and 3 PM.
			Teach protective measures such as the use of sunscreens and protective clothing when outdoors (see Box 4-3).
			Discourage the use of tobacco (e.g., pipe, snuff, chewing tobacco). If client is unable or unwilling to give up tobacco, encourage rotation of placement sites within the mouth.
			Provide appropriate skin cancer educational materials (see list on p. 48).
		Client and/or significant other will be able to demonstrate skin examination.	Teach monthly skin self-examination (see Figure 4-1).
	Knowledge deficit regarding home care of wound following the treatment regimen for lesions/neoplasms	Wounds, posttreatment, will heal without complications.	Instruct patient on wound care following biopsy, excision, or other treatment modality.
			Keep dressing clean and dry.
			Change dressing if needed, using sterile technique.
			Report bleeding, redness, or drainage to physician (Tucker et al, 1988).

Discharge planning and patient education

Emphasis should be on prevention and early detection and treatment of lesions. The primary preventive measure patients can take is protecting their skin from the sun (Box 4-3). They can play an important role in the early detection of skin lesions by routine self-examination of their skin. Older adults with poor vision or diminished flexibility may require assistance in performing a thorough examination that follows the step-by-step instructions in Figure 4-1. In addition to giving patients general information about skin cancer (Box 4-4), it is also im-portant to teach them about the dangers of photosensitizing drugs and to answer their questions about the use of sunscreens.

Evaluation

Client recovers from surgery or other procedure without complications.
Client practices monthly self-examination and reports any skin changes detected.
Client uses measures for prevention of skin cancer.
Client avoids the use of tobacco.

Patient Education

Sun Protection Recommendations

Avoid getting sunburned. Persons of all skin types and races can sunburn, but fair-skinned persons burn more easily.

Do not consider tanning healthy. Do not try to get a suntan, and avoid tanning booths.

Avoid the midday sun (10 AM to 3 PM) when the ultraviolet radiation is most intense.

Wear protective clothing such as a broad-brimmed hat, long sleeves, long pants; however, be aware that clothing alone does not provide complete protection.

Use sunscreen daily (if going outside), even on a cloudy day because clouds do not block ultraviolet radiation.

Select and use a broad-spectrum sunscreen appropriate for your skin type. Apply to sun-exposed areas 45 minutes before going outside and reapply periodically after perspiring heavily or swimming. If using cosmetics on face, apply sunscreen first.

Use a lip balm that contains a sunscreen. Beware of reflection from sand, snow, and water, which will intensify the radiation.

Avoid sun if using photosensitizing drugs.

Avoid para-aminobenzoic acid (PABA) sunscreens if allergic to procaine, sulfonamides, or hair dyes because of cross sensitization.

Facts about skin cancer from the American Academy of Dermatology

What is skin cancer?

Skin cancer is a malignant condition caused by uncontrolled growth of cells in one of the layers of the skin.

Are all skin cancers the same?

No, there are several different kinds of skin cancer, distinguished by the types of cells the tumors resemble. The three most common types of skin cancer are basal cell carcinoma, squamous cell carcinoma, and malignant melanoma.

How prevalent is skin cancer?

An estimated 450,000 Americans get skin cancer each year, making it the most prevalent form of cancer in the United States. More than one in seven Americans will develop some form of skin cancer. An estimated 300,000 to 400,000 cases of basal cell carcinoma and another 80,000 to 100,000 cases of squamous cell carcinoma occur annually. Basal cell is the most prevalent skin cancer.

What do basal cell carcinomas look like?

Basal cell carcinomas usually appear as slowly growing, raised, translucent, pearly nodules, which if untreated may crust, ulcerate, and sometimes bleed. They occur most often on the head, neck, hands, and trunk.

Is basal cell carcinoma a serious disease?

Basal cell carcinoma can cause considerable damage if allowed to invade the skin to underlying structures. It does not spread to other organs through the bloodstream, as some cancers do, and it grows slowly.

What do squamous cell carcinomas look like?

Squamous cell carcinomas usually are raised, red or pink, opaque nodules or warty growths that ulcerate in the center. They typically develop on the rim of the ear, the face, lips, mouth, hands, and other sun-exposed areas of the body.

Box 4-4.

Facts about skin cancer from the American Academy of Dermatology—cont'd

Are squamous cell carcinomas serious?

Yes, squamous cell carcinomas will increase in size, occasionally developing into large ulcerating, mushroomlike tumors. This form of skin cancer can spread to other parts of the body, and between 1500 and 2000 deaths result each year.

What is the most serious form of skin cancer?

Malignant melanoma is responsible for 75% of all skin cancer deaths. If untreated it can spread throughout the body. It is estimated that in 1987 malignant melanoma will affect 25,800 people and will cause 5800 deaths.

How can I recognize malignant melanoma?

Melanoma generally begins as a mottled, light brown to black, flat blemish with irregular borders. The blemish is usually at least ¼ inch in diameter and may turn shades of red, blue, and white, crust on the surface, and bleed. Melanomas often occur in moles, frequently appearing on the upper back, torso, lower legs, head, and neck.

What are my chances of getting malignant melanoma?

Although malignant melanoma is relatively rare, the incidence is increasing at a faster rate than for any other form of cancer, except lung cancer in women. Since 1980, the incidence has risen 75%, and if the present trend continues, by the year 2000, 1 person in 90 will develop malignant melanoma.

What causes skin cancer?

Prolonged and/or intermittent overexposure to ultraviolet radiation from the sun is the primary cause of skin cancer. Ninety percent of all skin cancers occur on parts of the body that are unprotected by clothing and in individuals who spend long hours in the sun. Less common causes include overexposure to x-rays or certain chemical carcinogens such as arsenic.

Who gets skin cancer?

Although skin cancer can affect anyone, the following people are at greater risk:
  Individuals with fair skin who sunburn easily
  Individuals who work outdoors or otherwise allow themselves considerable exposure to sunlight-

(There also is some evidence that bursts of high-intensity sun radiation, such as severe sunburn, may be particularly important in malignant melanoma.)
  Individuals who have multiple dysplastic nevi (unusual moles) (These people are at a higher risk for developing malignant melanoma.)
  Individuals who have a family history of skin cancer
  Individuals who suffer from genetic diseases characterized by sunlight intolerance (e.g., albinism) (This risk is related to nonmelanoma cancers.)
  Individuals who live in the South and Southwest, where the sun's rays are more intense.

Can skin cancer be prevented?

Yes, experts believe that the majority of skin cancers could be prevented if individuals would take simple precautions against the sun's ultraviolet radiation.

Can skin cancer be cured?

Yes, when detected in time, most skin cancers can be treated successfully. Dermatologists recommend regular self-examinations and annual physician examinations to detect changes in existing moles or blemishes.

How are skin cancers treated?

A variety of effective treatment options are available, including the following:
  Excisional surgery—A physician removes the entire growth and a small border of normal skin.
  Electrodesiccation—Cancerous tissue is destroyed by high-frequency current applied through a needle electrode.
  Moh's surgery—Thin layers of cancerous growth are removed and examined under a microscope.
  Cryosurgery—Cancerous tissue is destroyed by the application of intensely cold liquid nitrogen.
  Radiation therapy—High-energy x-rays or another source of radiation is directed at the cancer site to destroy the malignant tissue.
  Topical chemotherapy—Creams, ointments, or lotions containing the anticancer agent 5-fluorouracil (Fluorouracil, Adrucil) are applied directly to the skin. This therapy is useful in treating certain precancerous lesions.

From Facts about skin cancer (1987). Medical Times 115(12):92-93. Reprinted with permission.

Figure 4-1. Technique for self-examination of the skin. (From Friedman RJ, Rigel DS, and Kopf AW [1985]. Early detection of malignant melanoma, CA 35[3]:20-23. Reprinted with permission.)

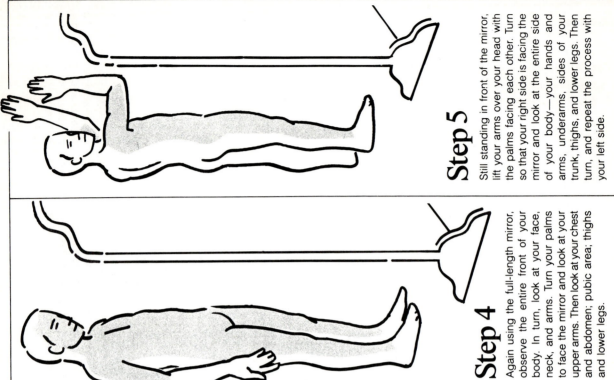

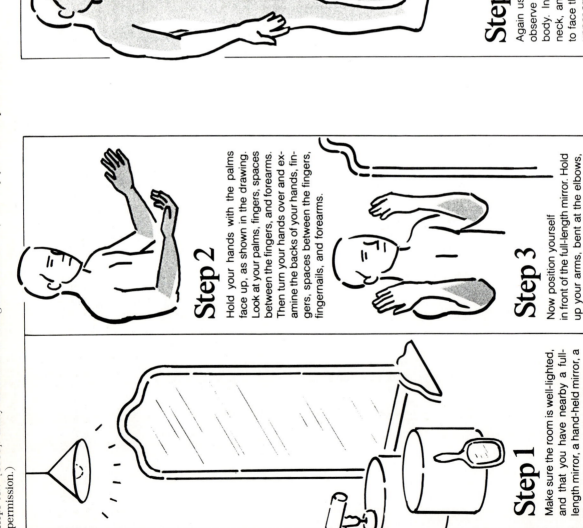

Step 1

Make sure the room is well-lighted, and that you have nearby a full-length mirror, a hand-held mirror, a hand-held blow dryer, and two chairs or stools. Undress completely.

Step 2

Hold your hands with the palms face up, as shown in the drawing. Look at your palms, fingers, spaces between the fingers, and forearms. Then turn your hands over and examine the backs of your hands, fingers, spaces between the fingers, fingernails, and forearms.

Step 3

Now position yourself in front of the full-length mirror. Hold up your arms, bent at the elbows, with your palms facing you. In the mirror, look at the backs of your forearms and elbows.

Step 4

Again using the full-length mirror, observe the entire front of your body. In turn, look at your face, neck, and arms. Turn your palms to face the mirror and look at your upper arms. Then look at your chest and abdomen; pubic area; thighs and lower legs.

Step 5

Still standing in front of the mirror, lift your arms over your head with the palms facing each other. Turn so that your right side is facing the mirror and look at the entire side of your body—your hands and arms, underarms, sides of your trunk, thighs, and lower legs. Then turn, and repeat the process with your left side.

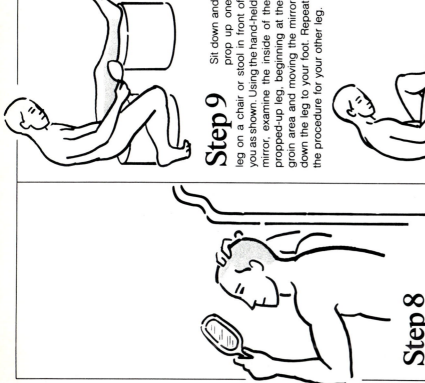

Step 9

Sit down and prop up one leg on a chair or stool in front of you as shown. Using the hand-held mirror, examine the inside of the propped-up leg, beginning at the groin area and moving the mirror down the leg to your foot. Repeat the procedure for your other leg.

Step 10

Still sitting, cross one leg over the other. Use the hand-held mirror to examine the top of your foot, the toes, toenails, and spaces between the toes. Then look at the sole or bottom of your foot. Repeat the procedure for the other foot.

Step 8

Use the hand-held mirror and the full-length mirror to look at your scalp. Because the scalp is difficult to examine, we suggest you also use a hand-held blow dryer turned to a cool setting, to lift the hair from the scalp. While some people find it easy to hold the mirror in one hand and the dryer in the other, while looking in the full-length mirror, many do not. For the scalp examination in particular, then, you might ask your spouse or a friend to assist you.

Step 7

Now pick up the hand-held mirror. With your back still to the full-length mirror, examine the back of your neck, and your back and buttocks. Also examine the backs of your arms in this way. Some areas are hard to see, and you may find it helpful to ask your spouse or a friend to assist you.

Step 6

With your back toward the full-length mirror, look at your buttocks and the backs of your thighs and lower legs.

PHOTOSENSITIZING DRUGS

Some drugs, including many that are taken routinely by older persons, cause photosensitivity reactions of the skin when the person taking them is exposed to UVA radiation. There are two types of photosensitivity reaction: (1) a photoallergy that causes urticaria, bullae, and/or sunburn, which is not dose-related, and (2) phototoxicity, which is an exaggerated reaction to UVA, is dose-related, and causes severe sunburn. If a person has had a photosensitivity reaction, sunscreens containing PABA or PABA esters should be avoided.

SUNSCREENS

Sunscreens offer protection from ultraviolet rays and are measured in terms of a sun protection factor (SPF) for UVB, the most damaging of the rays. The MED (minimal erythema dose) times the SPF equals the number of minutes an individual can be in the sun without burning. For example, a person with skin type I (with MED of 10), using a sunscreen of 15 SPF could stay in the sun 150 minutes (10×15) without burning. In essence, the number of SPF of a sunscreen means that a person can stay in the sun that many times longer without burning. It must be remembered, however, that the SPF is for the average individual, and the older adult is less resistant to the damaging rays of the sun. It is unrealistic to expect older adults to stay indoors and give up the pleasures of outdoor recreation such as walking, gardening, and golfing, but they need to be more cautious. See Table 4-1 for the suggested SPF for each skin type.

There are three major types of chemical sunscreens:
Para-aminobenzoic acid (PABA) or PABA esters (e.g., padimate A and padimate O)
Non-PABA sunscreens (e.g., benzophenones, cinnamates, salicylates, and anthranilates)
Combination sunscreens (Wolfe and Davidson, 1989)
PABA and PABA esters are extremely effective in absorbing UVB radiation, and salicylates, benzophenones, cinnamates, and anthranilates offer some protection against UVA as well as UVB. Therefore PABA or PABA esters used in combination with the non-PABA screens result in a very effective and substantive sunscreen. The substantivity of a sunscreen is its ability to be absorbed by and remain active in the stratum corneum. To allow time for absorption, one should apply sunscreens 30 to 45 minutes before going outdoors. Alcohol solutions and gels are more substantive than emollients.

The FDA has approved over 21 different agents as safe and effective sunscreens, but those just listed are the most widely used (Pathak, 1987). There are also physical sunscreens (sunblockers), which are opaque and totally block the rays (e.g., zinc oxide and titanium oxide). They are messy and cosmetically unpleasant, and are used primarily on selected areas such as the nose, lips, or tops of ears.

SKIN CANCER EDUCATION MATERIALS

American Cancer Society—(404) 320-3333
  "Fry Now, Pay Later," #901
  "Facts on Skin Cancer," #825
  "Early Detection of Malignant Melanoma," #1523 (Professional Education)
  "Melanoma/Skin Cancer—You Can Recognize the Signs," #904
  "The Diagnosis and Management of Common Skin Cancers," #2558 (Professional Education)
  "Why You Should Know About Melanoma," #922
  Video: "A Report on Skin Cancer," by Dr. Frank Field, 13 minutes
  Slides: "Good News About Skin Cancer," #P72
National Cancer Institute—(800) 4-CANCER
  "Progress Against Cancer of the Skin," #88-310
  "What You Need to Know About Skin Cancer," #89-1564
  "What You Need to Know About Melanomas," #89-1563
  "About Dysplastic Nevi"
  Posters on moles and melanoma
  Slides of normal and dysplastic moles (professional education)
  Video loan: "Prevention of Malignant Melanoma, A program for Melanoma Prone Families"

REFERENCES

American Cancer Society (1989). Cancer facts and figures. New York, The Society.

Balin AK and Lin AN (1989). Skin changes as a biological marker for measuring the rate of human aging. In Balin AK and Kligman AM, editors: Aging and the skin, New York, Raven Press.

Berliner H (1986). Aging skin, Am J Nurs 86(11):1259-1261.

Epstein JH (1989a). Photocarcinogenesis, skin cancer, and aging. In Balin AK and Kligman AM, editors: Aging and the skin, New York, Raven Press.

Epstein S (1989b). Oral lesions. In Newcomer VD and Young E Jr, editors: Geriatric dermatology: Clinical diagnosis and practical therapy, New York, Igaku-Shoin.

Fenske NA, Grayson LD, and Newcomer VD (1989). Common problems of the aging skin, Patient Care 23(7):225-234.

Friedman RJ, Rigel DS, and Kopf AW (1985). Early detection of malignant melanoma, CA 35(3):130-151.

Fry L, editor (1985). Skin problems in the elderly, New York, Churchill Livingstone.

Gilchrest BA (1986). Geriatric skin problems, Hosp Pract 21(9):55-65.

Goldman MP (1989). Skin tags (acrochordons) and colonic polyps. In Newcomer VD and Young EM Jr, editors: Geriatric dermatology: Clinical diagnosis and practical therapy, New York, Igaku-Shoin.

Green MH, Clark WH Jr, Tucker MA, Elder DE, et al (1985). Acquired precursors of cutaneous malignant melanoma: The familial dysplastic nevus syndrome, N Engl J Med 312:91-97.

Herten RJ (1989). Seborrheic keratoses and other benign keratoses. In Newcomer VD and Young EM Jr, editors: Geriatric dermatology: Clinical diagnosis and practical therapy, New York, Igaku-Shoin.

Hirsch P (1989). Nevi and melanoma. In Newcomer VD and Young EM Jr, editors: Geriatric dermatology: Clinical diagnosis and practical therapy, New York, Igaku-Shoin.

Kligman LH (1989). Skin changes in photoaging: Characteristics, prevention and repair. In Balin AK and Kligman AM, editors: Aging and the skin, New York, Raven Press.

Kligman LH and Balin AK (1989). Aging of human skin. In Balin AK and Kligman AM, editors: Aging and the skin, New York, Raven Press.

Marks R (1989). Epidermal aging. In Balin AK and Kligman AM, editors: Aging and the skin, New York, Raven Press.

Pathak MA (1987). Sunscreens and their use in the preventive treatment of sunlight-induced skin damage, J Dermatol Surg Oncol 13(7):739-750.

Roses DF, Gumport SL, Harris MN, and Copf AW (1989). The diagnosis and management of common skin disorders, New York, American Cancer Society (professional education publication).

Schleper JR (1984). Cancer prevention and detection: Skin cancer, Cancer Nurs 7(1):67-84.

Schwartz RA and Howard LS Jr (1987). Epithelial precancerous lesions. In Fitzpatrick TB et al, editors: Dermatology in general medicine, ed 3, New York, McGraw-Hill.

Stegman SJ (1986). Basal cell carcinoma and squamous cell carcinoma: Recognition and treatment, Med Clin North Am 70(1):95-107.

Strick RA (1989). Basal cell and squamous cell carcinoma. In Newcomer VD and Young EM Jr, editors: Geriatric dermatology: Clinical diagnosis and practical therapy, New York, Igaku-Shoin.

Tucker SM, Canobbio MM, Paquette EV, and Wells MF (1988). Patient care standards: Nursing process, diagnosis, and outcome, ed 4, St Louis, The CV Mosby Co.

Weiss SR (1989). Actinic keratoses. In Newcomer VD and Young EM Jr, editors: Geriatric dermatology: Clinical diagnosis and practical application, New York, Igaku-Shoin.

White MJ and Polk HC Jr (1986). Therapy of primary cutaneous melanoma, Med Clin North Am 70(1):71-85.

Wolfe DP and Davidson TM (1989). Sunscreens. In Newcomer VD and Young EM Jr, editors: Geriatric dermatology: Clinical diagnosis and practical application, New York, Igaku-Shoin.

BIBLIOGRAPHY

Anders JE and Leach EE (1983). Sun versus skin, A J Nurs 83(7):1015-1050.

Cancer prevention and detection in the cancer screening clinic (1988). Houston, The University of Texas MD Anderson Cancer Center.

Gilmore GD (1989). Sunscreens: A review of the skin cancer protection value and educational opportunities, School Health 59(5):210-213.

Hogstel M (1989). Integumentary system. In Burggraf V and Stanley M, editors: Nursing the elderly: A care plan approach, Philadelphia, JB Lippincott Co.

CHAPTER 5

Vision and Hearing

Mildred O. Hogstel

Much of communication occurs through the sensory system. Effective communication is very important to people as they become older because contact with others helps to maintain self-esteem and self-worth as well as prevent loneliness and depression. However, problems frequently occur in the sensory system, especially the eyes and ears, as people age. If not diagnosed and treated, other major problems occur, for example, decreased mobility and fewer social contacts. The most important problems that affect the sensory system in older adults are given in Table 5-1.

Table 5-1. Common problems affecting vision and hearing

Sense	Problem
Vision	Presbyopia
	Cataracts
	Glaucoma
	Macular degeneration
	Floaters and flashes
	Ectropion
	Entropion
Hearing	Presbycusis
	Ménière's disease

PRESBYOPIA

Presbyopia normally occurs in most people between the ages of 40 and 45. This is the time when many individuals find that they need to wear glasses for the first time to read and see close objects well.

▶ PATHOPHYSIOLOGY, SIGNS, AND SYMPTOMS

The crystalline lens of the eyes become more rigid and less elastic. "The ciliary muscles become weaker, and the lens cannot bulge to accommodate for near vision" (Malasanos, Barkauskas, and Stoltenberg-Allen, 1990, p. 242). The individual begins to hold reading material at a distance in order to see it clearly.

▶ DIAGNOSTIC PROCEDURES

A complete eye examination is needed, especially to test for acuity for close vision.

▶ MEDICAL MANAGEMENT

Glasses with bifocal (e.g., for reading distance) or trifocal (e.g., for reading distance and computer terminal distance) lenses are prescribed.

▶ PROGNOSIS

The prognosis is excellent with correct and persistent use of prescription bifocal or trifocal glasses.

▶ NURSING MANAGEMENT—NURSING CARE PLAN
Presbyopia

Assessment

SUBJECTIVE DATA
"My arms are not long enough to read this book."
"I believe I must need glasses."

OBJECTIVE DATA
Does not have 20/20 vision on a hand-held eye chart at 14 inches from eyes
Cannot read newspaper at 14 inches from eyes

<table>
<tr><td rowspan="2" style="writing-mode:vertical">N U R S I N G   C A R E   P L A N</td><td>Nursing diagnosis</td><td>Expected outcome</td><td>Nursing interventions (rationale)</td></tr>
<tr><td>Sensory/perceptual alterations (visual) related to decreased elasticity of the lens of the eye</td><td>Patient will have 20/20 vision to read 14 inches from eyes with bifocal prescription glasses.</td><td>Encourage patient to see an ophthalmologist for a complete eye examination at once and every 2 years thereafter.
Remind client to wear glasses whenever close vision is needed.
Provide printed information/instruction sheet (Box 5-1).</td></tr>
</table>

Evaluation

Patient has 20/20 vision for close objects with prescription glasses.

Patient wears glasses consistently when needing close vision.

Box 5-1.

Aging and your eyes

Poor eyesight is not inevitable with age. Some physical changes occur during the normal aging process that can cause a gradual decline in vision, but most older people maintain good eyesight into their 80s and beyond.

Older people generally need brighter light for such tasks as reading, cooking, or driving a car. In addition, incandescent light bulbs (regular household bulbs) are better than fluorescent lights (tubular overhead lights) for older eyes.

Certain eye disorders and diseases occur more frequently in old age, but a great deal can be done to prevent or correct these conditions. Here are some suggestions to help protect your eyes:

- Have regular health checkups to detect such treatable diseases as high blood pressure and diabetes, both of which may cause eye problems.
- Have a complete eye examination every 2 or 3 years since many eye diseases have no early noticeable symptoms. The examination should include a vision (and glasses) evaluation, eye muscle check, check for glaucoma, and thorough internal and external eye health exams.
- Seek more frequent eye health care if you have diabetes or a family history of eye disease. Make arrangements for care immediately if you experience signs such as loss or dimness in vision, eye pain, excessive discharge from the eye, double vision, or redness or swelling of the eye or eyelid.

Common eye complaints

Presbyopia (prez-bee-oh'pe-uh)—a gradual decline in the ability to focus on close objects or to see small print—is common after the age of 40. People with this condition often hold reading materials at arm's length, and some may have headaches or "tired eyes" while reading or doing other close work. There is no known prevention for presbyopia, but the focusing problem can be easily compensated for with glasses or contact lenses.

Floaters are tiny spots or specks that float across the field of vision. Most people notice them in well-lighted rooms or outdoors on a bright day. Although floaters are normal and are usually harmless, they may be a warning of certain eye problems, especially if associated with light flashes. If you notice a sudden change in the type or number of spots or flashes, call your doctor.

Dry eyes occur when the tear glands produce too few tears. The result is itching, burning, or even reduced vision. An eye specialist can prescribe special eyedrop solutions ("artificial tears") to correct the problem.

Excessive tears may be a sign of increased sensitivity to light, wind, or temperature changes. In these cases, protective measures (such as sunglasses) may solve the problem. Tearing may also indicate more serious problems, such as an eye infection or a blocked tear duct, both of which can be treated and corrected.

From U.S. Department of Health and Human Services, Public Health Service, National Institutes of Health.   *Continued.*

Eye diseases common in the elderly

Cataracts are cloudy or opaque areas in part or all of the transparent lens located inside the eye. Normally, the lens is clear and allows light to pass through. When a cataract forms, light cannot easily pass through the lens, and this affects vision. Cataracts usually develop gradually, without pain, redness, or tearing in the eye. Some remain small and do not seriously affect vision. If a cataract becomes larger or denser, however, it can be surgically removed. Cataract surgery (in which the clouded lens is removed) is a safe procedure that is almost always successful. Cataract patients should discuss with their doctor the risks and benefits of this elective procedure. After surgery, vision is restored by using special eyeglasses or contact lenses or by having an intraocular lens implant (a plastic lens that is implanted in the eye during surgery).

Glaucoma occurs when there is too much fluid pressure in the eye, causing internal eye damage and gradually destroying vision. The underlying cause of glaucoma is often not known, but with early diagnosis and treatment it can usually be controlled and blindness prevented. Treatment consists of special eyedrops, oral medications, laser treatments, or in some cases surgery. Glaucoma seldom produces early symptoms and usually there is no pain from increased pressure. For these reasons, it is important for eye specialists to test for the disease during routine eye examinations in those over 35.

Retinal disorders are the leading cause of blindness in the United States. The retina is a thin lining on the back of the eye made up of nerves that receive visual images and pass them on to the brain. Retinal disorders include senile macular degeneration, diabetic retinopathy, and retinal detachment.

- Senile macular degeneration is a condition in which the macula (a specialized part of the retina responsible for sharp central and reading vision) loses its ability to function efficiently. The first signs may include blurring of reading matter, distortion or loss of central vision (for example, a dark spot in the center of the field of vision), and distortion in vertical lines. Early detection of macular degeneration is important since some cases may be treated successfully with laser treatments.
- Diabetic retinopathy, one of the possible complications of diabetes, occurs when small blood vessels that nourish the retina fail to do so properly. In the early stages of the condition, the blood vessels may leak fluid, which distorts vision. In the later stages, new vessels may grow and release blood into the center of the eye, resulting in serious loss of vision.
- Retinal detachment is a separation between the inner and outer layers of the retina. Detached retinas can usually be surgically reattached with good or partial restoration of vision. New surgical and laser treatments are being used today with increasing success.

Low-vision aids

Many people with visual impairments can be helped by using low-vision aids. These are special devices that provide more power than regular eyeglasses. Low-vision aids include telescopic glasses, light-filtering lenses, and magnifying glasses, along with a variety of electronic devices. Some are designed to be hand-held; others rest directly on reading material. Partially sighted individuals often notice surprising improvements with the use of these aids.

For more information

The following organizations can send you more detailed information on eye care and eye disorders.

Office of Scientific Reporting, National Eye Institute, Bldg 31, Rm 6A32, Bethesda, MD 20205. This Institute, part of the Federal government's National Institutes of Health, conducts and supports research on eye disease and the visual system. They can send you a list of free brochures on eye disorders.

National Society to Prevent Blindness, 79 Madison Ave, New York, NY 10016. The Society has several free pamphlets on specific diseases affecting the eyes. To receive a free copy of their publication *The Aging Eye: Facts on Eye Care for Older Persons*, send them a self-addressed stamped envelope. They also have a *Home Eye Test for Adults* which is available for $1.00 (to cover the cost of postage and handling).

American Foundation for the Blind, 15 West 16th St, New York, NY 10011. This organization can send you a list of their free publications on vision.

Vision Foundation, 2 Mt Auburn St, Watertown, MA 02172. The Foundation has published a *Vision Inventory List*, which includes information on special products and services for visually impaired people. There is no charge for the *List*.

Two professional societies gather, study, and publish eye care information: American Optometric Association, Communications Division, 243 North Lindbergh Blvd, St Louis, MO 63141; and American Academy of Ophthalmology, 1833 Fillmore, PO Box 7424, San Francisco, CA 94120. Write to them for free information on eye care for the elderly.

Publications

"Keeping an Eye on Glaucoma" is a reprint from the June 1979 issue of the *FDA Consumer*. It is available free from the Food and Drug Administration, 5600 Fishers Ln, Rockville, MD 20857. Please send your request on a postcard.

Cataracts: A Consumer's Guide to Choosing the Best Treatment is a large-print book available for $3.50 from the Public Citizen's Health Research Group, 2000 P St, NW, Suite 708, Washington, DC 20036.

CATARACTS

Cataracts are one of the few normal physiological changes in the aging process and are the primary cause of blindness in older adults. All individuals will develop some degree of cataracts at some point in their lives. Cataracts usually begin to develop at about age 65, although some individuals develop cataracts as early as 50 years of age and some do not have major visual deficits because of cataracts even after the age of 100. About 95% of people aged 85 and over have some degree of lens opacity (Lewis and Collier, 1987, p. 344). The incidence increases with advancing age.

▶ PATHOPHYSIOLOGY, SIGNS, AND SYMPTOMS

A cataract occurs when the normally transparent lens of the eye begins to harden and become cloudy. The lens is located behind the pupil (Figure 5-1). When the lens becomes cloudy, less light can pass through to the retina at the back of the eye, resulting in blurred vision. The following are typical symptoms of cataracts:

Blurred, cloudy, hazy, fuzzy, or dim vision
Double vision
Decreased color perception
Seeing spots
Seeing halos around objects
Decreased night vision
Sensitivity to bright lights
Needing more light to see
Frequent changes in eyeglass prescriptions

These symptoms usually develop slowly over a period of years, although some develop more rapidly. Also, cataracts do not develop at the same rate in each eye.

The primary cause of cataracts is a physiological change that occurs in the aging process. However, other factors *that contribute to the formation of cataracts are diabetes, hypertension, kidney disease, physical or chemical eye injuries, some medications, and possibly extended exposure to ultraviolet lights, sunlight, intense heat or radiation.*

▶ DIAGNOSTIC PROCEDURES

Diagnosis is made by a complete eye examination, especially fundoscopy examination by an ophthalmologist or other qualified health practitioner. Cataracts may be visible without an ophthalmoscope in persons with dark pupils but may not be visible at all in persons with light-colored pupils.

▶ MEDICAL MANAGEMENT

Cataracts can be corrected only by surgical removal. Nothing else can be done to prevent or treat cataracts. Surgery is recommended when vision has been impaired enough to interfere with activities of daily living such as reading and driving. The patient and the ophthalmologist together usually decide when the surgery is necessary. Most cataract surgery is performed on an outpatient basis, not only for the convenience of the client but also because Medicare will not pay for hospitalization for this type of surgery unless medically necessary (e.g., need for general anesthesia). Local anesthesia is used, a small incision is made right above the pupil, and the entire lens is removed. In the most recently developed surgical technique, a very small incision is made, the lens material is broken into fragments by ultrasound vibrations, and the fragments are then suctioned out of the eye through a hollow-point needle. An artificial intraocular lens can then be folded in half and inserted through the small incision, which usually requires only one stitch to close.

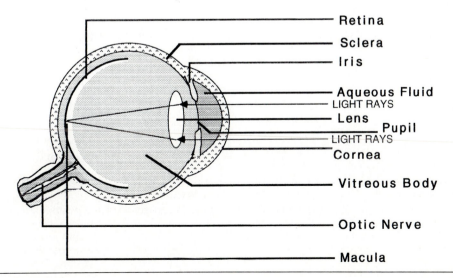

Figure 5-1. Normal eye.

▶ **PROGNOSIS**

The prognosis is excellent with the use of a contact lens, specially fitted cataract eyeglasses, or an intraocular lens, *depending on the type of surgery performed. Dramatic recovery and improvement of sight can be expected with an intraocular lens.*

▶ **NURSING MANAGEMENT—NURSING CARE PLAN**
Cataracts

Assessment

SUBJECTIVE DATA
"I cannot read or see as well as I used to."

OBJECTIVE DATA
Opaque lens is visible on external or internal eye examination.

	Nursing diagnoses	Expected outcomes	Nursing interventions (rationale)
N U R S I N G C A R E P L A N	Sensory/perceptual alterations (visual) related to a hard and cloudy lens	Patient will have cataract surgery when appropriate.	*Preoperative* Assess visual acuity in both eyes and assist as needed. Provide a safe environment (e.g., use side rails, and place call light and personal belongings within reach). Administer preoperative medications as ordered for sedation. *Postoperative* Avoid external pressure to the eye and increased intraocular pressure. Prevent squeezing the eyelids, vigorous laughing, bending over, lifting, sneezing, coughing, and straining to have bowel movement. (A stool softener or laxative may be needed.) Check with physician regarding special precautions (will depend on type of surgery). Have patient use an eye shield or patch at night. Position patient for comfort and as ordered by the physician. Have patient wear glasses during the day to prevent accidental touching of the eye. Apply cold compresses to the eye for discomfort and administer scheduled eye drops as ordered.
	Anxiety related to outcome of surgery	Patient will express fears and anxiety about surgery.	Encourage expression of fears about surgery. Listen. Explain procedures related to surgery (e.g., local anesthesia, sounds and sights of the operating room).
	Knowledge deficit related to postoperative care	Patient will understand how to administer eye drops safely. Patient will know how to care for eyes at home and what to do if complications occur.	Teach patient about postoperative care (e.g., instilling eye drops). Give postoperative instructions in concise, clear bold print to the patient and/or family member accompanying the patient home (see Box 5-2).

Nursing Care Plan—Cataracts—cont'd

Nursing diagnoses	Expected outcomes	Nursing interventions (rationale)
		Include a 24-hr telephone number to call in case of emergency.
		Tell patient to call the emergency number if he or she experiences severe pain or pressure in the eye, loss of vision, any other unusual symptom.
		Teach patient about aftereffects of surgery (scratching effect on eyelids for 2 or 3 days; inflammatory process may cause some transitory pain).
		Provide printed information/instruction sheet (see Box 5-1).
Potential for injury related to altered visual acuity	Patient will not fall, run into objects, or have an automobile accident before or after surgery.	Teach patient about the need for assistance for a few days after surgery, especially driving (distance and steps may appear distorted without lens transplant).
		Teach patient to tip head to avoid looking through bifocal lens.
Dressing/grooming self-care deficit related to inability to see color of clothes or face well enough to apply cosmetics	Patient will dress and groom self appropriately when vision returns.	Teach patient about effects of corrective lenses on vision.
		Teach patient about differences in applying makeup and dressing after surgery. (Objects may appear larger—not with the use of intraocular lenses—and colors may be distorted.)
Impaired communication related to inability to read letters, cards, newspapers	Patient will increase contact and communication with others after surgery.	Encourage patient to contact family and friends orally and in writing.

Discharge planning and patient/family education

Teach about postoperative care and give printed material to take home (for example, Box 5-2).

Teach use of eye drops if needed.

Evaluation

No complications of surgery or injuries due to distorted vision have occurred.

Patient has become accustomed to lens implant, contact lens, or corrective glasses.

Vision is gradually improved.

Patient is maintaining normal daily functioning.

Patient has support of family and friends.

Box 5-2.

Patient Education

Home Care Following Cataract Surgery

Do Not

Rub or touch your eyes
Squeeze your eyelids
Bend over
Lift heavy objects
Strain in any way
Sneeze, cough, laugh
Drive until you see the doctor after surgery

Do

Lie on back in reclining position or on side opposite surgery
Use eye shield while sleeping
Wear glasses during the day
Wear sunglasses with side shields during the day when outdoors
Apply cold cloth over closed eye for pain
Apply eye drops as ordered
   Do not touch tip of eye dropper
   Apply while flat in bed
   Tilt head back
   Pull down lower lid gently
   Place exact number of drops ordered in
     lower lid

Close eye and press gently inner eye next to nose

Note (if intraocular lens not inserted)

Your new cataract glasses may cause some distortions in your sight
   Objects look larger
   Distance looks farther away
   Side vision is decreased so move head
     to look to side
   Colors look different
   Steps appear distorted—bend head
     and look through top of glasses

These changes will be less noticeable in several weeks

Call 000-0000 any time of the day or night if you have
   Severe pain in eye
   Pressure in eye
   Loss of vision
   Other problems

Return to the clinic _____

The above is one sample. Instructions will vary considerably according to the individual surgeon and type of surgery performed.

GLAUCOMA

Glaucoma is the second leading cause of blindness in older people. Because there are few, if any, symptoms, it can cause blindness before the person is aware of any problem. Glaucoma affects 9% of those age 70 and older and is more common in blacks, persons with a family history of the problem (Purvis, 1990, p. 99), and women (Keith, 1987, p. 353). Quite often glaucoma and cataracts occur simultaneously in older people, causing the possibility of more complications with cataract surgery.

▶ **PATHOPHYSIOLOGY, SIGNS, AND SYMPTOMS**

Glaucoma is caused by inadequate drainage of aqueous fluid in the anterior portion of the eye (see Figure 5-1).

This fluid (approximately 4 to 5 ml/day) is secreted daily by the ciliary body and flows through the pupil to provide nutrients to the lens (Keith, 1987, p. 353). The trabecular meshwork and canal of Schlemm absorb/eliminate the fluid. When the fluid cannot leave the eye at the rate at which it is produced because of anatomic changes in the trabecular meshwork or canal of Schlemm, pressure within the eye increases and damages the optic nerve as well as other parts of the eye, eventually causing blindness.

There are three major types of glaucoma:

Primary open-angle glaucoma—Sometimes known as chronic simple wide angle, this type is the most common and develops slowly over a period of years; it is due to degenerative changes in the trabecular meshwork or canal of Schlemm.

Primary angle-closure glaucoma—Sometimes referred to as acute narrow angle, this type occurs suddenly as a result of complete blockage of the trabecular meshwork and can cause immediate loss of vision.

Secondary glaucoma—This condition is caused by other eye problems such as hemorrhage, inflammation, tumors, or trauma (Keith, 1987, pp. 353-354).

There are no early symptoms of primary open-angle glaucoma. The client cannot feel pressure in the eyes. However, as the disease progresses, the following symptoms may occur:

Loss of peripheral vision (tunnel vision)
Dull eye pain, especially in the morning
Difficulty adjusting to darkness
Halos seen around lights
Headaches without a cause
Frequent change in glasses (if >40 years of age) (Keith, 1987, p. 354)

Persons with the following characteristics are at high risk for open-angle glaucoma:

Have a blood relative with glaucoma
Have diabetes
Have had an eye injury
Have had eye surgery
Are black
Use cortisone medication (Glaucoma patient guide, 1984, p. 6)

Symptoms of primary angle-closure glaucoma are more sudden and specific. These may include the following:

Sudden severe pain in the eyes
Headache
Nausea and vomiting
Abdominal pain
Colored halos around lights
Sudden blurred vision

Decreased light perception
Eyes red
Cornea appears steamy (Keith, 1987, p. 354)

Persons with the following characteristics are at high risk for angle-closure glaucoma:

Have a blood relative with angle-closure glaucoma
Are very farsighted
"[H]ave an unusually shallow anterior chamber . . ."
Have had surgery for angle-closure glaucoma in one eye (Glaucoma patient guide, 1984, p. 20)
Have used mydriatic ophthalmic drugs for open-angle glaucoma (do not dilate pupils in an eye exam in persons with open-angle glaucoma)
Have used atropine or atropinelike medications (can precipitate an acute attack of closed-angle glaucoma)

▶ DIAGNOSTIC PROCEDURES

Everyone over 40 years of age should have a complete eye examination, including measurement of intraocular pressure, every 1 to 2 years. Glaucoma is diagnosed by the following:

History of eye problems
Other family members with glaucoma
Testing of visual acuity
Tonometry to determine eye pressure (average pressure is about 17, but pressure is very individualized; a higher pressure may not cause damage in some people while a lower pressure may)
Testing of visual fields to determine any loss of peripheral vision

▶ MEDICAL MANAGEMENT

Primary open-angle glaucoma: Prescription of eye medication is based on the patient's age, physical condition, and coexisting medical problems. Drugs commonly used are dipivefrin (Propine), pilocarpine, and physostigmine. They increase the outflow of aqueous humor from the anterior chamber. Others, such as acetazolamide (Diamox) and timolol (Timoptic) decrease production of aqueous humor. Timolol should not be used for older people who have congestive heart failure, abnormal heart rhythms, asthma, or emphysema. In these cases, pilocarpine is a better choice (Wolfe, Fugate, Hulstrand, and Kamimoto, 1988, p. 457). If medication does not decrease the intraocular pressure, surgery such as the following may be necessary:

Argon laser trabeculoplasty
Trabeculectomy
Cyclocryotherapy
Sclerotomy (Keith, 1987, p. 356)

Primary angle-closure glaucoma: Emergency treatment with medications is needed to relieve eye pressure and pain. If the medications do not relieve the pressure and pain, the following types of surgery may be necessary:

    Peripheral laser iridotomy
    Peripheral iridectomy (a small section of the iris is excised so the fluid can drain out into the drainage channels) (Keith, 1987, p. 356)

▶ PROGNOSIS

The prognosis is good if the glaucoma is detected in a very early stage and prescription eye medications are ordered and used consistently. It will be necessary for persons with glaucoma to use the eye medications for the rest of their lives. When vision is lost because of glaucoma, there is no treatment to restore it.

▶ NURSING MANAGEMENT—NURSING CARE PLAN
Glaucoma

Assessment

SUBJECTIVE DATA
Generally none (the client is usually not aware of any problem)
Possibly eye pain

OBJECTIVE DATA
Elevated intraocular pressure
Decreased peripheral vision when visual fields are tested

	Nursing diagnoses	Expected outcomes	Nursing interventions (rationale)
N U R S I N G C A R E P L A N	Sensory/perceptual alterations related to decreased peripheral vision	Patient will have no further loss of vision.	Test peripheral vision Teach to turn head to side to see if needed.

	Noncompliance (not using eye medications consistently and correctly) related to lack of understanding of the disease and importance of the medications	Eye medications will be used according to the ordered dose and time for the remainder of the patient's life.	Teach patient about the following:
			  Glaucoma as a disease
			  Eye medications ordered; check side effects (e.g., burning, redness, temporary blurring of vision)
			  Method of instilling eye drops
			  Need to see ophthalmologist at least once a year
			Provide printed information/instruction sheet (see Box 5-1).

	Pain related to increased intraocular pressure (especially of primary angle-closure glaucoma)	Eye pain/headache will cease after eye medications are started (or after surgery if indicated).	Administer eye drops and other drugs to relieve pain (if primary angle-closure glaucoma). Provide safe postoperative eye surgery care if surgery is required.

	Potential for infection (eye) related to method of using eye drops	No eye inflammation or infection will occur.	Teach patient about signs of infection:
			  Redness
			  Drainage
			  Blurred vision
			Tell patient to call physician if the above symptoms appear.

Discharge planning and patient/family education
Teach about need for eye medications.
Teach how to use eye medications safely.

Evaluation
No further peripheral vision loss has occurred.
No postoperative complications occurred (if surgery was necessary).
Patient has no eye pain, headaches, or infection in the eyes.
Patient can verbalize the dangers of glaucoma if treatment is not continued and the purpose of eye medications used.
Patient continues to use eye drops as ordered.
Patient sees an ophthalmologist at least once a year.

MACULAR DEGENERATION

Macular degeneration is another eye problem that primarily affects older adults, especially those past age 90. It is often referred to as age-related macular degeneration (AMD). Although it does not cause total blindness, it causes difficulty in reading and other activities that require close vision.

▶ PATHOPHYSIOLOGY, SIGNS, AND SYMPTOMS

The macula is a very small area in the retina at the back of the eye (see Figure 5-1). The light rays that enter through the cornea and lens of the eye meet at the macula. When the macula is damaged, the image on the retina is affected so that central vision becomes blurred. Peripheral vision remains intact. The disease may progress rapidly or slowly, and it usually affects one eye first and then the other.

Factors that cause the macula to be damaged and/or destroyed include the following:

Breakdown or thinning of tissue due to the aging process, called involutional macular degeneration (70% of cases)

Rupture and leakage of abnormal blood vessels in scar tissue at the back of the eye, called exudative macular degeneration (10% of cases)

Injury, infection, inflammation

Hereditary factors (Macular degeneration, 1987, pp. 2-3)

Symptoms of macular degeneration (Figure 5-2) are as follows:

Difficulty reading, sewing, and performing other activities that require close central vision

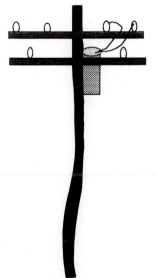

Straight Lines Look Distorted.

Figure 5-2. Symptom of macular degeneration.

Decreased color vision
Center vision that becomes blurred, distorted, dark, or empty
Wavy appearance of straight lines on paper or in the environment (e.g., flag pole)

▶ DIAGNOSTIC PROCEDURES

Diagnosis is determined by the following:
Comprehensive internal eye examination with ophthalmoscope
Grid test (looking at graph paper to determine degree of central vision loss) (Box 5-3)

Box 5-3.

Amsler grid test for macular degeneration

How can I test my own vision?

You can easily test yourself or help other people test themselves for possible signs of AMD with the Amsler Grid Chart. Simply look at the dot in the middle of the grid while keeping one eye covered. Be sure to test each eye separately. If the lines near the dot appear wavy or distorted, this could be a symptom of AMD or another visual problem. Such symptoms should be discussed with an eye doctor as soon as possible. This self-test does not replace an examination by an eye care professional.

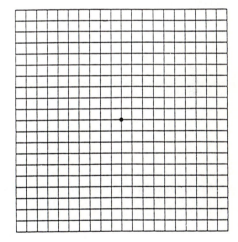

Instructions

1. Place the grid on the wall at eye level.
2. View it from 12 inches.
3. If you wear glasses for reading, you should wear them for the test.
4. Test one eye at a time.
5. Look at the center dot.
6. Tell your doctor if you can't see all the lines or if some lines appear wavy.

From Age-related macular degeneration (AMD) AB05 50M 3/89R, 1979. This information was used with permission from the National Society to Prevent Blindness.

Color vision test (e.g., Rosenbaum Pocket Vision Screener)

Fluorescein angiogram (after dye is injected in arm, photos of the retina and macula are taken to determine abnormalities) (Macular degeneration, 1987, pp. 4, 5)

▶ **MEDICAL MANAGEMENT**

There is no specific treatment or cure for involutional macular degeneration. Laser photocoagulation may prevent the spread of exudative macular degeneration if performed early in the course of the disease before the macula is damaged severely. The laser beam seals leaking membranes and destroys new blood vessels that contribute to the scarring of the macula (Macular degeneration, 1987, p. 6).

▶ **PROGNOSIS**

It is fortunate that macular degeneration alone will not cause complete blindness because the individual can usually manage fairly well with retained peripheral vision and the help of low-vision optical aids (see Box 5-4).

Box 5-4.
Low-vision optical aids

Magnifying devices
  Hand held
  Glasses
  Flat bars
Telescopic lenses for distance vision
Microscopic lenses for close vision
High-intensity reading lamps
Closed-circuit television
Computers
Large-print books, newspapers, magazines, checks (ask at a bank), telephone dials, clocks, watches, oven timers, playing cards, bingo cards, dominoes
Signature guide
Self-threading sewing needles
Talking clocks and wrist watches

▶ **NURSING MANAGEMENT—NURSING CARE PLAN**
Macular Degeneration

Assessment

SUBJECTIVE DATA
"I cannot see to thread this needle."

OBJECTIVE DATA
Abnormal appearance of macula on fundoscopy examination

	Nursing diagnoses	Expected outcomes	Nursing interventions (rationale)
N U R S I N G C A R E P L A N	Sensory alteration (visual) related to damaged macula	Patient will learn to adjust to loss of vision. Patient will obtain and use low-vision aids.	Teach patient about the use of low-vision optical aids. Give patient information about low-vision optical aids (see Box 5-4).
	Knowledge deficit (effects of macular degeneration) related to difficulty understanding the complexities of the eye	Patient will learn about macular degeneration. Patient will see ophthalmologist at least once a year.	Teach patient about macular degeneration. Encourage patient to see ophthalmologist yearly and when any problems occur. Provide printed information/instruction sheet (see Box 5-1).
	Anxiety related to fear of blindness	Patient will recognize that total blindness will not occur.	Encourage patient to express concerns about eye problems.

Evaluation
Patient has obtained several low-vision aids.

Patient describes eye condition reasonably well.
Patient realizes that total blindness will not occur.

FLOATERS AND FLASHES

Floaters appear as small specks or spots when looking at a clear sky or light background. They may look like dots, circles, lines, or cobwebs. Floaters often occur after age 50 as the result of vitreous gel that pulls away from the retina and floats in the vitreous fluid. They are more common in people who are nearsighted and those who have had cataract surgery.

Floaters are sometimes bothersome to the individual, but they are usually harmless unless there is a sudden increase in the number, there are flashes of light, or partial vision is lost in one eye. Any of these symptoms could mean that a retinal tear or detachment is occurring, and the individual should see an ophthalmologist as soon as possible for a comprehensive eye examination and treatment that usually requires laser surgery to prevent further damage. The most common cause of retinal detachment is shrinkage of vitreous humor with age, resulting in a tear of the retina. The liquid vitreous humor enters and causes separation of the layers of the retina. Aphakia (removal of the lens without replacement as in cataract surgery) is also a cause.

Patients who experience new symptoms of floaters or flashes, or a sudden increase in the presence of floaters or flashes, should be referred to an ophthalmologist as soon as possible for a comprehensive eye examination to determine whether there is damage to the retina. The nurse should teach patients about the cause, symptoms, and how to live with floaters and flashes after it has been determined that there is no retinal damage. For example, patients should be taught that looking up and down is more effective than looking back and forth in getting the floaters out of the way of vision (Floaters and flashes, 1989). Patients should be given a printed information/ instruction sheet (see Box 5-1).

ECTROPION AND ENTROPION

Ectropion and entropion are two external eye conditions that occur in older adults, especially those in their late 80s and 90s. If not treated, they can cause much discomfort to the older person as well as complications such as excessive tearing (ectropion) or corneal irritation (entropion). Ectropion occurs as a result of gravity in the aging process when "the lids may be loose or lax and roll outward. . . . [B]ecause the puncta cannot effectively drain the tears, *epiphora* (tearing) results" (Malasanos, Barkauskas, and Stoltenberg-Allen, 1990, p. 245). In entropion, the eyelids "roll inward because of lid spasm or the contraction of scar tissue. . . . [B]ecause the lashes are pulled inward they may produce corneal irritation" (Malasanos, Barkauskas, and Stoltenberg-Allen, 1990, p. 245).

Both of these conditions can be repaired by relatively minor surgery performed by a qualified ophthalmologist on an outpatient basis. Recovery is usually complete and symptoms subside.

Nurses should be alert to both ectropion and entropion when observing and assessing older patients who complain of excessive tearing or scratchy eyes.

PRESBYCUSIS (AND OTHER HEARING LOSSES COMMON IN OLD AGE)

Another common aging change is a decrease in the ability to hear, especially high-pitched tones. This change begins to occur at about age 65, although some individuals experience hearing loss at an earlier age and many older people never have a hearing loss. Hearing loss is *not* a normal part of the aging process; thus the cause of any loss should be determined so that treatment can be given if possible.

▶ **PATHOPHYSIOLOGY, SIGNS, AND SYMPTOMS**

There are three major types of hearing loss:
   Conductive loss—due to blockage in the sound-conducting system of the external or middle ear (e.g., otosclerosis or impacted cerumen, which is a common problem in older people)
   Sensorineural loss—due to damage or loss in the inner ear, auditory nerve, or brain, which do not receive the right signals or send the correct information to the brain
   Combination of conductive and sensorineural loss
   Presbycusis is caused by a sensorineural loss, affects both ears, and is more common and more severe in men than in women. Presby means elder and akousis means hearing.
   Other causes of hearing loss besides the aging process include the following:
   Excessive environmental noise over many years (e.g., due to occupation)
   Infection in the ear
   Side effects of medications (e.g., aspirin and some antibiotics)
   Head injury
   Stroke
   Heart or kidney disease
   Diabetes
   Emphysema
   Hereditary factors (Have you heard?, 1984, pp. 5-6)
Common symptoms experienced by the patient include the following:
   Inability to hear and understand normal voice tones
   Inability to hear television sounds at the same volume as someone with normal hearing
   Inability to hear the ticking of a watch when held close to the ear
   Misinterpretation of sounds and words (unfortunately this problem often causes family members or health care workers to assume older people are confused,

disoriented, or paranoid when, in fact, they simply have not heard the words correctly)

Asking others to repeat what they said

Inability to carry on a conversation with another person when the television is on or when in a crowded room where many people are talking

Inability to hear the telephone or doorbell

Behaviors the family or health care provider might observe in the older person with decreased hearing include the following:

Having the volume on the television or radio very high

Tilting the head so that one ear is closer to the person speaking

Using the hand to cup around one ear to hear better

Watching the speaker's lips closely

Speaking loudly as if the other person cannot hear

Not responding when a question is asked or giving a wrong response to the question

Having a puzzled or depressed look on the face

▶ DIAGNOSTIC PROCEDURES

Any older person who is experiencing any degree of hearing loss should be evaluated first by an otologist or otolaryngologist to determine the exact type and degree of hearing loss. This examination will include a complete external and internal ear examination to determine factors that may be causing the hearing loss. Auditory acuity will also be evaluated by voice, watch tick, tuning fork, and/or audiometer. It may be that the hearing loss is due to impacted cerumen, infection, or damage to the tympanic membrane rather than presbycusis.

▶ MEDICAL MANAGEMENT

Cochlear implants, which require surgery, have been approved by the U.S. Food and Drug Administration for persons who have severe hearing loss affecting the quality of their life. Many older people have benefited from this type of surgery.

Box 5-5.

Hearing devices

Hearing aids (multiple types are available)
    Attached to glasses
    Within the ear
    Behind the ear
    Body type
    Canal hearing aids
Telephone, television, radio amplifiers
Captioned television
Teletypewriters
Doorbell and telephone that light as well as ring
Flashing smoke detectors and alarm clocks
Burglar alarms that light up as well as sound

If there is no cause for the hearing loss that can be treated by medication or surgery, a hearing device may be recommended (Box 5-5). It is important that older people do not purchase a hearing device until they know whether it will help their type of hearing loss. All hearing aids amplify sound, but recently developed aids can produce more of the sounds desired (e.g., speech) and prevent background noise from being so loud.

▶ PROGNOSIS

Usually the hearing loss with presbycusis is gradual, and the older person learns to adjust over time to decreased hearing. Because there are varying degrees of hearing loss, there is much more of an adjustment for some people than for others. The older person with a major hearing loss often has decreased feelings of worth and self-esteem and becomes socially isolated, withdrawn, and depressed. Many hearing devices are available that will aid those with mild to moderate hearing loss so that they can continue a normal full life.

▶ NURSING MANAGEMENT—NURSING CARE PLAN
  Presbycusis

Assessment

SUBJECTIVE DATA
"WHAT DID YOU SAY?"

OBJECTIVE DATA
Has television on very loud
Tilts head to right side
Asks for each question to be repeated twice

	Nursing diagnoses	Expected outcomes	Nursing interventions (rationale)
N U R S I N G C A R E P L A N	Sensory alterations (auditory) related to sensorineural hearing loss	Patient will obtain and learn to use the most appropriate hearing devices available (see Box 5-5).	Discuss with patient the advantages and disadvantages of and resources for obtaining the various types of hearing devices.
	Impaired social interaction related to difficulty communicating with others	Patient will continue to speak to family, friends, and neighbors while learning to use hearing devices.	Help the patient learn to use hearing devices obtained when communicating with family members and others. Teach the patient to use other skills that will enhance communication (Box 5-6). Provide printed information/instruction sheet (Box 5-7).
	Social isolation related to low self-esteem	Patient will continue to visit friends and attend social activities.	Encourage patient to visit friends and neighbors and to attend social activities.
	Anxiety and fear related to inability to be aware of dangers in the environment (robbery, fire)	Patient will feel more secure and comfortable with newly installed house safety devices that alert to fire or break-ins.	Help the patient obtain and test the special security safety devices for hearing-impaired persons.

Discharge planning and patient/family education
Teach about hearing devices (see Box 5-5).
Teach patient how to improve communication skills (see Box 5-6).
Teach family how to communicate with older persons with hearing loss.
Teach about safety devices for the home for hearing-impaired persons.
Encourage to participate fully in communicating with family and friends.

Evaluation
Individual and environmental hearing devices have been obtained and are in use.
Hearing devices have helped the patient continue to communicate with others.
Patient has resumed visiting friends and attending social activities.
Patient feels secure in his or her own home.

Box 5-6.

Patient Education

Skills to Improve Communication When There Is Hearing Loss

Listen carefully.

Do not do all the talking.

Watch the other person's lips and face.

Do not be afraid to tell others you did not hear.

Ask the following of the other person:
  Not to shout because shouting makes words less clear and may cause pain

Not to mumble but to speak up or slow down

To decrease the background noise (e.g., turn off the television)

Not to speak with something in the mouth or with the hands over the lips

To give clues about what is being discussed

To state your name before making a statement or asking a question

Adapted from Have you heard? (1984). American Association of Retired Persons, 1909 K Street, NW, Washington, DC 20049.

Box 5-7.

Hearing and the elderly

It is easy to take good hearing for granted. In the world of the hearing impaired, words in a conversation may be misunderstood, musical notes might be missed, and a ringing doorbell may go unanswered. Hearing impairment ranges from difficulty understanding words or hearing certain sounds to total deafness.

Because of fear, misinformation, or vanity, some people will not admit to themselves or anyone else that they have a hearing problem. It has been estimated, however, that approximately 30% of adults age 65 through 74 and about 50% of those age 75 through 79 suffer some degree of hearing loss. In the United States alone, more than 10 million older people are hearing impaired.

If ignored and untreated, hearing problems can grow worse, hindering communication with others, limiting social activities, and reducing constructive use of leisure time. People with hearing impairments often withdraw socially to avoid the frustration and embarrassment of not being able to understand what is being said. In addition, hearing-impaired people may become suspicious of relatives and friends who "mumble" or "don't speak up."

Hearing loss may cause an older hearing-impaired person to be wrongly labeled as "confused," "unresponsive," or "uncooperative." At times, the feelings of powerlessness and frustration experienced by elderly individuals trying to communicate with others result in depression and withdrawal.

While older people today are, in general, demanding greater satisfaction from life, those with hearing impairments often find the quality of their lives diminished. Fortunately, help is available, in the form of surgery, treatment with medicines, special training, a hearing aid, or an alternate listening device.

Some common signs of hearing impairment

- Words are difficult to understand.
- Such sounds as the dripping of a faucet or the high notes of a violin cannot be heard.
- A hissing or ringing background noise is heard continually.
- Another person's speech sounds slurred or mumbled.
- Television programs, concerts, and social gatherings are less enjoyable because much goes unheard.

From U.S. Department of Health and Human Services, Public Health Service, National Institutes of Health.

Box 5-7.
Hearing and the elderly—cont'd

Diagnosis of hearing problems

If you are having trouble hearing, see your doctor for treatment or referral to a hearing specialist. By ignoring the problem, you may be overlooking a serious medical condition. Hearing impairments may be caused by exposure to excessively loud noises over a long period of time, viral infections, vascular incidents (such as heart conditions or stroke), head injuries, certain drugs, tumors, excessive ear wax, heredity, or age-related changes in the ear mechanisms. In view of the importance of good hearing, seeking medical help is certainly worthwhile.

In some cases, the diagnosis and treatment of a hearing problem may take place in the family doctor's office. More complicated cases may require the help of specialists known as *otologists* or *otolaryngologists*. These specialists are doctors of medicine or doctors of osteopathy with extensive training in ear problems. They will conduct a thorough examination, take a medical history, ask about hearing problems affecting other family members, and order any other necessary laboratory tests. Many times they will then refer the patient to an *audiologist*. Audiologists specialize in the identification, prevention, and management of hearing problems and in the rehabilitation of people with hearing loss. They do not prescribe drugs or perform surgery, but they can recommend and sometimes dispense hearing aids. To test hearing, the audiologist uses an audiometer, a device which electronically generates sounds of different pitches and loudness. The testing is painless and within a short time the degree of hearing impairment can be determined and a course of treatment recommended.

Types of hearing loss

Presbycusis (pronounced prez-bee-ku'sis) is a common type of hearing loss in older people. Changes in the delicate workings of the inner ear lead to difficulties understanding speech, and possibly an intolerance for loud sounds, but not total deafness. Thus, "don't shout—I'm not deaf!" is frequently heard from elderly persons with this type of hearing impairment.

Every year after age 50 we lose some of our hearing ability. The decline is gradual and progressive so that by age 60 or 70 as many as 25% of the elderly are noticeably hearing impaired. Just as the graying of hair occurs at different rates, presbycusis develops differently from person to person.

Although presbycusis is usually attributed to aging, it does not affect everyone and some researchers view it as a disease. Environmental noise, certain drugs, improper diet, and genetic makeup may contribute to this disorder. Although the condition is permanent, there is much a person can do to function well despite the impairment.

Conduction deafness is another form of hearing loss sometimes experienced by the elderly. It involves blockage or impairment of the mechanical movement in the outer or middle ear so that sound waves are not able to travel properly through the ear. This may be caused by packed ear wax, extra fluid, abnormal bone growth in the ear, or infection. People with this problem often find that voices and other sounds seem muffled, but their own voices sound louder than normal. As a result, they often speak softly. Depending on the cause, flushing of the ear, medicines, or surgery will prove successful in most cases.

Central deafness is a third type of hearing loss that occurs in the elderly, although it is quite rare even in this age group. It is caused by damage to the nerve centers within the brain. Sound levels are not affected, but understanding of language usually is. The causes include extended illness with a high fever, lengthy exposure to loud noises, use of certain drugs, head injuries, vascular problems, or tumors. Central deafness cannot be treated medically or surgically, but for some, special training by an audiologist or speech therapist can be beneficial.

Treatment

Examination and test results from the family doctor, ear specialist, and/or audiologist will determine the most effective treatment for a specific hearing problem. In some cases, medical treatment such as flushing the ear canal to remove packed ear wax or surgery may restore some or all of hearing ability.

At other times, a hearing aid may be recommended. A hearing aid is a small device designed to amplify sounds. Although hearing aids are not recommended for all hearing difficulties, some persons can benefit from a properly used device. Before you can buy a hearing aid, you must either obtain a written statement from your doctor (stating that your hearing impairment has been medically evaluated and that you might benefit from a hearing aid) or sign a waiver stating that you do not desire a medical evaluation.

Should a hearing aid be the recommended form of treatment for you, there are several things you should know about buying one. As an informed consumer you should shop for a hearing aid just as for any other product. There are many models on the market, offering different kinds of help for different kinds of problems. Hearing tests can determine the nature of the hearing problem, but only you can judge the comfort, convenience, and quality of sound of an aid. Remember, too, that you are not only buying a product, but a set of services which include any necessary adjustments, counseling in the use of the aid, maintenance, and repairs throughout the warranty period. Before deciding where to buy your aid, consider the quality of service as well as the quality of the merchandise.

Continued.

Box 5-7.

Hearing and the elderly—cont'd

When buying a hearing aid keep in mind that the most expensive hearing aid may not be the best for you. You may find one that sells for less and offers you more satisfaction. Buy an aid with only those features you need. Also, be aware that the controls for many of the special features are tiny and may be difficult to adjust. Choose an aid you can operate easily. Many hearing aid dealers (usually called "dispensers") offer a free trial period of up to 30 days so that you may wear the aid before making a decision. It is a good idea to take advantage of the trial period since it often takes at least a month to become comfortable with a new hearing aid. Your dispenser should have the patience and skill to help you through the adjustment period.

At times, people with certain types of hearing impairments may need special training. One form, speech-reading, trains a person to receive visual clues from lip movements as well as facial expressions, body posture and gestures, and the environment. Auditory training may include hearing aid orientation, but it is also designed to help hearing-impaired persons identify their specific communication problems and to better handle them. Although neither speech-reading nor auditory training can improve damaged hearing, they can reduce the handicapping effects of hearing impairment by making the best use of the hearing ability that remains. If needed, counseling is also available so that hearing-impaired elderly are able to maintain a positive self-image while understanding their communication abilities and limitations.

Cost

Because hearing impairments have so many causes, it is important to be examined by your doctor as soon as you suspect a problem with your hearing. Too often, people with hearing problems fail to get medical attention until the condition is beyond help. Unfortunately, the high cost of hearing health care contributes to this neglect. Medicare will pay for the diagnosis and evaluation of hearing loss if requested by a physician, but it will often not pay for the means to correct it. In some states Medicaid covers some costs of a hearing aid. Before buying an aid you may want to contact one of the organizations listed in this box. Many local chapters are able to provide information concerning Medicaid coverage of hearing aids.

If you have problems hearing

- See your doctor to determine the cause of your hearing problem. Ask if you should see a specialist.
- Don't hesitate to ask people to repeat what they have just said.
- Try to limit background noise (stereo, television, etc.).
- Don't hesitate to tell people that you have a hearing problem and what they can do to make communication easier.

If you know someone with a hearing problem

- Speak slightly louder than normal. However, shouting will not make the message any clearer, and may sometimes distort it. Speak at your normal rate, but not too rapidly. Do not overarticulate. This distorts the sounds of speech and makes use of visual clues more difficult.
- Speak to the person at a distance of 3 to 6 feet. Position yourself near good light so that your lip movements, facial expressions, and gestures may be seen clearly. Wait until you are visible to the hearing-impaired person before speaking. Avoid chewing, eating, or covering your mouth when speaking.
- Never speak directly into the person's ear. This prohibits the listener from making use of visual clues.
- If the listener does not understand what was said, rephrase the idea in short, simple sentences.
- Arrange living rooms or meeting rooms so that no one is more than 6 feet apart and all are completely visible. In meetings or group activities where there is a speaker presenting information, ask the speaker to use the public address system.
- Treat the hearing-impaired person with respect. Include the person in all discussions about him or her. This helps to alleviate the feelings of isolation common in hearing-impaired persons.

For your reference

If you would like further information about hearing problems, you may contact the organizations listed below. Please be sure to state clearly what type information you would like to receive.

American Academy of Otolaryngologists (Head and Neck Surgery), Inc, 1101 Vermont Ave, NW, Washington, DC 20005. The Academy is a professional society of medical doctors specializing in diseases of the ear and related areas. They can provide information on hearing and balance disorders.

American Speech-Language-Hearing Association, 10801 Rockville Pike, Dept AP, Rockville, MD 20852 (or call 1-[800] 638-8255 for the National Association for Hearing and Speech Action). Either organization can answer questions or mail information on hearing aids or hearing loss and communication problems in the elderly. They can also provide a list of certified audiologists in each state.

Office of Scientific and Health Reports, National Institute of Neurological and Communicative Disorders and Stroke, Bldg 31, Rm 8A06, Bethesda, MD 20205. The Institute is the focal point within the Federal government for research on hearing loss and other communication disorders. Ask for the Institute's pamphlet *Hearing Loss: Hope Through Research.*

Self Help for Hard of Hearing People *(Shhh)*, 4848 Battery Lane, Dept E, Bethesda, MD 20814. *Shhh* is a nationwide organization for the hard of hearing. Their national office publishes a bimonthly journal reporting the experiences of those with hearing impairments as well as new developments in the field of hearing loss. A number of publications and reprints are available for the hard of hearing.

From U.S. Department of Health and Human Services, Public Health Service, National Institutes of Health.

MÉNIÈRE'S DISEASE

Ménière's disease is not very common but is a major problem for some older people, especially women. Because one of the typical symptoms is sudden dizziness, the patient may fall and fracture a bone, thus causing other major problems for a person who already has poor balance and is at high risk for the complications of a fracture.

▶ PATHOPHYSIOLOGY, SIGNS, AND SYMPTOMS

Ménière's disease involves the inner ear. Excess endolymph or edema in the cochlea (Figure 5-3) causes pressure within the labyrinth. The cause of the excess fluid is not known. The three characteristic symptoms are vertigo (individual feels the environment is whirling about), tinnitus, and hearing loss. Other symptoms are unsteadiness, nausea and vomiting, and spasmodic eye movements.

▶ DIAGNOSTIC PROCEDURES

Diagnosis is made by history given by the client, audiogram, vestibular tests, electronystagmography, neuro-logical exam, and x-rays of the internal auditory canal (Keith, 1987, p. 367).

▶ MEDICAL MANAGEMENT

Treatment may include decreased fluid intake, a low-sodium diet, and medication such as a diuretic (to remove the excess fluid) and antihistamines. Other medications may be given (e.g., diazepam and meclizine [Antivert]) to control the vertigo and help relieve the severe tinnitus. Treatment is often ineffective. The major complication is total loss of hearing. "Surgical decompression of the endolymphatic sac is done to reduce the pressure on the cochlea hair cells and to prevent further damage and sensorineural hearing loss," and labyrinthectomy may be necessary (Keith, 1987, p. 367).

▶ PROGNOSIS

Severe repeated attacks are frustrating to the client. There is generally no complete cure. Often the client must learn to live with the disease. Medications relieve the symptoms during an acute attack and surgery may be necessary.

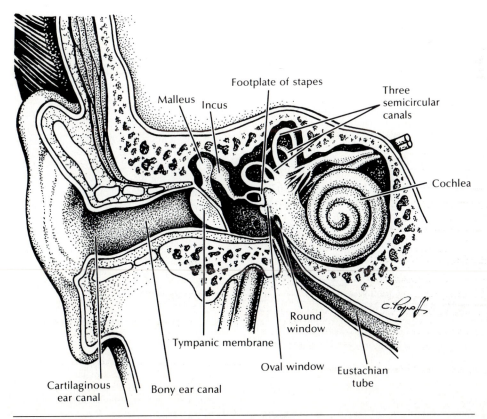

Figure 5-3. External auditory canal, middle ear, and inner ear. (From Malasanos L, Barkauskas V, and Stoltenberg-Allen K [1990]. Health assessment, ed 4, St Louis, Mosby–Year Book, Inc.)

▶ NURSING MANAGEMENT—NURSING CARE PLAN
Ménière's Disease

Assessment

SUBJECTIVE DATA

"I feel like the room is whirling around me."
"I can't keep my feet flat on the floor."
"I feel sick at my stomach."

OBJECTIVE DATA

Unable to hear watch tick at 12 inches from ear.
Vomited 30 ml of clear fluid.

N U R S I N G C A R E P L A N	Nursing diagnoses	Expected outcomes	Nursing interventions (rationale)
	Potential for injury related to severe vertigo	Patient will learn to sit or lie down as soon as vertigo begins.	Teach patient what to do during an acute attack: Sit or lie down. Stay in a quiet darkened room. Limit movement. Be prepared to vomit.
	Anxiety related to loud ringing in ears	Patient will take medications as prescribed when severe tinnitus occurs.	Administer medications as prescribed for anxiety and tinnitus.
	Knowledge deficit related to cause of problem and treatment	Patient will understand the causes and treatment of the disease. Patient will learn to live with the disease.	Explain the possible causes and proposed treatment to the patient. Assess degree of hearing loss at regular intervals.
	Sensory alteration (auditory) related to pressure of fluid on cochlea in inner ear	Patient will obtain and learn to use hearing devices when hearing loss occurs.	Help patient obtain and learn to use hearing devices when needed.

Evaluation

Patient has not fallen or been injured in any way during an acute attack.
Patient takes medications as prescribed.

Patient can explain the disease and treatment, and has learned to live with the disease.
No major hearing loss has occurred.

EDUCATIONAL MATERIALS

Aging and your eyes (1983). Age Page, National Institute on Aging, Bethesda, Md., U.S. Department of Health and Human Services, Public Health Service, National Institutes of Health.

Aging and vision (Publication FAL 909 2-87/20M). American Association of Retired Persons, 1909 K Street, NW, Washington, DC 20049.

Age-related macular degeneration (AB05 50M 3/89R). National Society to Prevent Blindness, 500 East Remington Road, Schaumburg, IL 60173.

American Foundation for the Blind. Toll-free hotline: (800) 232-5463.

Cataract: what it is and how it is treated (Publication G-4). National Society to Prevent Blindness, 500 East Remington Road, Schaumburg, IL 60173.

Cochlear Implant Hotline: (800) 458-4999 (Voice TDD).

Floaters and flashes (Revised February 1989). American Academy of Ophthalmology, PO Box 7424, San Francisco, CA 94120-7424.

Glaucoma patient guide (Publication G-2). National Society to Prevent Blindness, 500 East Remington Road, Schaumburg, IL 60173.

Growing older with good vision (Publication LSI 75M 9/87). National Society to Prevent Blindness, 500 East Remington Road, Schaumburg, IL 60173.

Have you heard? Hearing loss and aging (PF 3006/4 [389] D12219).

American Association of Retired Persons, 1909 K Street, NW, Washington, DC 20049.

Hearing and the elderly (1983). Age Page, National Institute on Aging, Bethesda, Md., U.S. Department of Health and Human Services, Public Health Service, National Institutes of Health.

Living with low vision (Publication LV2/1187). American Optometric Association, 243 N Lindbergh Blvd, St Louis, MO 63141.

Macular degeneration (October 1987). American Academy of Ophthalmology, PO Box 7424, San Francisco, CA 94120-7424.

National Society to Prevent Blindness. Toll-free hotline: (800) 221-3004.

So your doctor said, "You have a cataract" (Form No. 540-138 [R3/88]). Cooper Vision C/LCO, 3190 160th Avenue, SE, Bellevue, WA 98008-5496.

The eyes have it (Publication PF3687 [789] D12460). American Association of Retired Persons, 1909 K Street, NW, Washington, DC 20049.

REFERENCES

Floaters and flashes (revised February 1989). San Francisco, American Academy of Ophthalmology.

Glaucoma patient guide (1984). Publication G-2, Schaumberg, Ill, National Society to Prevent Blindness.

Have you heard? Hearing loss and aging (1984). Publication PF

3006/4 (389) D12219. Washington, DC, American Association of Retired Persons.

Lewis SM and Collier IC (1987). Medical-surgical nursing, ed 2, New York, McGraw-Hill.

Keith CF (1987). Problems of vision and hearing. In Lewis SM and Collier IC, editors: Medical-surgical nursing, New York, McGraw-Hill.

Macular degeneration (1987). San Francisco, American Academy of Ophthalmology.

Malasanos L, Barkauskas V, and Stoltenberg-Allen K (1990). Health assessment, ed 4, St Louis, Mosby–Year Book, Inc.

Purvis A (1990). A real "vision thing," Time, p 99, April 23.

Wolfe SM, Fugate L, Hulstrand EP, and Kamimoto LE (1988). Worst pills best pills, Washington, DC, Public Citizen Health Research Group.

BIBLIOGRAPHY

Phipps WJ, Long BC, Woods NF, and Cassmeyer VL (1991). Clinical manual of medical-surgical nursing, ed 2, St Louis, Mosby–Year Book, Inc.

Tucker SM, Canobbio MM, Paquette EV, and Wells MF (1988). Patient care standards: Nursing process, diagnosis, and outcome, St Louis, Mosby–Year Book, Inc.

CHAPTER 6

Cardiovascular System

Lisa L. Havens
Joycelyn W. Weaver

Cardiovascular disease is a frequent occurrence in the older population. The changes that occur with age make the older population more at risk for cardiovascular disease and cause them to respond differently to the disease and its treatment modalities.

THE AGING HEART

In looking at the usual changes that occur in the heart as a person ages, it is important to remember (1) that it is difficult to separate aging effects from disease effects on the heart and (2) that many factors affect cardiovascular function during a person's lifetime. These factors include environmental factors, lifestyle factors, and the function of other organ systems that affect the heart (Weisfeldt, 1986). The most generally accepted lifestyle cardiac risk factors include heredity, male sex, black race, older age, high cholesterol level, hypertension, diabetes, cigarette smoking, obesity, sedentary lifestyle or lack of regular exercise, and stress (American Heart Association, 1988).

As the heart ages, it normally develops structural changes that alone usually do not result in cardiac dysfunction. The heart size is not significantly decreased or increased as one ages. Because of general physical deconditioning common in the older person, the myocardium may decrease in size as a result of lack of use (Martin, 1989).

The connective tissue of the cardiac valves undergoes myxomatous degenerative changes with aging. This results in stretching and enlargement of all valves, but especially the mitral valve. The chordae tendineae also lengthen and thin out. Degenerative changes in the cardiac valves result in scarring and valvular calcification in some cases. This calcification can result in regurgitation and obstruction of the affected valve (Killen, 1988).

The conduction system of the heart is damaged as a result of aging. The conduction system shows fewer sinus node or pacemaker cells as the heart ages, especially after the age of 60 (Porth, 1986). Scarring or calcification of the atrioventricular node, the bundle of His, and the main bundle branches may occur, resulting in conduction system arrhythmias (Killen, 1988).

The vessels of the heart show increased stiffness with age. This stiffness, or loss of elasticity, results in the heart ejecting into a stiffer, more resistant structure. The aorta not only has decreased elasticity with age but also has increased wall thickness. These structural changes in the heart vessels increase pulse wave velocity, aortic resistance, peripheral resistance, and systolic blood pressure (Weisfeldt, 1986).

In addition to the structural changes that occur with aging, several physiologic changes occur. Decreased cardiovascular sensitivity to beta-adrenergic stimulation occurs, resulting in a slower heart rate and decreased inotropic (force of myocardial contraction) and arterial vasodilatory responses to catecholamines (Weisfeldt, 1986). The cardiac output, which is the volume of blood the heart ejects per minute, is determined by multiplying the stroke volume by the heart rate. Factors affecting cardiac output are preload, afterload, compliance, and contractility. Because the force of the heart's contraction decreases with age, the resistance that the ventricles pump against increases (which increases afterload), the amount of elasticity of the myocardium decreases (which increases preload), and the heart rate decreases. This results in a decreased cardiac output in the older population, which means that less cardiac reserve is available. Cardiac reserve is the heart's ability to increase its pumping capacity. Usually these changes do not dramatically affect the daily life of the individual. Rather, the impact is significant during times of stress or illness when cardiac reserve is needed. In response to the stressor, the heart rate increases, but with a slower response rate and

70

a slower return to the resting heart rate (Brenner, 1987; Eichner, 1989; Martin, 1989).

ISCHEMIC HEART DISEASE

Ischemic heart disease can be defined as an impairment in the myocardium related to an inequality between myocardial oxygen requirements and the available coronary blood supply (Steingart and Scheuer, 1986). The major cause of ischemic heart disease is coronary artery disease. Coronary artery disease is the process in which the following occur:

1. Fatty materials accumulate in the artery.
2. As the fat builds up, the lining of the artery forms scar tissue in the wall of the artery.
3. This scarred area calcifies, forming an atheroma, which narrows the artery even more.
4. Because of the abundance of capillaries in the atheroma, the atheroma bleeds and clots form that enlarge the atheroma.
5. Platelets aggregate to the atheroma.
6. As this process repeats itself, the artery becomes narrower and a thrombus can form, resulting in complete occlusion of the artery (DeAngelis, 1985).

Myocardial ischemia is a manifestation of pathological changes in the coronary arteries.

Symptomatic evidence of coronary artery disease is prevalent in the older population, demonstrated in the form of angina pectoris and myocardial infarction. The older patient commonly has complications of myocardial infarction, especially congestive heart failure (Wenger, 1990).

ANGINA PECTORIS

▶ PATHOPHYSIOLOGY, SIGNS, AND SYMPTOMS

In the majority of the older population, angina (chest pain or chest discomfort) is the first sign of coronary artery disease. Angina is caused by an inadequate supply of oxygen to the heart muscle. The pain that results is temporary. A situation that places additional stress or demands on the heart often precipitates the onset of angina. Other possible causes of angina are the following: coronary artery spasm, valve disorders, hypertension, anemia dysrhythmias, congestive heart failure, hemodynamic instability, hyperthyroidism, and any condition that results in a transient imbalance of the oxygen supply and demand for the myocardium. Because of the transient nature of angina, actual cell death does not occur (DeAngelis, 1985; Martin, 1989).

Transient myocardial ischemia may manifest itself in the form of angina or angina-associated symptoms, or the client may lack any apparent symptoms (Coodley, 1990). Angina pain is usually located in the substernal area but may radiate to the arms, jaw, neck, shoulder,

or epigastric area. The sensation of pain is usually described as a feeling of burning, squeezing, heaviness, suffocation, tightness, or pressure. Angina-associated symptoms may be described as diaphoresis, shortness of breath, fatigue, heart palpitations, or anxiety. Anginal pain is usually relieved with rest, removal of the precipitating factor, and/or nitroglycerin.

▶ DIAGNOSTIC PROCEDURES

Diagnostic procedures are presented in Table 6-1.

▶ MEDICAL MANAGEMENT

Medical management of the older patient with angina usually begins with drug therapy. The medications used for angina include nitrates, beta-blockers, and calcium channel blockers. The action of the nitrates is primarily to relax the smooth vascular muscle, resulting in rapid systemic and coronary vasodilation. The end result is improved blood flow to the myocardium. Nitrates can be administered through the following routes: sublingual, oral, topical, and intravenous. Beta-blockers decrease oxygen demands of the myocardium by decreasing the heart rate and therefore are effective for the relief and prevention of ischemia. Calcium channel blockers decrease heart rate, force of contraction, and arterial resistance and increase coronary blood flow by vasodilation of the coronary arteries. Calcium channel blockers are especially useful for angina caused by coronary artery spasms. If drug therapy is not successful in relieving angina, revascularization may be considered. The patient

Table 6-1. Diagnostic procedures for angina pectoris

Test	Comments
History	Have patient describe events leading to angina, describe pain (type, location, duration, and relieving factors). Identify risk factors, past medical history.
Laboratory tests	Test cardiac enzymes to rule out myocardial infarction. Do a complete blood count (to check for anemia) and a lipid profile.
Electrocardiogram	During angina, T wave inversion may be present and is indicative of ischemia. ST segment elevation or depression is indicative of injury. Compare with previous ECG.
Stress test, cardiac catheterization, nuclear imaging studies	If stress test is positive (1-mm ST segment depression), consider cardiac catheterization or nuclear imaging studies.

may be considered for percutaneous transluminal coronary angioplasty (PTCA) or a coronary artery bypass graft (CABG). CABG surgery in the older patient is associated with higher morbidity and mortality. The treatment goal for angina is to provide the patient/family with an acceptable quality of life (Coodley, 1990; De-Angelis, 1985; Martin, 1989; Steingart and Scheuer, 1986; Valle and Lemberg, 1989; Wenger, 1990).

Silent myocardial ischemia has been shown to occur frequently in the older adult. Silent ischemia results from lack of adequate blood supply rather than increased demand placed on the heart. Silent ischemia is diagnosed primarily by exercise testing and ambulatory electrocardiographic monitoring (Holter monitor).

▶ PROGNOSIS

Drug therapy can be effective in reducing the frequency and duration of silent ischemia. Silent ischemia has a poor prognosis for patients who have coronary artery disease (Coodley, 1990).

MYOCARDIAL INFARCTION

▶ PATHOPHYSIOLOGY, SIGNS, AND SYMPTOMS

A myocardial infarction occurs when the ischemia is severe enough to result in actual necrosis, or death, of the myocardial cells. Myocardial infarction results from lack of blood supply to the myocardium (Martin, 1989). In older adults, myocardial infarction is often precipitated by other associated medical problems, such as infection, bleeding, or hypotension, rather than solely by coronary artery disease (Eichner, 1989). Signs and symptoms include the following: chest pain that is prolonged and is usually described by the patient as different from angina pain, generally as more severe; chest pain that is unrelieved by rest or nitroglycerin; nausea/vomiting; anxiety; denial of event; diaphoresis, clammy skin; pallor; dyspnea; orthopnea; dysrhythmias; syncope; dizziness; fatigue; and an impending feeling of doom (DeAngelis, 1985). The presenting signs and symptoms of a myocardial infarction in older adults are often atypical. There is an increased frequency of unrecognized myocardial infarctions in this age group. Among the reasons for this are the following: (1) older adults are more likely to experience silent ischemia; (2) they are experiencing cardiac changes as a result of aging, such as conduction system disorders; and (3) they are more likely to develop a non–Q wave infarction. All of these factors limit the diagnosis of myocardial infarction by the electrocardiogram (Coodley, 1990; Eichner, 1989; Valle and Lemberg, 1989). Also, in the older adult the cardiac enzyme (CK) may increase only slightly in the presence of a myocardial infarction. This may be due to decreased muscle mass. Isoenzymes will reflect actual myocardial necrosis (Valle and Lemberg, 1989).

▶ DIAGNOSTIC PROCEDURES

Diagnostic procedures are presented in Table 6-2.

Table 6-2. Diagnostic procedures for a myocardial infarction

Test	Comments
Patient history	Ask questions regarding onset of pain; other signs/symptoms; duration, location, and characteristics of pain.
Physical exam	Look for S_4, friction rub, murmurs, rales, S_3, irregular pulse, diaphoresis, dyspnea, cyanosis, and apprehension.
Laboratory tests	Test cardiac enzymes and isoenzymes (Table 6-3).
Electrocardiogram	Depending on the stage of the myocardial infarction, ST or T wave changes may be seen. Pathological Q waves are diagnostic. In non–Q wave myocardial infarction reciprocal changes may be seen.
Stress test, nuclear imaging test, cardiac catheterization, and/or echocardiogram	

Data compiled from DeAngelis (1985), Gary (1988), Valle and Lemberg (1989).

Table 6-3. Enzyme results indicative of a myocardial infarction

Enzyme	Isoenzyme	Onset (hr)	Peak (hr)	Return to normal
CPK		6-8	24	72-96 hr
	CPK-MB	4-8	18-24	72 hr
LDH		24-48	72-96	10 days
	LDH_1	12-24	24-48	72-96 hr
AST		8-12	18-36	72-96 hr

Data compiled from Springhouse Corporation (1990).

▶ MEDICAL MANAGEMENT

The goal of medical management for a myocardial infarction is management of presenting problems, preventing and/or limiting its size, and prevention or early detection of potential complications. Medication therapy may include the following: thrombolytic agents, nitrates, calcium channel blockers, antiarrhythmics, anticoagulants, sympathomimetic drugs (stimulate sympathetic nervous system), vasodilators, and beta-blockers (DeAngelis, 1985; Schlant et al, 1988).

▶ PROGNOSIS

Complications from a myocardial infarction occur more often in the older adult. They can include dysrhythmias, congestive heart failure, cardiogenic shock, persistent pain, extension of the myocardial infarction, pericarditis, thromboemboli, papillary muscle dysfunction, rupture of the ventricle or septum, ventricular aneurysm, and psychological complications (Coodley, 1990; Killen, 1988; Valle and Lemberg, 1989; Wenger, 1990). The occurrence of these complications is what contributes to the increased length of hospital stay and the increased morbidity and mortality for the older patient who develops a myocardial infarction.

▶ NURSING MANAGEMENT—NURSING CARE PLAN
Angina and Myocardial Infarction

The information in this section applies to both angina and myocardial infarction.

Assessment

SUBJECTIVE DATA
Ask patient's description of pain and events.

OBJECTIVE DATA
Assess patient, vital signs, laboratory tests, and ECG.

	Nursing diagnoses	Expected outcomes	Nursing interventions (rationale)

N U R S I N G C A R E P L A N	Alteration in comfort
	Radiating or nonradiating chest discomfort related to an imbalance in myocardial oxygen supply and demand caused by angina or myocardial infarction
		Patient will experience relief of chest discomfort.	Assess and document the location, duration, precipitating events, associated signs/symptoms, relieving factors, and severity of chest discomfort to describe type of pain. (The severity of pain can be described on a scale of 0 to 10, with 10 being the worst pain and 0 being pain-free.)
			Assess patient's cardiac risk factors for ischemic heart disease.
			Intervene to minimize myocardial oxygen supply and demand imbalance.
			  Instruct patient to minimize activity level during acute phase (bed and chair rest and bedside commode) to minimize oxygen demands.
			  Utilize oxygen therapy as ordered to maximize oxygen supply.
			  Instruct patient to avoid activities that could cause Valsalva response (straining to have a bowel movement and holding breath while moving).
			  Avoid large meals because they will cause a need for increased blood supply to the gastrointestinal system.

Continued.

Nursing Care Plan—Angina and Myocardial Infarction—cont'd

Nursing diagnoses	Expected outcomes	Nursing interventions (rationale)
Alteration in comfort—cont'd		Avoid caffeine and nicotine because caffeine stimulates the myocardium and can result in increased myocardial oxygen use. (Nicotine causes vasoconstriction and can decrease the blood supply.)
		Administer medications as ordered to relieve pain. (Avoid the intramuscular route because this can elevate the CPK, and absorption of medications intramuscularly can be reduced during episodes of ischemia.)
		Document patient's response to medications, including vital signs before and after administration of medications.
		Assist patient during episodes of chest pain (back rub, relaxation strategies, calm, quiet environment, reassurance, and diversional activities).
	Patient will notify the nurse of recurrent chest discomfort.	Instruct patient to notify the nurse immediately of recurrent chest discomfort.
		Instruct patient regarding importance of a progressive exercise program and home care prior to discharge.
Potential or actual decreased cardiac output related to dysrhythmias, decreased myocardial contractility, and/or increased myocardial oxygen demand	Patient will demonstrate hemodynamic stability, as evidenced by stable blood pressure, adequate urine output, appropriate level of consciousness, absence of chest pain, and ECG within normal limits.	Place patient on cardiac monitor, and continually assess heart rate and rhythm.
		If dysrhythmias develop, evaluate the patient to see whether symptoms are present (hypotension, chest pain, change in level of consciousness, and/or decreased in urine output).
		Give medications as ordered. Be sure to check patient's vital signs/rhythm before and after medication to evaluate effectiveness.
		Encourage bed rest with progressive activity.
		Assist patient with activities of daily living.
		Maintain a calm, quiet environment.
		Administer medications as ordered, and evaluate their effectiveness.
		Assess patient for signs/symptoms of decreased cardiac output (decreased blood pressure, decreased urine output, decreased or absent pulses, decreased level of consciousness, crackles in lungs, decreased

Nursing Care Plan—Angina and Myocardial Infarction—cont'd

Nursing diagnoses	Expected outcomes	Nursing interventions (rationale)
Anxiety related to fear of unknown, unfamiliar environment, and potential or actual threat to physical integrity	Patient/family will be able to express anxiety, fear, and concerns.	heart rate, change in rhythm, S_3 or S_4 heart sounds, change in vital signs, pale skin, cyanosis, restlessness, and/or increased central venous pressure). Encourage the patient/family to verbalize anxiety, fears, concerns, and questions. Use flexible visiting hours to allow the family to be available to offer support to the patient.
	Patient/family will demonstrate a decrease in anxiety and fear.	Teach stress-reducing behaviors. Refer to social worker, chaplain, or other members of the health care team as necessary. Allow for adequate sleep periods. Orient patient to hospital routines, visiting hours, and care being given. Demonstrate a caring attitude. Provide a calm environment. Provide support to the patient.
	Patient/family will utilize effective coping behaviors.	Assess patient/family's level of anxiety and coping mechanism. Encourage active participation in care and rehabilitation program.

Discharge planning and patient/family education
Teach about the following:
   Orientation to unit
   Coping behaviors
   Diagnostic test procedures
   Stress identification (Guzetta and Dossey, 1984; Ulrich, Canale, and Wendell, 1986)
   Basic cardiac function
   Disease process (angina and myocardial infarction)
Prepare patient/family for any procedures/care being done.
Teach the following before discharge:
   Necessary activity guidelines (bed rest to minimize workload on the heart) (Brenner, 1987; Thompson, McFarland, Hirsch, et al, 1989; Ulrich, Canale, and Wendell, 1986).
   Risk factors (Box 6-1)
   Medication guidelines
   Home care (Box 6-2)
   How to take pulse (Box 6-2)
   Stress reduction

Evaluation
Patient experiences prompt relief of chest discomfort.
Patient is hemodynamically stable.
Patient is using effective coping mechanism.

Box 6-1.

Risk factors for cardiac disease

Heredity (especially heart disease at a relatively young age)
Male sex
Black race
Older age
High cholesterol level
Hypertension
Diabetes
Cigarette smoking
Obesity
Sedentary lifestyle
Lack of regular exercise
Stress

Box 6-2.

Patient Education

Myocardial Infarction

If you develop chest pain, the first thing you need to do is to lie down and take your nitroglycerin. You may repeat nitroglycerin every 5 minutes up to three times. If you still have chest pain, make arrangements to be taken to the hospital.

Some other things that you may experience when having a heart attack are excess perspiration, shortness of breath, nausea, indigestion, weakness, dizziness, and a feeling that something bad is going to happen.

Take all medications as ordered by your doctor.

Keep all appointments with your doctor.

Learn to take your pulse. Your pulse is the number of times your heart beats per minute. You can feel a pulse over a large artery. Place a watch with a second hand where you can easily see it. Place your index and middle finger on the inside of your wrist, just past the thumb. Do not use your thumb to count your pulse. Once you can feel your pulse, count the number of times you feel it within 60 seconds. The normal heart beat is 60 to 100 per minute.

Follow your diet as instructed.

Follow your exercise plan as instructed. Exercise should be approved by your doctor and be a gradual process.

CONGESTIVE HEART FAILURE

Heart failure is one of the most common manifestations of heart disease in older adults.

▶ **PATHOPHYSIOLOGY, SIGNS, AND SYMPTOMS**

Heart failure is the inability of the heart to pump the needed amount of oxygenated blood to meet the metabolic requirements of the body. Congestive heart failure (CHF) is a state in which the left ventricle is unable to maintain a cardiac output sufficient to meet the needs of the body. One can have acute or chronic CHF. Acute CHF has a sudden onset and could occur after an acute myocardial infarction or after a cardiac arrest situation. Chronic CHF usually develops over a longer period of time when a damaged chamber of the heart gradually enlarges and contractility decreases (Impallomeni, 1988). In left-side CHF congestion occurs mainly in the lungs as a result of the backing up of blood into the pulmonary circulation. Right-side CHF causes elevated pressure and congestion in the systemic circulation. If the left ventricle fails and is unable to pump out the necessary amount of blood, this blood builds up in the left ventricle, backs up into the left atrium, and then moves into the pulmonary circulation (left-side CHF). Acute pulmonary edema is the presence of excess fluid in the lung, either in the interstitial spaces or in the alveoli (Wilson, 1989).

The precipitating events for left-side CHF can be as follows: atherosclerotic heart disease, acute myocardial infarction, tachycardia, bradycardia, cardiomyopathy, increased circulating volume, aortic stenosis or insufficiency, mitral insufficiency, coarctation of the aorta, atrial or ventricular septal defect, cardiac tamponade, or constrictive pericarditis (DeAngelis, 1985; Jessup, Lakatta, Leier, and Santinga, 1990; Stanley, 1986).

The precipitating events for right-side CHF include left-side CHF, atherosclerotic heart disease, acute myocardial infarction, tachycardia, bradycardia, pulmonary embolism, fluid overload, excess sodium intake, chronic obstructive pulmonary disease, pulmonary hypertension, right ventricular failure, mitral stenosis, atrial or ventricular septal defect, and pulmonary outflow stenosis

(DeAngelis, 1985; Jessup, Lakatta, Leier, and Santinga, 1990; Thompson, McFarland, Hirsch, et al, 1989; Underhill, Woods, Sivarajan, and Halpenny, 1982).

The precipitating factors for acute pulmonary edema can be acute left ventricular failure, myocardial infarction, aortic stenosis, severe mitral valve disease, hypertension, congestive heart failure, circulatory overload, drug hypersensitivity, pulmonary embolism, lung injuries, stroke or head injury, infection, and fever (DeAngelis, 1985; Thompson, McFarland, Hirsch, et al, 1989; Underhill, Woods, Sivarajan, and Halpenny, 1982; Wilson, 1989).

When the heart is damaged, the body uses three compensatory mechanisms to increase cardiac output and venous return to the heart: (1) increased sympathetic activity, (2) renal retention of fluid, and (3) increased stretch of the heart muscle (Jessup, Lakatta, Leier, and Santinga, 1990).

Increased sympathetic activity results in increased heart rate, increased contractility, and vasoconstriction. Within a few hours of heart failure the kidneys secrete an increased amount of renin. Renin acts upon angiotensin to produce angiotensin I. Angiotensin I is converted to angiotensin II in the lungs. Angiotensin II causes arterial vasoconstriction, which increases peripheral vascular resistance and maintains blood pressure. Angiotensin II also stimulates secretion of aldosterone from the adrenal gland. Aldosterone promotes reabsorption of sodium and chloride in the kidney. Retention of sodium and water produces expansion of the blood volume.

The stretch of the myocardial fibers is increased to improve contractility. Over time, these fibers cannot stretch any more and hypertrophy can result. It is when these compensatory mechanisms fail that signs and symptoms of CHF can be observed.

The clinical signs and symptoms of left- and right-side CHF are listed in Table 6-4.

The most common clinical signs and symptoms of acute pulmonary edema are cough, pink-tinged, frothy sputum, extreme dyspnea and orthopnea, extreme anxiety and panic, noisy breathing (wheezes and crackles), cyanosis, diaphoresis, distended neck veins, and tachycardia (DeAngelis, 1985; Wilson, 1989).

Left-side CHF is more common and can lead to right-side CHF. The pathophysiology is as follows:

1. A diseased left ventricular myocardium cannot pump blood returning from the lungs into the systemic circulation. This condition decreases cardiac output.
2. Pressure increases in the lungs as a result of accumulation of blood in the lungs. If the pressure exceeds pulmonary capillary oncotic pressure (30 mm Hg), fluid will leak into the pulmonary interstitial space, resulting in pulmo-

Table 6-4. Clinical signs and symptoms of left-side and right-side congestive heart failure

Left-side	Right-side
Anxiety	Hepatosplenomegaly
Shortness of breath, dyspnea	Dependent pitting edema
Cough with frothy sputum	Jugular venous distension
Tachycardia	Bounding pulses
Basilar rales (crackles)	Oliguria
Bronchial wheezes	Dysrhythmias
Cyanosis or pallor	Increased central venous pressure
Diaphoresis	Anorexia, nausea
Hypoxia	Nocturia
S_3 heart sound	Weakness
Insomnia	
Increased pulmonary artery diastolic pressure and pulmonary artery capillary wedge pressure	
Palpitations	
Fatigue	
Restlessness	
Pulmonary edema	
Hyperventilation	
Pulmonary hypertension	
Pulsus alternans	

Data compiled from Impallomeni (1988), Jessup, Lakatta, Leier, and Santinga (1990), Thompson, McFarland, Hirsch, et al (1989), Underhill, Woods, Sivarajan, and Halpenny (1982), Wilson (1989).

nary edema. Oxygen–carbon dioxide exchange is compromised.
3. As pressure increases in the lungs, pressure increases in the right heart as a result of backflow pressure on the pulmonary circulation.
4. The right heart cannot pump its blood into the pulmonary system because of this backflow of pressure.
5. Venous return to the right heart is reduced.
6. Pressure continues to back up, and systemic circulation and body organs become congested with blood (DeAngelis, 1985; Jessup, Lakatta, Leier, and Santinga, 1990).

▶ **DIAGNOSTIC PROCEDURES**

Diagnostic findings are presented in Box 6-3.

Congestive heart failure can be divided into different classes depending on the limitations it places on the patient's activity level. Class I places no limitations on physical activity. Class II places slight limitations on physical activity; the patient with Class II CHF is usually comfortable at rest, but ordinary physical activity results in fatigue, palpitations, dyspnea, or angina. Class III CHF places marked limitations on physical activity; the

---

Box 6-3.

Diagnostic findings for congestive heart failure or pulmonary edema

Cardiomegaly on chest x-ray
Ventricular gallop (S_3)
Tachycardia
Distended neck veins
Upper abdominal pain (hepatosplenomegaly)
Abnormal liver function tests
Nocturia
Anorexia, nausea
Pulmonary edema on chest x-ray

Data compiled from Impallomeni (1988), Jessup, Lakatta, Leier, and Santinga (1990), Thompson, McFarland, Hirsch, et al (1989), Underhill, Woods, Sivarajan, and Halpenny (1982).

patient with Class III CHF is usually comfortable at rest, but less than ordinary physical activity causes fatigue, palpitations, dyspnea, or angina. Patients with Class IV CHF are unable to carry on any physical activity without discomfort; signs and symptoms of cardiac insufficiency or angina may be present at rest, and with any physical activity, discomfort increases. Once a patient develops Class IV CHF, the life expectancy is usually less than 6 months.

▶ **MEDICAL MANAGEMENT**

The medical management of CHF or acute pulmonary edema may include monitoring for dysrhythmias, bed rest with semi-Fowler's position, oxygen, monitoring intake and output, fluid restriction, limiting sodium intake, checking weight daily, close monitoring of laboratory values, and hemodynamic monitoring via a Swan-Ganz catheter. Medications commonly used in these patients include positive inotropic drugs to improve contractility, negative chronotropic drugs to decrease heart rate, vasodilators, diuretics to promote excretion of water, and morphine. Morphine causes vasodilation, decreased venous return to the heart, decreased pain, decreased anxiety, and decreased myocardial oxygen demand.

▶ **PROGNOSIS**

The complications of CHF can be progressive deterioration of cardiac and pulmonary function, serious cardiac arrhythmias, digitalis toxicity, pneumonia, and fluid and electrolyte imbalance. The treatment goal is to avoid these complications. Acute pulmonary edema is a life-threatening situation and is a true medical emergency. The goal is to improve ventilation and to reduce pulmonary congestion.

▶ **NURSING MANAGEMENT—NURSING CARE PLAN**
Congestive Heart Failure

Assessment

SUBJECTIVE DATA
Question the patient regarding symptoms, the course of the illness, and precipitating events.

OBJECTIVE DATA
Monitor ECG rhythm; assess heart and breath sounds, jugular venous distension, peripheral edema, vital signs, laboratory values, intake and output, and nonverbal signs of shortness of breath.

N U R S I N G C A R E P L A N	Nursing diagnoses	Expected outcomes	Nursing interventions (rationale)
	Decreased cardiac output related to decreased contractility, increased afterload, and increased preload	Patient will demonstrate hemodynamic stability as evidenced by stable blood pressure, adequate urine output, appropriate level of consciousness, absence of chest pain, and normal ECG.	Monitor and assess ECG rhythm and report arrhythmias. Encourage bed rest with progressive activity as tolerated to conserve energy and decrease oxygen demand. Assist patient with activities of daily living, and encourage family to be involved in care of the patient. Administer medications as ordered and evaluate effectiveness. Monitor for digitalis toxicity. (As an individual ages, renal blood flow decreases; with the onset of congestive heart failure, this decreased renal blood flow is

Nursing Care Plan—Congestive Heart Failure—cont'd

Nursing diagnoses	Expected outcomes	Nursing interventions (rationale)
		worsened. Since digoxin is primarily excreted by the kidneys, the digoxin level needs to be closely monitored [Stanley, 1986].)
		Monitor for signs/symptoms of decreased cardiac output (decreased blood pressure, decreased peripheral pulses, decreased urine output, altered level of consciousness, pallor, cyanosis, cold, clammy skin, and increased heart rate).
Alteration in oxygenation related to impaired gas exchange due to increased pulmonary capillary pressure	Gas exchange improves as evidenced by decreased shortness of breath, arterial blood gases within normal limits, and breath sounds that are clear bilaterally.	Monitor intake and output. Elevate the head of the bed to improve ventilation. Administer oxygen therapy as ordered. Monitor arterial blood gases, oxygen saturation. Administer medications as ordered and evaluate effectiveness. Assess breath sounds frequently to determine changes in congestion and state of ventilation. Explain all care and procedures to patient and family to minimize anxiety. Maintain a calm, quiet, restful environment.
Fluid volume excess related to right/left ventricular failure	Volume excess is lessened as evidenced by decreased weight, decreased edema, and improved ventilation.	Monitor intake and output. (Intake of fluid and/or sodium may be restricted.) Check weight daily to determine loss or gain of fluid. (Weigh patient on same scale and at the same time of day for increased accuracy.) Inspect patient for jugular venous distension. Assess heart sounds and breath sounds to determine increased or decreased congestion. Monitor laboratory values such as fluid balance profile and electrolytes.

Discharge planning and patient/family education

Explain to patient and family about how and why congestive heart failure develops.

Instruct patient and family about signs and symptoms to report, such as increased shortness of breath, exertional dyspnea, orthopnea, nocturnal dyspnea, weight gain, chest pain, increased weakness.

Instruct patient about medications—purpose, dose, frequency, and possible side effects.

Plan individualized activity program.

Consult with dietitian as needed for dietary instructions regarding low-sodium diet (DeAngelis, 1985; Impallomeni, 1988; Jessup, Lakatta, Leier, and Santinga, 1990; Rideout and Monemuro, 1986; Stanley, 1986; Thompson, McFarland, Hirsch, et al, 1989; Underhill, Woods, Sivarajan, and Halpenny, 1982; Wilson, 1989).

Provide guide for home care (see Box 6-4).

Evaluation

Patient is adequately oxygenated.

Patient is hemodynamically stable.

Box 6-4.

Patient Education

Congestive Heart Failure

Follow your salt-restricted diet. Do not add salt at the table. Avoid foods with a lot of salt.

Take all medications as ordered by your doctor. Do not let your medications run out.

Keep all appointments with your doctor.

Weigh yourself every day. It is important to weigh at the same time every day on the same scale. It is usually a good idea to weigh yourself before breakfast. If you gain 2 to 3 pounds over a few days, you need to report this to your doctor. An increase in your weight could be a warning sign for congestive heart failure.

Notify your doctor of increased urination at night, swelling in your ankles and legs, worsening shortness of breath, and a cough that does not go away.

VALVULAR HEART DISEASE

▶ PATHOPHYSIOLOGY, SIGNS, AND SYMPTOMS

Valvular heart disease is a term used to describe diagnoses involving pathology of the valves of the heart that are characteristic of stenosis associated with obstruction of blood flow or of valvular breakdown associated with regurgitation of blood. The two most common types of valvular disorders are valvular insufficiency and stenosis. Valvular insufficiency exists when the valves fail to close completely and blood is allowed to back-flow (also known as valvular regurgitation). Valvular stenosis is a thickening and hardening of the valve that narrows its opening. This limits the amount of blood flow through the heart.

Another disorder associated with the mitral valve is prolapse. Mitral valve prolapse is the most common of the valvular diseases; it is believed to affect approximately 40% of the adult population (Guzetta and Dossey, 1984). During systole, one or both leaflets of the valve (most commonly the posterior) billow upward and back into the left atrium.

The origin of valvular heart disease can usually be traced to either congenital or acquired disorders. Congenital disorders include conditions such as mitral valve stenosis and prolapse, and pulmonary stenosis. Examples of acquired disorders include those resulting from the effects of rheumatic fever and endocarditis. Trauma, myocardial infarction, and cardiomyopathy are other exam-

ples. When the integrity of the valves is disrupted by disease or injury, valve dysfunction occurs.

Clinical signs and symptoms vary with the type of disorder and its severity. Many people with mitral stenosis are asymptomatic for years because of the slow, gradual development of the stenosis. When the stenosis becomes significant enough to cause symptoms, it commonly causes complaints of fatigue, dyspnea (most common), palpitations, and chest pain. Atrial fibrillation is not an uncommon experience for these people. With mitral regurgitation, symptoms rarely occur unless there is an underlying abnormality involved. If the cardiac output falls, for example, symptoms such as fatigue, orthopnea, and exertional dyspnea occur. When there is known pulmonary vascular hypertension with associated right heart failure, mitral regurgitation sufferers may exhibit distended neck veins, ascites and hepatic congestion, and ankle edema.

With mitral valve prolapse many people are asymptomatic but some exhibit symptoms such as dyspnea, fatigue, chest pain, and palpitations. The most common symptom is chest pain that mimics angina. The difference is that this type of pain is not relieved by nitroglycerin or rest.

Aortic valve stenosis rarely produces symptoms until 40 to 50 years of age. Cardiac output is usually normal at rest but cannot be maintained during exercise. The most common symptom is dyspnea on exertion. Angina and syncope may also occur with physical activity. Persons with aortic regurgitation usually do not experience symptoms until compensatory mechanisms of the left ventricle fail to keep them asymptomatic. Usually the first noticeable symptoms are an increased awareness of the heartbeat (especially when lying on the left side), palpitations, and neck vein pulsations.

▶ DIAGNOSTIC PROCEDURES

Diagnostic studies useful in determining the presence of valvular heart disease include electrocardiogram (ECG), echocardiogram, chest x-ray, radionucleotide studies, and cardiac catheterization.

In mitral stenosis, ECG studies show right ventricular (RV) hypertrophy, left atrial (LA) enlargement, and a notched P wave. With mitral regurgitation, ECG studies show atrial fibrillation, left ventricular (LV) hypertrophy, and an enlarged left atrium. With aortic stenosis and regurgitation, ECG studies show LV hypertrophy. Conduction defects are often found with aortic stenosis.

Echocardiogram studies convert sound waves to moving pictures. With mitral stenosis, decreased leaflet excursion can be seen. In mitral regurgitation, LA enlargement can be detected. Findings with aortic stenosis reveal LV wall thickening, and with regurgitation LV dilation may be seen.

Chest x-ray will often reveal pulmonary venous congestion and RV enlargement in mitral stenosis. It may also detect pulmonary edema and LV enlargement. With mitral regurgitation, LV enlargement is also seen along with LA enlargement and pulmonary congestion. In aortic stenosis and regurgitation, chest x-rays help detect aortic valve calcification and dilation of the aorta. LV enlargement is also seen in aortic regurgitation. Radionucleotide studies are useful in that they help to determine exercise ejection and resting fractions.

Cardiac catheterization is a most valuable diagnostic procedure because it gives very precise information as to the state of the heart in each individual chamber. Pressures in key areas of the cardiopulmonary vasculature are obtained. Usual findings in mitral stenosis reveal increased LA pressure, increased pulmonary capillary wedge pressure, and a low cardiac output. In mitral regurgitation, increases in the left ventricular end-diastolic pressure (LVEDP) and left atrial pressure (LAP) are found. In both aortic stenosis and regurgitation, LVEDP is increased. With aortic regurgitation, pulse pressure and LAP are also increased. Angiography with

contrast dye will confirm and reveal the extent of regurgitation.

▶ MEDICAL MANAGEMENT

Medical management involves various approaches that are individualized on a case by case basis. Dietary management requires a low sodium intake, especially if signs of pulmonary congestion are present. Pharmacologic management includes the use of diuretics and digitalis for heart failure, antiarrhythmics when indicated, antibiotics prophylactically when invasive procedures are performed, and anticoagulants for patients with atrial fibrillation. Cardioversion is also a consideration for those people who are symptomatic with atrial fibrillation or who are at risk for embolism formation.

Percutaneous transluminal valvuloplasty (PTV) is a nonsurgical option for dilation of a stenosed valve. This technique has been used for dilation of peripheral arteries and coronary arteries for some time with good results. In patients who are not considered good surgical candidates but medical treatment is not adequate to alleviate symptoms, PTV has been used with success in adults with stenosis of calcified mitral or aortic valves. The procedure is done in the cardiac catheterization laboratory. A right femoral artery approach is used for aortic valvuloplasty and a right femoral vein approach is used for mitral valvuloplasty. Other advantages of PTV include the following: there is no sternotomy incision, it can delay or eliminate the need for surgery, the hospital stay is short, usually no blood transfusion is needed, and there is no anesthesia.

Surgery is usually indicated only when all other modalities are no longer able to relieve symptoms or when cardiac failure is inevitable without surgical intervention. Surgical correction may involve the replacement of the valve with a pig valve or a homograft (a human heart valve from a donated heart). Prosthetic valves are no longer used as commonly as they were in the past.

▶ PROGNOSIS

The prognosis for those who suffer from valvular heart disease varies with the extent of the disease and the age and general health of the individual. The overall success rate for surgical repair of diseased valves is quite high. Persons who are not good surgical candidates often do well with activity modification, but again the overall health is a critical factor in determining the effects on lifestyle.

▶ NURSING MANAGEMENT—NURSING CARE PLAN
Valvular Heart Disease

Using data from the person's history and the presenting physical signs and symptoms will help in the formation of an optimal plan of care for the person with valvular heart disease.

Assessment

SUBJECTIVE DATA

Dyspnea on exertion

Complaints of fatigue, palpitations, and sometimes chest discomfort or pain

OBJECTIVE DATA

Atrial fibrillation is occasionally observed on the ECG. Neck vein pulsations, increased blood pressure, and increased respirations on exertion are often seen.

	Nursing diagnoses	Expected outcomes	Nursing interventions (rationale)
N U R S I N G C A R E P L A N	Alteration in comfort related to chest pain, shortness of breath, and palpitations	Patient will be free from the discomfort related to chest pain, shortness of breath, and palpitations.	Administer medications such as propranolol, quinidine, and procainamide (assists in the management of palpitations that result from premature ventricular contractions [PVCs] and supraventricular tachycardia). Teach patient to do the following: Regulate daily activities on a schedule that allows for adequate periods of rest between activities. Climb stairs slowly, and stop and rest at the first sign of dyspnea. Complete all tasks that are limited to one area before going to another area. Spread activities and tasks out over the day or over several days. Use relaxation techniques to help relieve pain and shortness of breath.
	Anxiety and fear related to the threat to health status	Fears will be reduced to a manageable level.	Assess readiness. Allow for verbalization of fears and concerns.
	Decreased cardiac output related to valvular insufficiency	Patient will maintain adequate cardiac output and be as symptom-free as possible.	Establish a baseline cardiovascular assessment to determine the level of activity tolerance and the response to prescribed therapy. Establish planned rest periods, and pace activities according to tolerance. Stress the importance of close medical supervision and the importance of regular checkups.

Discharge planning and patient/family education

Help patient to understand drug regimen and to follow it as prescribed.

Instruct on daily exercise program to ensure that patient does not overexert but maintains his or her health at an optimum level.

Teach patient the disease mechanism.

Foster optimism and offer realistic assurances.

Evaluation

Patient verbalizes fears and comes to the realization that he or she can be active and relatively free of discomfort by proper regulation of activities.

Patient has maximum activity tolerance.

Patient is free of the discomfort associated with overexertion.

PERIPHERAL VASCULAR DISEASE

▶ PATHOPHYSIOLOGY, SIGNS, AND SYMPTOMS

Peripheral vascular disease (PVD) is a term used to describe certain pathologies of the vascular system. PVD can involve the arterial system and/or venous system. It generally has an insidious onset, and the diagnosis is not usually made until the disease has progressed enough to produce symptoms. The disorder occurs as a result of atherosclerosis and/or arteriosclerosis occurring simultaneously with the normal aging process of the vascular system (Esberger and Hughes, 1989).

The pathology begins with an atheromatous plaque that sets up on the intimal lining of the vessel. The lesion then progresses to a fibrous plaque. Beginning as early as age 3 to 10 years, this process continues for 20 to 30 years before a person becomes symptomatic. Once symptomatic, partial obstruction has usually occurred. The condition is then viewed as chronic, and the term arteriosclerosis applies. Calcification occurs in the medial layer of the vessel and accounts for the stiffening of the vessel. This condition interferes with normal flow of blood through the vessel, and occasionally thrombus formation occurs. A thrombus is believed to be caused by formation of a blood clot on this disturbed intimal surface of the vessel.

In people with PVD, of which arteriosclerosis is a common form, the most frequent presenting symptom is complaint of pain in the involved extremity. This pain is a result of decreased blood flow distal to the obstruction. Arterial occlusion can be acute or chronic. In an acute arterial occlusion the onset of pain is sudden and peaks quickly. The sufferer often reports extremity weakness immediately after the severe pain, and sometimes the extremity gives way, causing a fall to occur. Another characteristic of this phenomenon is that the pain often subsides very quickly.

In chronic arterial occlusion the most common symptom is intermittent claudication. Claudication can be described as a tightness or a cramping, burning sensation that is relieved by rest. Intermittent claudication is pain that occurs with exercise and is relieved by rest. Another type of pain characteristic of chronic arterial occlusion is ischemic rest pain. This usually occurs at night. The person is awakened suddenly by severe foot pain and must get up and walk around or massage the affected foot to obtain relief. It is believed that circulation to the extremity is improved simply by virtue of gravity improving perfusion pressure to the extremity as it is lowered.

In peripheral venous disease the symptoms are less painful than in arterial disease. Varicose veins and thrombophlebitis are venous diseases that are common in the older population. Elevation of the extremity usually relieves the symptoms of varicose veins, which cause the legs to feel heavy and easily fatigued.

▶ DIAGNOSTIC PROCEDURES

The types of diagnostic studies are based on whether the physician suspects an arterial or venous disorder. Doppler ultrasonography is a transcutaneous technique in which sound waves are used to evaluate blood flow through peripheral arteries and veins. In plethysmography wave forms are produced that are used to measure fluid volume differences in various regions or organs of the body. Other diagnostic procedures such as angiography involve the injection of a radiocontrast dye into a vessel to make it visible on x-ray. In arteriography the dye is injected into an artery to locate an occlusion or aneurysm. A venogram calls for injection of the dye into a vein and is commonly performed to diagnose deep vein thrombosis. Another diagnostic study, digital subtraction angiography (DSA), provides direct arterial visualization without invasive puncture of the vessel. Ultrasonography and computerized tomography (CT) scans are also used as evaluation tools for diagnosing vessel disease.

▶ MEDICAL MANAGEMENT

Medical management of persons with PVD directs its goals of treatment toward modification of risk factors, prophylactic protection of affected extremities, and in some cases pharmacologic therapy. Risk factor modification includes complete cessation of smoking, lowering serum lipid levels, controlling hypertension and diabetes, and reducing weight and stress factors. Protection of the affected extremities includes avoidance of chemical or mechanical trauma. Properly fitting shoes, meticulous cleaning, grooming of toenails, and daily inspection of the skin are paramount. The benefits of pharmacologic therapy have been somewhat controversial. However, Trental (pentoxifylline) has been approved by the Food and Drug Administration for the treatment of intermittent claudication. It is the only drug approved for this condition (Doyle, 1986). Other treatments include the thrombolytic agents streptokinase and urokinase, percutaneous transluminal angioplasty (PTA), laser thermal angioplasty (LTA), and lastly surgical intervention.

▶ PROGNOSIS

The prognosis for PVD depends on risk factors involved, patient compliance with the health care program, and the extent of damage prior to the initiation of treatment.

▶ NURSING MANAGEMENT—NURSING CARE PLAN
Peripheral Vascular Disease

Effective nursing care of persons with PVD demands keen assessment skills. Questions commonly asked include the following: "When do your legs hurt?" "Describe the pain—Is it sharp, sudden or gradual in on- *set?" "What relieves the pain?" "Is there swelling or discoloration of the extremity?"*

Caring for people with PVD is a challenge.

Assessment

SUBJECTIVE DATA

Complaints of leg pain and extremities that are cold to the touch

Complaints of periodic swelling or discoloration of extremities

OBJECTIVE DATA

Extremities cold to the touch

Weak or absent pulses

Edema of the lower extremities

	Nursing diagnoses	Expected outcomes	Nursing interventions (rationale)
N U R S I N G C A R E P L A N	Alteration in comfort related to painful extremity	Patient will have increased comfort and decreased episodes of pain.	Encourage a progressive exercise program that begins slowly and gradually increases. (Walking exercise can be gradually increased over time and will help promote the development of collateral circulation.) Offer the use of analgesics for increased comfort.
	Alteration of peripheral tissue perfusion	Tissue perfusion will improve to its optimum.	Teach the patient to avoid crossing the legs either at the knee or at the ankle, especially for an extended period of time. The use of knee-flexing devices on beds should be strongly discouraged. Explain the need to decrease or avoid completely the use of nicotine because it is known to be a powerful vasoconstrictor.
	Alteration in skin integrity	Skin integrity will be maintained with normal color and temperature and no ulcerations.	Teach patient to do the following: Avoid constrictive clothing or bed linens. Observe bony prominences for areas that may be rubbed by clothing, bed rails, or tight-fitting shoes. Keep environment comfortably warm. Avoid use of adhesive tapes directly on the skin.

Discharge planning and patient/family education

Teach patient the following:

To avoid wearing clothes that are constrictive and to avoid the use of adhesive tape

The importance of wearing shoes that fit well and do not rub the feet when walking

To wear cotton socks

That good hygiene and daily inspection of the skin are most important

Show the patient and family members how to check pe- *ripheral pulses and the signs and symptoms of altered tissue perfusion (i.e., cold and/or mottled extremity, swelling of the extremity).*

Instruct the patient to report any changes, abnormalities, or ulceration immediately to the physician. (A limb with compromised circulation is at high risk for bacterial infections.)

Encourage the patient to space daily activities and take frequent rest periods.

Explain the importance of alternate activity and rest to

the family and obtain their cooperation in promoting this behavior.

Give home care instructions (see Box 6-5).

Evaluation

Patient has a working knowledge of the disease process.

Patient has a working knowledge of a planned activity program that is attainable and promotes the development of collateral circulation.

Patient verbalizes knowledge of early recognition of the signs and symptoms of complications of the disease.

Any problems will receive early treatment.

Many of the older population tend to accept discomfort and disability as an inevitable occurrence that comes with growing old. However, with early recognition of the signs and symptoms of disease processes such as PVD, prompt initiation of treatment, and education that is geared toward self-care and living a full life, many older persons can live longer, healthier, more self-sufficient lives.

Box 6-5.

Patient Education

Peripheral Vascular Disease

Be aware of the signs and symptoms of poor circulation, and report them to your physician immediately:

Extremity is cool to touch.

Extremity is bluish or unusually pale in color.

Extremity tingles or becomes painful at rest, or pain is brought on consistently by exertion.

There is swelling of the extremity.

A scratch or cut fails to heal in a reasonable amount of time, or foul drainage is noted.

Exercise in moderation only under the supervision of the physician and the prescribed exercise program.

Locate and mark areas where peripheral pulses can be felt. Patient or family should check pulses daily or as needed and report any changes or loss of pulses.

Care for your skin:

Wear clothes that do not bind or constrict. Clothes should fit very loosely.

Avoid the use of adhesive tape on the skin.

Wear cotton socks and shoes that fit well and do not rub the feet.

Keep nails groomed and clean. Clean between toes and report any signs of infection noted. Lambs wool may be placed between the toes to prevent rubbing.

Avoid extremely hot or cold temperatures.

HYPERTENSION

Hypertension, also called high blood pressure, is a common finding among the older population. Generally a resting systolic blood pressure that is consistently above 160 mm Hg and a diastolic blood pressure that is consistently above 90 mm Hg is considered to be hypertension. Normal adult blood pressure may be defined as a systolic blood pressure of 140 mm Hg or lower and a diastolic blood pressure of 90 mm Hg or lower. Pressures that remain consistently between these two sets of parameters are described as borderline hypertension (Porth, 1986).

According to the American Heart Association, approximately 35 million Americans have hypertension. That is about one in every six adults. It is estimated that another 25 million have borderline hypertension and that half of those persons are unaware of their hypertension.

▶ PATHOPHYSIOLOGY, SIGNS, AND SYMPTOMS

The progressive course of hypertensive disease is insidious, and individuals often remain asymptomatic for years. Hypertension is usually not detected until significant organ damage occurs. It is difficult to predict who will develop high blood pressure because the causes of hypertension cannot be determined in approximately 90% of all cases (Guyton, 1982). When this is the situation, it is known as primary or essential hypertension. The remaining 10% of hypertension appears to be secondary to some other underlying disease process. Among some of the known causes of secondary hypertension are kidney disorders, adrenal gland tumors (pheochromocytoma), coarctation of the aorta, Cushing's syndrome, renovascular hypertension, and primary aldosteronism.

The aging process itself tends to contribute to the development of hypertension. As a person ages, the linings of arterial vessels lose their elastic properties. This increased rigidity of the peripheral vessels, and the aorta, is caused by the loss of the elastic fibers in the tunica media. There is an increase in the amount of calcium and collagen deposits in the tunica media and formation of atheroma in the tunica intima (Porth, 1986). This increases the pressure of the blood against the walls of the vessels. Other vascular changes include increased peripheral resistance, decreased baroreceptor sensitivity, and a reduction in renal blood flow.

The signs and symptoms of hypertension depend largely on the category of the disease itself, either primary or secondary. Primary hypertension is often asymptomatic and is discovered by chance on routine exam or during screening sessions. Suboccipital headache, which frequently occurs in the morning, is a common symptom of hypertension but is not reliable alone. Fatigue, nervousness, and irritability are also associated signs and symptoms. If the heart is involved, there may be dyspnea, edema, palpitations, or angina. As the kidneys become involved, the person with hypertension may experience nocturia or other signs of renal damage such as elevated blood urea nitrogen (BUN) and creatinine. There may also be other symptoms such as blackouts and transient ischemic attacks that indicate central nervous system involvement. Physical examination may reveal changes in the retinas such as hemorrhages, exudate, and narrowing arterioles. In severe cases, papilledema may be found. Diagnostic examination often reveals cardiac enlargement, arrhythmias, and congestive heart failure.

▶ DIAGNOSTIC PROCEDURES

There are a few diagnostic tests that are useful in confirming hypertension. Laboratory tests include urinalysis to detect proteinuria and/or hematuria. Blood chemistry may reveal BUN levels of >20 mg/dl, creatinine levels of >1.5 mg/dl, and potassium levels of >5.0 mEq/L in renal failure and <3.5 mEq/L in primary aldosteronism. Left ventricular hypertrophy (LVH) and myocardial ischemia may be present on the electrocardiogram (ECG). Chest x-ray often shows cardiomegaly and aortic atherosclerosis. Renin levels are measured to identify patients with renovascular occlusive disease. An intravenous pyelogram (IVP) will suggest the presence of stenosed renal arteries.

▶ MEDICAL MANAGEMENT

Management is directed toward lowering blood pressure to normal for the patient's age and maintaining that therapeutic range. The goal is to alleviate symptoms and slow or halt the progression of vascular damage that results from hypertension. Dietary management, modified lifestyle, and pharmacologic treatment have produced a greatly improved outlook for those suffering from hypertensive disease.

Dietary management includes the restriction of sodium intake, usually limited to 2 to 6 g/day. Restriction may vary from moderate to strict reduction of sodium intake, depending on the severity of the hypertension. Reduction of alcohol and caffeine intake is strongly encouraged. Reduced intake of cholesterol and saturated fats is also recommended. Dietary counseling and sample dietary modification charts are most helpful, and people with hypertension should be afforded the opportunity to receive dietary instructions from a reliable source.

Modifications in lifestyle include weight control, regular exercise, stress reduction and management, and identification and modification of risk factors. In obese patients the recommended weight loss is approximately 5%, and in some cases more. A regular exercise program is desirable and should be prescribed or approved by a physician. Some common programs include cardiac rehabilitation exercises, aerobic exercise programs geared for specific age groups. Isometric exercises should be avoided because sustained muscle contraction has been shown to precipitate angina, cerebral hemorrhage, and congestive heart failure. Stress reduction and management are desirable because prolonged stress has been shown to potentiate hypertensive episodes. Identification of risk factors and behavior modification also contribute to successful management of hypertension. Reduction in the number of cigarettes smoked daily or complete cessation of smoking is beneficial to the patient, along with regular monitoring of the blood pressure.

Often behavior and dietary modification are enough to reduce blood pressure to acceptable ranges. However, when such measures do not sufficiently control hypertension, pharmacologic treatment may be instituted by the physician. Because older adults are especially sensi-

tive to the effects of drugs, hypertensive medications are initiated at a lower than therapeutic dose and gradually increased (Esberger and Hughes, 1989). Serum levels of the medications are monitored to detect toxicity, and the doses are adjusted until the desired therapeutic effect is attained.

In the past, the step method was used to treat hypertension (diuretics, thiazides, sympatholytics, and alpha-adrenergic agents). Diuretics promote excretion of sodium and water, resulting in decreased plasma volume and lower circulating volume and sodium levels. If diuretic therapy, which includes thiazides, loop diuretics, and potassium-sparing agents, does not achieve the desired results, sympatholytics are added to the therapy. Sympatholytics achieve their effect by reducing the sympathetic reflexes that cause increased heart rate and blood pressure. When a third type of medication is necessary, antihypertensive alpha-adrenergic agents are instituted to relax smooth muscle in arterial walls (Table 6-5). Other classes of medications used are calcium channel blockers.

The current approach is to individualize medical treatment according to age, race, and complicating factors (e.g., diabetes or congestive heart failure).

▶ **PROGNOSIS**

The prognosis for persons diagnosed with hypertension is good for those who are faithful to their medical and nursing plans of care. Having regular checkups by their physician, taking their medication as prescribed, and knowing the adverse side effects and what to report all contribute to a normal or near normal lifestyle.

Table 6-5. Common antihypertensive medications

Brand name	Generic name	Usual dose
Diuretics		
Thiazides		
Diuril	Chlorothiazide	0.5-1.0 g/day
Esidrix, Hydrodiuril	Hydrochlorothiazide	50-100 mg/day
Naturetin	Bendroflumethiazide	2.5-10.0 mg/day
Loop diuretics		
Edecrin	Ethacrynic acid	25-50 mg initially
Lasix	Furosemide	40-80 mg bid or tid
Potassium-sparing diuretics		
Aldactone	Spironolactone	100-400 mg bid or tid
Dyrenium	Triamterene	100-300 mg bid
Midamor	Amiloride	5-20 mg/day or bid
Beta-adrenergic blocking agents		
Blocadren	Timolol maleate	20-40 mg/day
Corgard	Nadolol	80-320 mg/day
Inderal	Propranolol	80-100 mg po bid, tid
Lopressor	Metoprolol tartrate	50-200 mg po qd or bid
Tenormin	Atenolol	50-100 mg/day
Visken	Pindolol	15-60 mg/day
Other agents		
Aldomet	Methyldopa	Up to 2 g/day po
Apresoline	Hydralazine	10-50 mg po qid
Capoten	Captopril	24-150 mg tid
Catapres	Clonidine	0.1-1.2 mg po bid
Hyperstat	Diazoxide	300-mg rapid IV push
Ismelin	Guanethidine	5-200 mg/day po
Nipride	Sodium nitroprusside	0.5-10 μg/kg/min IV
Alpha-adrenergic agents		
Minipress	Prazosin	Begin with 1 mg po and gradually increase to 10-15 mg/day
Regitine	Phentolamine	1-5 mg IV intermittently

Data compiled from Thompson, McFarland, Hirsch, et al (1989).

▶ **NURSING MANAGEMENT—NURSING CARE PLAN**
Hypertension

Once the diagnosis of hypertension has been made and treatment modalities have been decided upon, there is the issue of long-term maintenance of the treatment plan.

Nursing management begins with identification of actual or potential problems.

Assessment

SUBJECTIVE DATA
Complaints of fatigue and frequent headaches
In some cases complaints of blurred vision at times

OBJECTIVE DATA
Systolic and diastolic blood pressure are elevated.
Pulse may be bounding.

<table>
<tr><th rowspan="8">N U R S I N G C A R E P L A N</th><th>Nursing diagnoses</th><th>Expected outcomes</th><th>Nursing interventions (rationale)</th></tr>
<tr>
<td>Noncompliance related to denial of disease</td>
<td>Patient will understand the disease and treatment and comply with prescribed therapy.</td>
<td>Discuss the disease process with the patient and family in terms they can understand.
Utilize available teaching aids such as pictures, videotapes, and pamphlets.
Encourage questions and dialogue that might help to identify any misconceptions patient or family may have.
Help the patient and family identify ways changes can be made to reduce the known risk factors.</td>
</tr>
<tr>
<td>Powerlessness related to forced dependence on health care regimen</td>
<td>Patient will demonstrate participation in self-care activities within the limitations of prescribed therapy and activities.</td>
<td>Encourage and allow participation in determining a therapeutic plan (will enable patient to gain a sense of control over what is happening).
Identify fears and clarify misconceptions about the health care plan.</td>
</tr>
<tr>
<td>Alteration in systemic tissue perfusion related to increased peripheral vascular resistance</td>
<td>Patient will maintain adequate tissue perfusion that is evidenced by a blood pressure that declines toward and eventually is maintained at a range normal for age.</td>
<td>Observe the skin for discoloration and determine the baseline quality of peripheral pulses.
Monitor for any decrease in the pulses or change in color of the skin.
Avoid dependent positions of the extremities and avoid anything that might cause friction or bruising to the area.</td>
</tr>
</table>

Discharge planning and patient/family education

Teach the patient and family members to check blood pressure periodically at home and interpret the results.

Explain to family members the importance of allowing the patient to maintain as much independence as possible in performing his or her own care.

Offer positive feedback for all efforts on both the patient's and the family's accomplishments in self-care.

Assist the patient to identify and utilize available support systems and community resources that will assist in coping with the effects of hypertension (e.g., support groups, stress management classes).

Teach the rationale for, the side effects of, and the importance of taking the prescribed medications. Written information regarding the medications will serve as a reference after discharge.

Encourage regular visits to the physician and instruct the patient to bring all medication being taken each time he or she visits the physician. For most of the older population economics play a major factor in the area of compliance. Often inability to financially support their medication needs or find transportation to keep follow-up appointments is viewed as noncompliance. It is important to identify these needs early and make reasonable arrangements to issue effective treatment while at the same time containing costs.

Teach the patient to recognize and report signs and symptoms of diminished systemic tissue perfusion. For example, teach the patient to check for capillary refill and to report a capillary refill time greater than 3 seconds to the physician. Other reportable signs and symptoms include increased or labored respirations, an increase in blood pressure readings obtained when checking at home, decreased urine output, weak or absent pulses, discoloration of the skin, and restlessness or confusion.

Discourage smoking and encourage the person to adhere to prescribed dietary program.

Give patient education handout (see Box 6-6).

Evaluation

Patient accurately monitors the blood pressure to recognize abnormalities early.

Patient feels better with hypertension under control and complications minimized.

Optimum integrity of the peripheral circulation and skin condition is being maintained.

Box 6-6.

Patient Education

Hypertension

. Take all of the prescribed medication as the physician has ordered. DO NOT skip your medication.

Have your blood pressure checked regularly. Report your blood pressure readings to your physician if your systolic (upper number) pressure is greater than _____ or lower than _____, or if your diastolic (lower number) pressure is greater than _____ or lower than _____. For accurate results always rest for about 15 minutes before taking your blood pressure reading.

Maintain your prescribed diet. It is especially important to cut down on sodium (salt) intake.

Exercise is important, and you should follow an exercise program that is approved by the physician.

Rest is also very important. Avoid stress and fatigue, and get plenty of rest and relaxation.

Report any severe headache, dizziness, or ringing in the ears. These may be signs of an increasing blood pressure.

REFERENCES

American Heart Association (1988). An older person's guide to cardiovascular health, Dallas, The Association.

Brenner ZR (1987). Nursing elderly cardiac clients, Crit Care Nurse 7(2):78-87.

Coodley E (1990). Silent myocardial ischemia in the elderly, Geriatr Med Today 9:47-50.

DeAngelis R (1985). The cardiovascular system. In Alspach JG and Williams SM, editors: Core curriculum for critical care nursing, ed 3, Philadelphia, WB Saunders Co.

Doyle J (1986). Treatment modalities in peripheral vascular disease, Nurs Clin North Am 21(2):241-253.

Eichner RE (1989). The aging heart, functional and clinical implications, Geriatr Consultant 6:15-19.

Esberger K and Hughes S (1989). Nursing care of the aged. Norwalk, Conn, Appleton & Lange.

Gary L (1988). The twelve lead electrocardiogram, Dallas, Methodist Medical Center.

Guyton AC (1982). Human physiology and mechanism of disease, ed 3, Philadelphia, WB Saunders Co.

Guzetta C and Dossey B (1984). Cardiovascular nursing: body–mind tapestry, St Louis, The CV Mosby Co.

Impallomeni M (1988). Heart disease in later life, Health Visitor 61:309-310.

Jessup M, Lakatta E, Leier C, and Santinga J (1990). CHF in the elderly: Is it different, Patient Care 3:39-75.

Killen D (1988). Cardiac surgery in the elderly. In Adkins RB and Scott HW, editors: Surgical care for the elderly, Baltimore, Williams & Wilkins.

Martin F (1989). Cardiovascular changes. In Esberger K and Hughes S, editors: Nursing care for the aged, Norwalk, Conn, Appleton & Lange.

Porth C (1986). Pathophysiology: Concepts of altered health status, Philadelphia, JB Lippincott Co.

Rideout E and Monemuro M (1986). Hope, morale and adaptation in patients with chronic heart failure, J Adv Nurs 11:429-438.

Schlant RC, Collins J, Engle M, et al (1988). The yearbook of cardiology, Chicago, Mosby–Year Book, Inc.

Springhouse Corporation (1990). Cardiac emergencies, Springhouse, Pa, Springhouse.

Stanley M (1986). Helping an elderly patient live with CHF, RN 9:35-37.

Steingart R and Scheuer J (1986). Assessment of myocardial ischemia. In Hurst JW, editor: The heart, ed 6, New York, McGraw-Hill.

Thompson J, McFarland G, Hirsch J, et al (1989). Manual of clinical nursing, ed 2, St Louis, The CV Mosby–Year Book Inc.

Ulrich S, Canale S, and Wendell S (1986). Nursing care planning guides, Philadelphia, WB Saunders Co.

Underhill S, Woods S, Sivarajan E, and Halpenny C (1982). Cardiac nursing, Philadelphia, JB Lippincott Co.

Valle B and Lemberg L (1989). The senescent heart. Heart Lung 18(2):206-211.

Weisfeldt M (1986). Cardiovascular aging and adaptation to disease. In Hurst JW et al., editors: The heart, ed 6, New York, McGraw-Hill.

Wenger NK (1990). Rehabilitation of the elderly coronary patient, Geriatr Med Today 9(5):47-50.

Wilson D (1989). Acute pulmonary edema: How to respond to a crisis, Nursing 10:34-41.

CHAPTER 7

Respiratory System

Carol A. Stephenson

CHRONIC OBSTRUCTIVE PULMONARY DISEASE

Chronic obstructive pulmonary disease (COPD) is a set of chronic conditions of persistent expiratory airway obstruction. The two major diseases in this group are emphysema and chronic bronchitis. These diseases are predominantly caused by smoking, although hereditary factors and air pollution are implicated to a lesser extent. Many persons have a mix of chronic bronchitis and emphysema, but one disease usually predominates over the other. In addition, as people age some elasticity of the lungs and chest wall are lost. As a result, the work of breathing increases to some extent. However, this is not normally enough to interfere with respirations or activity (Steffl, 1984). COPD is not necessarily a disease of aging. Although many older adults develop it, it may also be severe in persons who are in their 50s. Once COPD is well developed, the prognosis for both older and younger patients is poor.

▶ PATHOPHYSIOLOGY, SIGNS, AND SYMPTOMS

Chronic bronchitis is an inflammatory disease of the airways. As the respiratory mucosa is irritated during years of smoking, the mucosa becomes edematous and large amounts of sputum are produced. The cilia are paralyzed or destroyed, which reduces the ability to clear the airway of sputum. Because the airways naturally enlarge on inspiration, some air can be taken into the lungs with each breath. However, when the airways close naturally and normally on expiration, the edematous mucosa and high sputum volume may occlude or nearly occlude the airway. As a result, expiration is difficult and incomplete. Classic signs of chronic bronchitis include coughing and producing sputum 3 months of the year for 2 consecutive years, frequent respiratory infections, gradually declining exercise tolerance, and gradually increasing dyspnea on exertion.

Emphysema is a disease of the alveoli rather than the airways. In this disease the alveoli are greatly enlarged and their architecture is destroyed. This damage has two major consequences: (1) exchange of respiratory gases is decreased, and (2) the elastic support of the airways is reduced so that the natural closure of the airways on expiration is greater, leading to total or near total closure of the airways on expiration. This results in the same symptoms as chronic bronchitis, except that the patient with emphysema does not produce sputum on a regular basis. There is a frequent, severe, nonproductive cough instead.

▶ DIAGNOSTIC PROCEDURES

Arterial blood gases (ABGs)—Patients with COPD usually show chronic hypoxia and often have hypercapnia (increased pCO_2). It is not unusual for the pCO_2 to be in the 50s (norm 35 to 45 mm Hg). Patients are often allowed to live with pO_2s in the 60s and 70s, partly because this is a basic adequate oxygenation level and partly because the normal pO_2 declines as a person ages.

Hemoglobin and hematocrit (H & H)—If a patient is chronically hypoxic, the body tends to produce extra red blood cells (RBCs) in order to carry more oxygen to the body cells. This is called polycythemia. When polycythemia is present, the hematocrit is elevated. The extra RBCs tend to make the blood more viscous, which can reduce circulation (especially to the extremities), increase cardiac workload, and predispose to thrombus formation.

Sputum examination—The most common cause of acute illness in the COPD patient is infection. When this occurs, the sputum will show evidence of the offending organism as well as a color change to yellow, green, or gray.

Chest x-ray (CXR)—Since patients with COPD cannot exhale properly, they trap air in their chests. A CXR will show a depressed or flattened diaphragm as the result of the air trapping. There will also be evidence of hyperinflated lungs. If an infection is present at the time of the CXR, this will also show on the film.

Pulmonary function tests (PFTs)—PFTs are not usually done when patients with COPD are acutely ill. However, they are valuable aids to diagnosis and monitoring of patient progress. These tests should be done at a time when the patient is rested and has an empty stomach. The tests will show a reduced FEV_1 (1-second forced expiratory volume) and peak flow, meaning that the patient cannot exhale air as rapidly or as completely as normal. There will also be an increased FRC (functional residual capacity), RV (residual volume), and TLC (total lung capacity), which indicate trapped air in the lungs.

▶ MEDICAL MANAGEMENT

Improve ventilation:

Administer xanthines and other bronchodilators (intravenous, oral, or topical; topical bronchodilators may be delivered by cartridge inhaler, unassisted nebulization, or IPPB [intermittent positive pressure breathing]), steroids (intravenous, oral, or inhaled), possibly anticholinergics (atropine inhaled).

Have patient avoid respiratory depressants.

Give oxygen therapy as indicated by ABGs (low flow— <5 L/min per nasal cannula).

Improve airway clearance:

Have patient maintain a high fluid intake. (If the patient has cardiac disease, fluids are needed to thin secretions, but diuretics may be necessary to avoid overload. Secretions cannot be thinned when patients are on fluid restriction.)

Use postural drainage and percussion during acute phases for all patients with COPD and daily all the time for patients with chronic bronchitis.

Have patient stop smoking (personal resolve to stop is needed; may be assisted by programs such as those provided by the American Cancer Society or the American Lung Association).

Aerosol therapy (inhalation of nebulized mist to increase airway moisture) may be used.

Prevent or treat infection:

Have patient avoid exposure to infection.

Teach patient early recognition and treatment of infection. (Box 7-1 lists situations that should prompt the patient to call the doctor.)

Treat infection early with appropriate antibiotics.

Improve strength and exercise tolerance:

Gradually increase patient's activity. Do not overdo on days when patient feels better than usual; patient will then need several days to rest up.

Teach patient how to use energy conservation techniques to accomplish more with the same or less energy expenditure.

Box 7-1.

When to call the doctor

You should always call your doctor or health care provider when:

- There is any change in your symptoms—
  - Shortness of breath, wheezing, or coughing increase.
  - Chest discomfort occurs or increases.
  - You have more difficulty than usual when sleeping because of respiratory symptoms.
  - The color, amount, or character of your sputum changes, or it is more difficult to cough up.
- You develop new symptoms—
  - Chills and/or fever
  - Sudden weight gain
  - Swelling of your feet
  - Reduced ability to exercise
- There is a question or problem regarding your medications—
  - You think you are having adverse effects from your medications.
  - You have questions about your medications.
  - You need a prescription refilled.
  - You are planning to take over-the-counter medications or drugs prescribed by another doctor.

Adapted from Stephenson C (1989). Respiratory changes. In Esberger KK and Hughes ST, editors: Nursing care of the aged, Norwalk, Conn, Appleton & Lange.

Ensure adequate nutrition, and encourage weight loss as needed.

Teach patient to rest properly when tired or short of breath. (If the patient is walking where there is no place to sit to rest, resting can be accomplished by forward lean standing [stand leaning forward from the hips with the forearms resting on an object of suitable height, e.g., stair rails, window ledge, or mailbox] or relaxed standing [lean back against the wall with the feet approximately 12 inches from the wall with the shoulders relaxed and the arms hanging loosely at the sides].)

Teach patient to use bronchodilator inhaler before activities that usually cause wheezing or shortness of breath.

Teach patient to use pursed-lip breathing with problematic activities (see Box 7-2).

Reduce depression and anxiety:

Gradually increase activity as above—encourage patient to see others and be active with them rather than remaining alone.

Provide counseling.

Avoid sedatives and tranquilizers.

Drug therapy

Table 7-1 summarizes the actions and effects of drugs used to treat respiratory disease.

▶ **PROGNOSIS**

Although COPD will not be obliterated by stopping smoking, the course of the disease will be slowed and the quality of life can be improved when the patient stops smoking and is adequately treated. Life span depends on the severity of the disease. Unfortunately, many older persons with severe COPD do not live into their 80s and 90s.

Box 7-2.

Teaching pursed-lip breathing

Pursed-lip breathing should be taught when the patient is relaxed and not in respiratory distress, in pain, or distracted.

Have the patient sit upright if possible.

Tell the patient to inhale slowly through the nose and exhale slowly through pursed lips. The nurse should count to two out loud as the patient inhales and then count to four as the patient exhales.

After doing the exercise with the nurse counting, tell the patient to count mentally as inhalation and exhalation are being done.

When the patient can comfortably maintain the rhythm of mentally counting and breathing, the exercise should be done with activity. For example, the patient could walk a few steps during the counted inspiration and stop to rest during expiration.

Gradually, the patient should be able to do all types of activities on inspiration, such as stair climbing, bed making, tying shoes, shaving, and exercising. During expiration, the patient should always stop to rest.

Instruct the patient to use pursed-lip breathing during any activities that normally cause dyspnea, or shortness of breath, and to gain control during episodes of respiratory distress. The patient should practice several times each day so that the technique can be easily used when necessary.

Table 7-1. Summary of major drug therapy for respiratory disease

Classification: BRONCHODILATORS
Major actions: Open the airway; bronchodilation; improve ciliary action.
METHYLXANTHINES (THEOPHYLLINES)
General information
Contraindication: Peptic ulcer.
At special risk for toxicity: Infants, debilitated, concurrent liver or heart disease.
Half-life is increased in CHF and decreased in smokers.
Intolerance to one xanthine does not necessarily mean intolerance to another.
Dose must be individualized and checked with blood levels. Draw blood for testing levels 1 hr before next scheduled dose. Therapeutic level: 11-20 mg/dl.
Low incidence of adverse effects
Common side effects: Polydipsia, dizziness, tachycardia, mild diuresis. These effects may be worsened by excess caffeine. Gastric discomfort common if po preparations are taken on empty stomach. Exception to giving with food: sprinkles.
Toxic effects: Nausea/vomiting, seizures, hematemesis, hypotension, coma, arrhythmias, flushing, headache, delirium.

Drug categories/types/names	Precautions/nursing implications

IV drugs
Aminophylline
  250-300 mg tid
PO liquids
Elixophylline, Somophylline
  100-200 mg 2-4 times/day
Dyphylline (Lufyllin)
PO tablets
Aminophylline tabs
  100-200 mg 4-6 times/day
	The IV and liquid preparation are the only xanthine preparations suitable for prn use.
	Must dilute IV drug well and deliver slowly.
	Minimum: dilute in 30 ml and run over 30 min. Is usually diluted more and run longer.
	pH of IV preparation makes it incompatible with many other IV drugs.
	
	Oral preparations must be taken regularly to maintain blood level. They are not prn drugs.

Adapted from Stephenson C (1989). Respiratory changes. In Esberger KK and Hughes ST, editors: Nursing care of the aged, Norwalk, Conn, Appleton & Lange, pp 234-235.

Continued.

Drug categories/types/names	Precautions/nursing implications

Theodur (Aminodur)
  100-200 mg 2-4 times/day
Oxtriphylline (Choledyl)
  200 mg q 8 hr
Bronkodyl
  100 mg 2-4 times/day
Sprinkles
(Theo-Dur Sprinkles)
  50-200 mg q 12 hr
	Do not chew or crush. Empty capsule contents onto one spoonful of apple-sauce, pudding, or similar food; swallow without chewing; follow with water or juice.
	Take 1 hr before or 2 hr after a meal.

Suppositories Aminophylline	Absorption erratic and unpredictable.

BETA-2 AGONISTS
General information
These are often used along with a xanthine preparation.
Cautions: Coronary insufficiency, hyperthyroidism, diabetes, hypertension.
General side effects: Nervousness, tremors, drowsiness, weakness, headache, nausea/vomiting, hypotension, tachycardia.
The oral preparations must be used regularly to maintain blood level.

Drug categories/types/names	Precautions/nursing implications
Subcutaneous Terbutaline (Brethine, Bricanyl) 0.25 mg q 8 hr	If tremors are extremely problematic, may reduce dose. Tremors often decrease with time.
Oral Terbutaline tabs (Brethine, Bricanyl) 2.3-5 mg 2-4 times/day	Tremors as described above decrease with time.
Metaproterenol (Alupent, Metaprel) 10-20 mg 3-4 times/day	Contraindications: pregnancy, under 12 years old, allergy.
Albuterol sulfate (Proventil Repetabs) 4-8 mg q 12 hr (Ventolin tabs) 2-4 mg 4 times/day	
Inhaled beta-2 agonists	**General information** May use on regular basis, prn for wheezing or dyspnea, or before activities that cause wheezing. Patient should be sitting or standing upright for use. Should not be overused.
Isoetharine (Bronkosol)	Dilute with 3 parts saline or water to use in nebulizer. Use every 4 hr. Should not be used with epinephrine but can be used alternately.
Metaproterenol (Alupent) inhaler	Lasts about 4 hr. Excess use can lead to paradoxical bronchoconstriction.
Albuterol (Proventil, Ventolin)	Lasts about 6 hr. Effects similar to terbutaline. Produces less tremor and nervousness than terbutaline. May cause unusual taste or irritation of mouth.
Isoetharine mesylate (Maxair)	Lasts about 5 hr.
Isoproterenol (Isuprel Mistometer Medihaler-Iso)	Lasts about 4 hr.
Isoetharine (Arm-A-Med Isoetharine Bronkometer)	Lasts 4-6 hr.
Terbutaline (Brethaire, Brethine)	Lasts 4-6 hr.
Sympathetic amines (adrenergic) Ephedrine (Bronchaid Tabs)	Alone, may be purchased over-the-counter (OTC) and is common component of combination drugs. Improves effect of xanthines.

Table 7-1. Summary of major drug therapy for respiratory disease—cont'd

Drug categories/types/names	Precautions/nursing implications
	Duration is short. Overdose results in rebound bronchospasm. Adverse effects: bronchial irritation and edema, dried secretions, mucus plugs, gastrointestinal stimulation and irritation, nausea, tachycardia, palpitations, hypertension, tremor, headache, flushing, anxiety, dizziness. High incidence of prostatic hypertrophy and urinary retention in older males.

Epinephrine (Adrenalin)
Nebulized forms:
  Micronephrine
  Vaponephrine
  Primatine (OTC)
  Bronkaid Mist (OTC)
	Duration extremely short. Repeat in about 20 min.
	High incidence of cardiovascular effects.
	Inhalers should not be used to treat acute episodes.

Classification: STEROIDS

Major actions: Antiinflammatory. Decrease airway obstruction and improve responsiveness to bronchodilators.

General information

Caution: Peptic ulcer, diabetes, cardiovascular disease, hypertension, TB, chronic infection, psychological disorders.

Short-term adverse effects: Stress ulcer, increased appetite.

Long-term adverse effects: Adrenal suppression, abnormal fat deposits, osteoporosis, growth suppression, myopathy, hypertension, peptic ulcer, cataracts, electrolyte imbalances, easy bruising, lower resistance to infection, increased appetite, altered mentation (euphoria, psychosis).

Skin test for TB before starting long course of steroids. Former TB patients on long-term steroids should also get INH.

Do not use alone—only with bronchodilators

If long term, give every other day or daily as a single dose early in the morning. Long-term patients are steroid dependent and must wear identifying bracelet. Dose must be increased in times of stress.

Do not discontinue suddenly. Must taper. Must overlap drugs if changing from po to inhaled drugs.

Signs of steroid withdrawal: Malaise, headache, nausea/vomiting, anorexia, backache, joint pain, emotional instability, increased allergic symptoms, bronchospasm.

Drug categories/types/names	Precautions/nursing implications
Intravenous Solu-Medrol 60-80 mg	Use q 6-8 hr for 48-72 hr in acute illness.
Oral Prednisone Prednisolone 5-60 mg daily or in divided doses	May use daily or in divided doses in acute illness. Try to use small doses daily or every other day if needed for long-term management.
Inhaled Beclomethasone dipropionate (Vanceril, Beconase, Beclovent)	Use 2-4 times/day for maintenance—not prn. Not effective in acute illness. Adverse effects of steroids do not apply since it is not systemically absorbed. Use about 3 min after bronchodilator inhaler—patient still in upright position. Always rinse mouth well after use to prevent opportunistic infection. Adverse effects possible: sore throat, thrush *(Candida)* of mouth. Increased nasal congestion or nasal polyps may occur after discontinuing drug.

Classification: ANTICHOLINERGICS

Major action: Reduce bronchospasm in some patients.

General information

For chronic use only—not initial drug or for acute illness.

All cautions and contraindications as for this category apply: Do not use in glaucoma, benign prostatic hypertrophy, bladder neck obstruction. Must be used regularly—not prn. General adverse effects: May dry secretions; nervousness, dizziness, headache, cough, dry mouth.

Drug categories/types/names	Precautions/nursing implications
Inhaled drugs Atropine Ipratropium bromide (Atrovent)	Usually use these drugs 4 times daily.

▶ **NURSING MANAGEMENT—NURSING CARE PLAN**
   COPD

Assessment

SUBJECTIVE DATA

Symptoms are insidious and include dyspnea on exertion or at rest, a reduced ability to participate in activities of daily living, poor appetite, poor judgment, confusion, irritability or restlessness, poor sleeping and orthopnea, and excess fatigue.

OBJECTIVE DATA

Reduced or distant breath sounds, increased resonance, crackles, and possibly rhonchi

Sputum production in chronic bronchitis and in times of infection

Wheezing in some patients with chronic bronchitis

	Nursing diagnoses	Expected outcomes	Nursing interventions (rationale)
N U R S I N G C A R E P L A N	Ineffective breathing pattern related to expiratory airway obstruction	Patient will have minimal or reduced dyspnea/orthopnea.	Administer oxygen as ordered (low flow). (Reduces difficulty of oxygenating body.) Elevate head of bed, and support arms as necessary. (The airways are more open and there is less pressure on the diaphragm when a person sits up; therefore breathing is easier. If respiratory distress is extremely serious, the person may need to use the tripod position; that is, lean on the elbows so as to elevate the shoulder girdle to reduce intrathoracic pressure and thus facilitate respiration.)
		Patient will use breathing techniques appropriately.	Teach breathing exercises, pursed-lip breathing and when to use (see Box 7-2). (Breathing exercises strengthen appropriately the muscles of breathing and improve breathing control. Pursed-lip breathing slows the respiratory rate in times of distress, which reduces work of breathing and improves respiratory control.)
	Impaired gas exchange related to expiratory airway obstruction	ABGs will be acceptable for patient.	Teach breathing exercises, pursed-lip breathing and when to use (see Box 7-2). (See previous entry for rationale.) Administer oxygen as ordered. (See previous entry.) Elevate head of bed; support arms as necessary. (See previous entry.)
	Ineffective airway clearance related to increased secretions	Sputum will be thin and easily coughed up.	Fluid intake should be at least 64 ounces daily, excluding milk—more if sputum thickens. (Milk thickens sputum. The best expectorant is water. Without water, it is impossible to thin the sputum enough for it to be easily expectorated. If the patient has a cardiac condition and fluid overload might be a problem, it is more effective to give the fluid and manage the fluid balance with diuretics than to restrict fluids.)

Nursing Care Plan—COPD—cont'd		
Nursing diagnoses	**Expected outcomes**	**Nursing interventions (rationale)**
	Patient will have no adventitious breath sounds.	Assess quantity and character of sputum. (The character of the sputum is a good guide to adequacy of fluid intake. If sputum thickens, as might occur early in an infection, increasing fluid intake will help to keep it thin and more easily expectorated.)
		Encourage patient to use cascade coughing (see Box 7-3). (Often, a single cough will not raise sputum high enough to be expectorated. A series of coughs as described in Box 7-3 can be more effective in airway clearance.)
		Use postural drainage and percussion during times of infection or daily for chronic bronchitis patients. (Postural drainage and percussion use gravity and percussion to aid in clearing the airways.)
		Assess respiratory status at least every 4 hours during acute phases of illness.
		Have patient turn, cough, and deep breathe at least every 2 hours.
		Teach relaxation exercises.
Reduced activity tolerance related to expiratory airway obstruction	Dyspnea will be minimal or reduced.	Use all actions that apply from previous entries.
	Activity tolerance will improve. Ability to perform activities of daily living and self-care will improve. (Be specific in expectations.)	Assess current activity tolerance, and set specific, reasonable goals for increase. (Many COPD patients are extremely debilitated and able to do little or no activity. Activity should be increased very gradually but consistently and on a daily basis. Improving activity will reduce the amount of oxygen required by body cells per unit of work, as well as improving quality of life and general outlook on life [Lewis and Collier, 1987].)
		Teach patient to recognize exercise termination points (see Box 7-4) and points when rest is necessary during exercise.
		Administer oxygen with activity if ordered (reduces respiratory work necessary to oxygenate the body).
		Teach to use pursed-lip breathing with activity (slows respiratory rate, improves control, and reduces dyspnea).
		Teach to use energy conservation techniques (allow increased activity, self-care, and quality of life with less dyspnea).

Continued.

Nursing Care Plan—COPD—cont'd

Nursing diagnoses	Expected outcomes	Nursing interventions (rationale)
Altered nutrition: less than body requirements, related to dyspnea, diaphragmatic pressure	Caloric intake will be appropriate (specify) for patient. Intake will include appropriate nutrient variety.	Have patient eat six small meals daily of light, highly nutritious foods. (Digestion takes a great deal of oxygen, which increases respiratory workload; large meals fill the stomach and abdomen and further compromise breathing.) Do not include gas-forming, fatty, or fried foods in diet. (These further fill the stomach and abdomen and press on the diaphragm.) Encourage good oral hygiene before meals. (Coughing and sputum production leave a foul taste in the mouth and depress the appetite; oral hygiene will enable the patient to enjoy meals more.) Plan inhaled bronchodilator and postural drainage treatments so that secretions do not interfere with eating. (Large amounts of secretions may be produced as the result of postural drainage and bronchodilator treatments; eating immediately after treatments would be hindered by the patient continuing to cough up sputum for some time after the treatments.) Obtain Meals-on-Wheels or other assistance as necessary. (Many debilitated patients are unable to shop for food and prepare nutritious meals for themselves. Outside assistance with nutrition is necessary. A varied, nutritious diet will improve respiratory muscle strength and general immunity and will boost energy.)

Discharge planning and patient/family education

Discharge planning for the patient with COPD should focus on breathing techniques, energy conservation, the knowledgeable use of drug therapy, nutrition, exercise, avoiding infections, and knowing when to call the doctor. The patient should be taught to take the pulse if this is necessary, and frequent rest should be emphasized.

The nurse should assess patient and family knowledge, beliefs, and practices regarding normal lung structure and function and the disease process. Information regarding problem areas should be incorporated into teach-

ing. Pathology should be related to the individual's symptoms. Explanations regarding drugs should include why the drug is taken, when it should be taken, adverse effects, and special information related to administration. Drug actions should be related to symptoms and pathology. Information in Boxes 7-1 through 7-5 should be provided to patients in a large-print, readable form.

Evaluation

Dyspnea/orthopnea is minimal or reduced.
Patient uses breathing techniques appropriately.

ABGs are acceptable for patient.
Sputum is thin and easily coughed up.
There are no adventitious breath sounds.
Activity tolerance is improving.
Patient increases performance of activities of daily living and self-care.
Caloric intake is appropriate (specify) for patient. Intake includes appropriate nutrient variety.
Patient uses medications and oxygen correctly and reports untoward effects.

Box 7-3.

How to teach cascade coughing

Rationale: A COPD patient should not force a cough because the disease and the cough together tend to cause premature airway closure and spasm. As a result, sputum cannot be coughed out and the patient will become more dyspneic and short of breath. A controlled or cascade cough enables the sputum to be slowly worked up and out of the airway without precipitating airway closure.

The patient should be sitting upright, be comfortable, and not be in distress when cascade coughing is taught. The patient should follow these directions when learning this type of coughing:

1. Using diaphragmatic breathing, take a slow, deep breath and hold it for a few seconds.
2. During the exhalation of this breath, cough several times with the mouth slightly open. Lean forward slightly when exhaling and coughing.
3. After the exhalation and coughs are finished, inhale the next breath by sniffing so as to avoid pushing secretions farther down in the airway.
4. Exhale slowly and cough as before.
5. Repeat the sequence as long as necessary until the airways are cleared.

Adapted from Stephenson C (1989). Respiratory changes. In Esberger KK and Hughes ST, editors: Nursing care of the aged, Norwalk, Conn, Appleton & Lange.

Box 7-4.

Guide to terminating exercise

Rationale: Many COPD patients terminate exercise soon after beginning because of shortness of breath or panic. They need to accept some shortness of breath as normal and have specific objective guides for decision making about exercise termination. They should be able to accurately count their pulse during exercise and use proper breathing and rest techniques during the exercise. If oxygen is ordered to be used for exercise, it should be used according to directions.

The COPD patient should stop exercising if any of the following occur:

Severe shortness of breath (more than is usual for this person while exercising)
Chest pain that is suggestive of angina or severe leg pain
Extreme fatigue
Dizziness or faintness
Lack of coordination, mental confusion, severe apprehension
Sudden onset of perspiration or cyanosis
Increase or decrease in heart rate of more than 15 beats/minute
Pulse rate over target pulse rate (the patient should know the exact target pulse rate)

Adapted from Stephenson C (1989). Respiratory changes. In Esberger KK and Hughes ST, editors: Nursing care of the aged, Norwalk, Conn, Appleton & Lange.

Box 7-5.

Patient Education

COPD

There are a number of things that you can do to make your daily life easier and more comfortable. These include the following:

Use relaxation techniques when you feel uncomfortable or tense.

Stick to your gradual, planned exercise program. Use pursed-lip breathing when you become short of breath.

Do your breathing exercises several times a day.

Eat small, light, nutritious, easily digested meals. Avoid fried, fatty, or gas-forming foods.

Drink at least 2 quarts of fluid a day, excluding milk. Increase your fluid intake if your sputum thickens.

Follow your doctor's orders for postural drainage and percussion.

Use your oxygen according to directions.

Avoid airway irritants and other breathing hazards: dust, fumes, perfumes, aerosol sprays, excessive heat or cold. Stay indoors during times of excess air pollution.

Use your inhaler before any activity that usually makes you wheeze or become short of breath.

Take your medicines exactly as ordered. Report adverse effects or the feeling that you need more of the medicine.

Notify the physician of any change in your condition (see Box 7-1).

Avoid persons with infections, especially respiratory infections.

Get your influenza and pneumonia immunizations.

Avoid taking over-the-counter medications without your doctor's permission.

Wear medical alert information at all times.

Energy conservation techniques will be helpful:

Never stand to work when you can sit.

Assemble all equipment before beginning a task.

Use lightweight appliances such as an electric broom rather than a vacuum cleaner.

Use slip-on shoes rather than those that tie.

Use a small shopping cart rather than carrying grocery bags.

Ask grocery clerks to divide groceries into several small bags rather than one large one.

Add individual instructions for patient/family to take home if desired:

ASTHMA

Asthma is an acute reversible (episodic) obstructive airway disease that involves inflammation and edema of the respiratory mucosa, excessive sputum production, and bronchospasm. There are many causes of asthma, the basic one of which is a genetic predisposition to irritable airways. Asthma attacks may be precipitated by many factors such as allergy, exercise, infection, exposure to irritants, pollution, or excessive heat or cold, emotional stress, and drugs (especially aspirin or beta-blockers). Between exacerbations of asthma, the lungs are theoretically normal or nearly so (West, 1987). Asthma affects persons of all ages and may appear at any time in adulthood without warning. In older individuals, it is often associated with chronic bronchitis.

▶ PATHOPHYSIOLOGY, SIGNS, AND SYMPTOMS

When an asthma attack occurs, the airways overreact to any of the various stimuli mentioned earlier. The inflamed respiratory mucosa becomes edematous, which obstructs the airways to some extent. The airway irritation stimulates the production of large amounts of sputum, which further obstructs the airways. Wheezing results from bronchospasm, or spasm of the muscles that encircle the airways. The airways continue to enlarge slightly on inspiration and close somewhat on expiration. The swollen mucosa, excess sputum, and bronchospasm further close the airways, causing air trapping, poor air exchange, increased work of breathing, and respiratory distress.

▶ DIAGNOSTIC PROCEDURES

Arterial blood gases (ABGs)—Early in the asthma attack, the ABGs will show hypoxemia and hypocapnia. As the person becomes hypoxic, he or she hyperventilates in an attempt to raise the pO_2. This blows off excess CO_2 and lowers the pCO_2 well below the normal 35 to 45 mm Hg. As the patient becomes fatigued over the course of an asthma attack, the ability to hyperventilate is diminished and the pCO_2 gradually rises. When the pCO_2 is at the high edge of normal, the patient is in danger of respiratory failure.

Sputum examination—The most common cause of acute illness in the asthmatic patient is infection. When this occurs, the sputum will show evidence of the offending organism as well as a color change to yellow, green, or gray.

Chest x-ray (CXR)—Because patients in acute asthma attacks cannot exhale properly, they trap air in their chests. A CXR will show a depressed or flattened diaphragm as the result of the air trapping. There will also be evidence of hyperinflated lungs.

Pulmonary function tests (PFTs)—PFTs are not usually done during an acute asthma attack. During remis-

sions, PFTs may be done to establish a baseline pulmonary status or to evaluate the results of drug therapy.

Serum IgE and eosinophil count—If the attack is due to an allergic reaction, these may rise.

▶ MEDICAL MANAGEMENT

(See COPD section for rationales.)

Prevent attacks when possible:

  Encourage healthy lifestyle—adequate nutrition and exercise.

  Have patient maintain a high fluid intake (64 ounces minimum, excluding milk).

  Administer bronchodilators (may need daily doses of oral and inhaled drugs), steroids (may need maintenance doses of inhaled steroid, or oral steroids, which are avoided if possible); some patients need cromolyn to prevent attacks.

  Have patient avoid over-the-counter medications, especially aspirin and sedatives.

  Tell patient to report symptoms of bronchospasm and infection early (see Box 7-1).

Manage the attack when it occurs:

  Improve ventilation by administering xanthines and other bronchodilators (intravenous, topical), steroids (intravenous during acute attack). Give oxygen therapy as indicated by ABGs.

  Improve airway clearance by keeping fluid intake high, using postural drainage and percussion, eliminating smoking.

Prevent or treat infection and attacks:

  Have patient avoid exposure to infections.

  Teach patient early recognition and treatment of infection.

  Have patient avoid respiratory irritants and allergens.

Improve strength and exercise tolerance:

  Ensure adequate nutrition, and encourage weight loss as needed.

  Tell patient to rest when tired or short of breath.

  Teach patient to use bronchodilator inhaler before activities that usually cause wheezing or shortness of breath.

  Have patient avoid respiratory depressants—sedatives, tranquilizers, narcotics.

Drug therapy

Drug therapy for asthma is basically the same as for COPD. If epinephrine is used to treat attacks, it should be used in addition to xanthines and the other treatments listed rather than used alone because epinephrine is very short acting and is a potent cardiac stimulant.

In addition, cromolyn may be used to prevent attacks. Cromolyn is a drug that stabilizes mast cells in an attempt to inhibit release of the bronchoconstrictors, histamine, and SRS-A (slow reacting substance of anaphylaxis), thereby suppressing an allergic response. It is useful only when taken prophylactically and is not useful during an asthma attack. It may be given orally or by nasal inhalation and must be taken regularly for several weeks before it is effective. The patient must learn to use the inhaler properly, which requires some coordination. Adverse effects may include headache, dizziness, sneezing, nasal stinging and burning, epistaxis, postnasal drip, nasal congestion, itchy, puffy eyes, dry mouth, *bitter aftertaste, nausea, allergic symptoms, and others less often (Govoni and Hayes, 1988).*

▶ PROGNOSIS

If untreated, severe asthma attacks can be fatal. If the attacks are prevented or properly treated, the patient should recover to a point of normal or near normal airway and lifestyle.

▶ NURSING MANAGEMENT—NURSING CARE PLAN
Asthma

Assessment

SUBJECTIVE DATA

Progressive development of wheezing, dyspnea, chest tightness, cough
Poor exercise tolerance
Respiratory distress

OBJECTIVE DATA

Obvious respiratory distress, hyperresonance, distant heart and breath sounds, wheezing, and the use of accessory muscles to breathe
As the attack progresses, the cough becomes dry because the patient becomes dehydrated and the sputum is impossible to cough up

Nursing diagnoses	Expected outcomes	Nursing interventions (rationale)
Ineffective breathing pattern related to expiratory airway obstruction	Patient will have minimal or reduced dyspnea/orthopnea.	Administer oxygen as ordered (low flow). (See COPD section for rationale.)
	Patient will use breathing techniques.	Elevate head of bed; support arms as necessary.
		Teach breathing exercises, pursed-lip breathing and when to use.
Impaired gas exchange related to expiratory airway obstruction	ABGs will be acceptable for patient.	Teach breathing exercises, pursed-lip breathing and when to use (see Boxes 7-1 and 7-2).
		Administer oxygen as ordered.
		Elevate head of bed; support arms as necessary.
		Reduce body oxygen demands through bed rest, minimal activity and stimulation, long rest periods.
Ineffective airway clearance related to increased secretions	Sputum will be thin and easily coughed up.	Keep fluid intake high, at least 64 ounces daily excluding milk—more if sputum thickens.
	Patient will have no adventitious breath sounds.	Assess quantity and character of sputum.
		Encourage patient to use cascade coughing (see Box 7-4).
		Perform postural drainage and percussion during times of infection.
		Assess respiratory status at least every 4 hours during acute illness.
		Have patient turn, cough, and deep breathe at least every 2 hours during acute illness.
	Patient will have minimal or reduced dyspnea.	Teach relaxation exercises.
		Use all actions described earlier that apply.

Side label (vertical): NURSING CARE PLAN

Nursing Care Plan—Asthma—cont'd

Nursing diagnoses	Expected outcomes	Nursing interventions (rationale)
Reduced activity tolerance related to expiratory airway obstruction	Activity tolerance will improve. Ability to perform activities of daily living and self-care will improve. (Be specific in expectations.)	Assess current activity tolerance, and set specific, reasonable goals for increase. Teach patient to recognize exercise termination points (see Box 7-4) and points when rest is necessary during exercise. Administer oxgen with activity if ordered. Teach patient to use pursed-lip breathing with activities that usually cause dyspnea or wheezing. Teach patient to use energy conservation techniques.
Altered nutrition; less than body requirements, related to dyspnea, diaphragmatic pressure	Caloric intake will be appropriate (specify) for patient. Intake will include appropriate nutrient variety.	Have patient eat six small meals daily of light, highly nutritious foods. Do not include gas-forming, fatty, or fried foods in diet. Encourage good oral hygiene before meals. Plan inhaled bronchodilator and postural drainage treatments so that secretions do not interfere with eating. Obtain Meals-on-Wheels or other assistance as necessary.

Discharge planning and patient/family education
Discharge planning for the patient with asthma will depend upon the degree of illness at the time of discharge. The asthma patient should follow a normally healthy lifestyle with good rest, exercise, and dietary habits. The patient is often taught to use a peak expiratory flow device to help predict or identify an impending attack and enable treatment to be sought early. Medications should be understood and taken as ordered. The information in Box 7-6 should be provided to patients in an easily readable form.

Evaluation
Evaluation of the outcomes of care for the asthma patient is generally the same as for the patient with COPD.

Box 7-6.

Patient Education

Asthma

There are a number of things that you can do to make daily life easier and more comfortable. These include the following:

Use relaxation techniques when you feel uncomfortable or tense.

Drink at least 2 quarts of fluid a day, excluding milk. Increase your fluid intake if your sputum thickens.

Get regular exercise every day.

Avoid airway irritants and other breathing hazards: dust, fumes, perfumes, aerosol sprays, excessive heat or cold. Stay indoors during times of excess air pollution.

Use your inhaler before any activity that usually makes you wheeze or become short of breath.

Take your medicines exactly as ordered. Report adverse effects or the feeling that you need more of the medicine.

Notify the physician of any change in your condition (see Box 7-1).

Avoid persons with infections, especially respiratory infections.

Get your influenza and pneumonia immunizations.

Avoid taking over-the-counter medications without your doctor's permission.

Wear medical alert information at all times.

Use your peak flow device each day. Report any major difference in airflow to your physician.

Add individual instructions for patient/family to take home if desired:

PNEUMONIA

Older persons are particularly prone to pneumonia, which is an inflammation or infection of the lungs. It can be classified as acute, subacute, or chronic, as infectious or noninfectious, as bacterial or nonbacterial, and as lobar, lobular (bronchopneumonia), or interstitial. The acute and subacute forms are most prevalent among older individuals. Pneumonia can also be classified by where it is acquired (in the hospital or in the community) (Stephenson, 1989).

▶ PATHOPHYSIOLOGY, SIGNS, AND SYMPTOMS

Bacteria are the causative organisms for about half of the cases of pneumonia. Other causes are viruses, fungi, and protozoa. Aspiration pneumonia and hypostatic pneumonia are two common and preventable types of pneumonia. Immunosuppressed patients are at higher risk for pneumonia than are other patients (West, 1990).

Pneumonia generally does not occur in persons with normal lung defenses (Patrick, Woods, Craven, et al, 1986). The severity of pneumonia depends greatly on host resistance and airway clearance. When pneumonia occurs, the acute, inflammatory response to the invading pathogen brings excess water and plasma proteins to the dependent areas of the lower lobes of the lungs. The alveoli are infiltrated by red blood cells, fibrin, and polymorphonuclear leukocytes. All of this material consolidates in the affected area, leading to engorgement of the alveolar spaces with fluid and blood. This alveolar edema fluid provides a perfect medium for bacterial growth and spreads throughout the alveoli. By this time, the lung tissue is red and engorged. At this point, increasing numbers of leukocytes infiltrate the alveoli, causing the tissue to have a solid, liverlike appearance. Of course, there is no air in the affected alveoli. The infection resolves as exudate is lysed and reabsorbed by the neutrophils and macrophages. Exudate is also carried away in the lymph (Bullock and Rosendahl, 1988).

▶ DIAGNOSTIC PROCEDURES

Four classic signs of pneumonia are usually required for a positive diagnosis: (1) new infiltrate on a chest x-ray (although a normal film may be present early in the disease) (Patrick, Woods, Craven, et al, 1986); (2) cough productive of purulent sputum; (3) leukocytosis (in most types of pneumonia in nonimmunosuppressed patients, there will be a pronounced leukocytosis with a left shift); and (4) fever. Other signs and symptoms are often pres-

ent, but these vary according to the type of pneumonia and the age and condition of the patient (Stephenson, 1989).

Other diagnostic tests for pneumonia include Gram stain of the sputum, cultures of blood and sputum, white blood cell (WBC) count with differential (viral pneumonia will not elevate the WBCs), viral serology (for viral pneumonia), and ABGs as a guide for oxygen therapy (Stephenson, 1989).

▶ MEDICAL MANAGEMENT

Identify and treat the causative organism appropriately. Once antibiotic or other appropriate treatment is begun, patients usually show improvement within 48 hours.

Provide adequate ventilation/oxygenation:
  Administer bronchodilators (systemic and inhaled).
  Give oxygen as indicated by ABGs.
  Reduce metabolic demands (bed rest, long rest periods, light diet, reduce fever).

Improve airway clearance through hydration (oral, intravenous, mist therapy), postural drainage and percussion, and suction as needed. Cough suppressants are contraindicated.

Relieve pain by using mild analgesia that will not depress respirations but will allow coughing and breathing without splinting.

Drug therapy

Antibiotics or antiviral drugs are central to therapy for pneumonia. The theophyllines, beta-2 agonists, and sometimes steroids are used for patients with pneumonia as described in drug therapy for COPD.

▶ PROGNOSIS

The prognosis for pneumonia varies greatly depending on the organism and its virulence, the condition and resistance of the patient, and whether early and adequate treatment is obtained. It is a leading cause of death among hospitalized patients (West, 1990). According to Patrick Woods, Craven, et al (1986), untreated, bacterial pneumonia can have fatality rates of 20% to 60%. With treatment, these rates drop to 5% to 10% for pneumococcal infections and near 30% for Klebsiella infections. Complications of pneumonia are not uncommon. These include a second type of pneumonia superimposed on the existing type, acute respiratory failure, shock, pulmonary edema, pleural effusion, sepsis, otitis media, herpes simplex, and gastrointestinal problems (Stephenson, 1989).

▶ **NURSING MANAGEMENT—NURSING CARE PLAN**
Pneumonia

Assessment

SUBJECTIVE DATA

Dyspnea, cough productive of green or yellow sputum, orthopnea, respiratory distress, lethargy, and severe chest discomfort with breathing

Fever, chills, headache, nausea, and vomiting are often present, and there may be arm or shoulder pain.

Older persons may not have the classic signs and symptoms of pneumonia. They may have little or no fever, although they may have chills, vomiting, and an altered level of consciousness, in addition to the subjective symptoms listed (Futrell, Brovendu, McKinnon-Mullet, and Browder, 1980).

OBJECTIVE DATA

Bronchial breath sounds, rales, rhonchi, and sometimes wheezing

Pleural friction rub or evidence of pleural effusion (dullness to percussion) may occur.

There may be signs of consolidation (especially in lobar pneumonia): increased tactile fremitus, whispered pectoriloquy, and egophony ("E to A" change).

It is not unusual for sputum to be rusty or blood streaked.

	Nursing diagnoses	Expected outcomes	Nursing interventions (rationale)
N U R S I N G C A R E P L A N	Actual infection due to disease process	WBC, differential, and viral serology will remain in normal.	Collect ordered blood and sputum specimens for culture *before* antibiotics or other specific drugs are begun. (Starting the drugs first will alter test results. See COPD section for rationales not listed here.)
		Respiratory secretions will be thin, clear, and odorless.	Encourage fluids as indicated. (Fluids are the best expectorant to thin secretions.)
			Monitor quantity and character of secretions as a guide to the efficacy of therapy. (The patient must be able to clean the secretions out of the lungs if the infection is to be resolved.
		Temperature will remain within normal range.	Monitor temperature at least every 4 hours. (Temperature is often high; monitoring keeps the health care team informed and enables prompt treatment. Fever increases the body's metabolism, thus increasing body oxygen need.)
			Administer antipyretics and other measures as needed.
		Potential for spread of infection will be minimized.	Follow careful aseptic technique. Use respiratory isolation as needed.
			Handle sputum and tissues properly. (Proper technique can reduce the spread of infection and the transmission of new organisms to the already ill patient.)
			Older, debilitated, or immunosuppressed patients should not share a room with a person who has pneumonia. (They are at particular risk for the disease.)

Nursing Care Plan—Pneumonia—cont'd

Nursing diagnoses	Expected outcomes	Nursing interventions (rationale)
Impaired gas exchange related to expiratory airway obstruction and large amounts of secretions	ABGs will be acceptable for patient.	Administer oxygen as ordered (improves bodily oxygenation). Elevate head of bed; support arms as necessary (improves diaphragmatic action, opens the airways, and allows the use of the shoulder girdle for inspiration if necessary). Reduce metabolic demands by means of bed rest, long rest periods, light diet, and reducing fever (reduces body oxygen need). Administer mild analgesia as ordered to facilitate respirations and coughing. (The patient who has severe chest pain with breathing and coughing will splint the chest during both activities.) Teach relaxation techniques to reduce discomfort.
Ineffective airway clearance related to increased secretions	Sputum will be thin and easily coughed up.	Encourage fluids as described previously—at least 2 to 3 L/day. Monitor and document sputum characteristics.
	Patient will have no adventitious breath sounds.	Assess respiratory status at least every 4 hours. Perform postural drainage and percussion to aid in clearing chest.
	Patient will have minimal or reduced dyspnea.	Have patient turn, cough, and deep breathe at least every 2 hours.
Altered nutrition (less than body requirements) related to dyspnea, fatigue, anorexia	Caloric intake will be appropriate (specify) for patient. Intake will include appropriate nutrient variety.	Have patient eat six small meals daily of light, highly nutritious foods. (Digestion takes much oxygen/energy.) Do not include gas-forming, fatty, or fried foods in diet. (These foods tend to cause pressure on diaphragm and hinder breathing.) Encourage good oral hygiene before meals. (Coughing and vomiting leave an unpleasant taste in the mouth and reduce appetite.) Plan inhaled bronchodilator and mist treatments and postural drainage treatments so that secretions do not interfere with eating.

Continued.

Nursing Care Plan—Pneumonia—cont'd

Nursing diagnoses	Expected outcomes	Nursing interventions (rationale)
Altered comfort related to disease process	Patient will state that pain is relieved. Splinting of respirations and cough will not occur.	Administer mild analgesia as ordered. Monitor levels of discomfort, splinting. Monitor response to analgesics. Monitor respiratory rate, depth, character. (Pain causes the patient to splint respirations and cough. The stress of pain also increases metabolism, which increases bodily oxygen needs. Analgesia should relieve the pain enough to facilitate breathing and coughing without depressing respirations.)

Discharge planning and patient/family education

Patients will need to plan for several weeks of continued recovery after hospital discharge. Explain importance of management, high fluid intake, extra rest, a nutritious diet, and avoidance of exposure to infections. Provide the information in Box 7-7.

Evaluation

WBC count, differential, and viral serology remain in normal range.

Respiratory secretions are thin, clear, odorless.

Temperature remains within normal range.

Potential for spread of infection is minimized.

ABGs are acceptable for patient.

Sputum is thin and easily coughed up.

Patient has no adventitious breath sounds.

Patient has minimal or reduced dyspnea.

Caloric intake is appropriate (specify) for patient.

Intake includes an appropriate nutrient variety.

Patient states that pain is relieved.

Splinting of respirations and cough do not occur.

Box 7-7.

Patient Education
Pneumonia

When you have had pneumonia, you need to plan for an extended recovery period at home.

Continue to eat light, nutritious foods, rest often, and exercise regularly but not so much that you become fatigued or short of breath.

You need to continue a minimum fluid intake of 2 liters of fluid (eight 8-ounce glasses), excluding milk, per day.

Take your medicines as prescribed. Do not take over-the-counter medications, especially those for rest and sleep or for cough suppression.

Avoid exposure to persons who have infections or who are ill.

Call your physician if you have any increase in respiratory distress, chest pain, amount of blood in your sputum, fever, or other symptoms.

Be sure to return to the physician's office for follow-up examinations as instructed.

Discuss the need for influenza vaccine and pneumonia vaccine with your physician.

Add individual instructions for patient/family to take home if desired:

LUNG CANCER

Lung cancer is now the number one cancer killer of both men and women. Cancers of the lung may be primary or secondary; that is, they may originate in the lung, or they may metastasize to the lung from other areas of the body, which is common. Primary lung cancer is a malignancy that originates in the lung. The most common risk factor for lung cancer is smoking, but air pollution has also been implicated. It is believed that the body's immunity or lack of it plays a role, since not everyone who smokes develops lung cancer. It is known that older people lose some of their immunity and that their ability to cough and clear the chest is diminished. Older people also tend to have longer smoking histories. For these reasons, the risk of lung cancer increases with age.

▶ PATHOPHYSIOLOGY, SIGNS, AND SYMPTOMS

About 95% of lung cancers originate in the airways and are, therefore, classified as bronchogenic cancers. Other lung cancers include squamous cell or epidermoid carcinoma, small cell or oat cell carcinoma, and bronchiolar or alveolar carcinoma (the adenomas). Other types of lung cancer may also occur, though less often. Regardless of the site of origin, the pathogenesis, signs, symptoms, and outcome of lung cancers are much the same. In general, the cancers form over a very long period of irritation from factors such as smoking. Early signs and symptoms usually do not occur, so lung cancers are often not detected until very late in the course of the disease.

▶ DIAGNOSTIC PROCEDURES

Chest x-ray (CXR)—The CXR will show the tumor if it is large enough to be visualized. If the cancer is detected early, the tumor is small and is called a coin lesion. This can usually be resected and a cure achieved. If the tumor is larger and has spread, total removal may not be possible. Often, the CXR will show a pneumonitis that has formed around the tumor and the tumor will show only when the pneumonitis has cleared. Evidence of pneumothorax, rib involvement, and pleural effusion may also show on the CXR.

Sputum cytology—Sputum is collected and examined for tumor cells because these cells are sometimes coughed up. Often they are not, and a biopsy is necessary.

Bronchoscopy—If the patient has hemoptysis for no apparent reason, bronchoscopy would be indicated along with a standard pulmonary workup.

Pulmonary biopsy—If possible, a biopsy of the lesion is taken via a bronchoscopy. If this is not possible, an open lung biopsy is necessary.

Pleural fluid exam—If pleural effusion is present, the fluid is removed and examined for tumor cells.

Other tests—Other tests that may be required are bronchograms, angiograms, lung scans, sedimentation rate (which may be elevated), and hemoglobin and hematocrit (which may be low). Pulmonary function tests (PFTs) may be done to help decide whether the patient can tolerate surgery. Once the cancer is diagnosed, other tests may be done to stage the disease and detect metastasis.

Arterial blood gases (ABGs)—ABGs may be done as a guide to oxygen therapy.

Pulmonary function tests (PFTs)—PFTs, described in the section on diagnostic tests for COPD, may be used to determine whether the patient can tolerate surgery and/or the loss of a significant amount of lung tissue.

▶ MEDICAL MANAGEMENT

Medical management of lung cancer depends on the desires of the patient and family, how advanced the cancer is when discovered, and whether the patient can tolerate surgery. Pain control and improvement of ventilation and oxygenation will be done for all patients. If surgery is chosen, it will often be followed by radiation therapy or chemotherapy. If the patient is frequently developing a pleural effusion, the fluid will be removed at intervals by thoracentesis. Eventually, the pleura may be sclerosed by infusing tetracycline or another sclerosing agent into the pleural space. This is a comfort measure that damages the pleura so much that it can no longer produce effusion fluid and thus interfere with breathing.

Drug therapy

Drug therapy will depend on the specific needs of the patient. Bronchodilators, fluid therapy, and oxygen therapy are often used. Although radiation therapy and chemotherapy may be used, they often extend the life span only by months, not years. Pain control and medical improvement of ventilation with drugs such as bronchodilators are always critical aspects of drug therapy for the patient with lung cancer.

▶ PROGNOSIS

Because lung cancer is often discovered very late, the prognosis is very poor. A large number of patients do not survive for 1 year after diagnosis. Because of this, some patients choose to receive only comfort measures rather than therapeutic treatment of the cancer. Many of these persons also have preexisting pulmonary disease, such as COPD, which worsens their prognosis.

▶ **NURSING MANAGEMENT—NURSING CARE PLAN**
Lung Cancer

Assessment

SUBJECTIVE AND OBJECTIVE DATA

Symptoms of lung cancer are usually very late in appearing. When they do appear, they are often nonspecific and include a worsening of existing cough and sputum production and/or symptoms of complications or metastasis such as dyspnea from the pleural effusion. There may be a pneumonia or pneumonitis that has formed around the tumor, weight loss, low-grade fever, or discomfort of the shoulder or arm. There may be symptoms of the tumor pressing on an airway (localized wheeze) or on the esophagus (dysphagia). Late signs include clubbing of the fingers, loss of the voice (vocal cord involvement), severe dyspnea and fatigue, and persistent headaches and nausea. If hemoptysis occurs for no apparent reason, it should always be cause for a bronchoscopy and pulmonary workup because lung cancer is a common cause of this condition.

	Nursing diagnoses	Expected outcomes	Nursing interventions (rationale)
N U R S I N G C A R E P L A N	Impaired gas exchange related to disease process	ABGs will be acceptable for patient.	Administer oxygen as ordered. Elevate head of bed; support arms as necessary. Reduce metabolic demands through bed rest, long rest periods, light diet, reducing fever. Administer analgesia as ordered to relieve pain and to facilitate respirations and coughing. (The patient who has severe chest pain with breathing and coughing will splint the chest.)
	Altered comfort related to disease process	Patient will state that pain is relieved. Splinting of respirations and cough will not occur.	Administer analgesia as ordered. Monitor levels of discomfort, splinting. Monitor response to analgesics. Monitor respiratory rate, depth, character. (Pain causes the patient to splint respirations and cough. The stress of pain also increases metabolism, which increases bodily oxygen needs. Analgesia should relieve the pain enough to facilitate breathing and coughing without depressing respirations.) Teach relaxation techniques to reduce discomfort.
	Ineffective airway clearance related to disease process, poor cough effort, fatigue, poor nutrition	Sputum will be thin and easily coughed up. Patient will have no adventitious breath sounds. Patient will have minimal or reduced dyspnea.	Encourage fluids—at least 2 to 3 L/day. Monitor and document sputum characteristics. Assess respiratory status at least every 4 hours. Have patient turn, cough, and deep breathe at least every 2 hours.
	Potential for infection related to reduced immunity	Respiratory secretions will be thin, clear, odorless.	Encourage fluids as indicated. (Fluids are the best expectorant to thin secretions.) Monitor quantity and character of secretions as a guide to whether infection is developing. (Cancer patients are in particular danger of infection. The patient must be able to clean the secretions out of the lungs if the infection is to be prevented.)

Continued.

Nursing Care Plan—Lung Cancer—cont'd

Nursing diagnoses	Expected outcomes	Nursing interventions (rationale)
Potential for infection related to reduced immunity—cont'd	Temperature will remain within normal range.	Monitor temperature at least every 4 hours. Administer antipyretics and other measures as needed.
Altered nutrition: less than body requirements, related to dyspnea, fatigue, anorexia	Caloric intake will be appropriate (specify) for patient. Intake will include an appropriate nutrient variety.	Have patient eat six small meals daily of light, highly nutritious foods. Do not include gas-forming, fatty, or fried foods in diet. Encourage good oral hygiene before meals. (Coughing and vomiting leave an unpleasant taste in the mouth and reduce appetite. Often, the oral mucosa is excoriated and uncomfortable when chemotherapy or radiation therapy is being given.) Plan inhaled bronchodilator and mist treatments and postural drainage treatments so that secretions do not interfere with eating. Give antimetics before meals to combat nausea.
Powerlessness, hopelessness, anxiety, ineffective individual coping related to attitude to disease process	Patient will discuss feelings that are present. Patient will utilize appropriate support systems, support persons, and coping strategies.	Listen. Assure patients that they have a right to their own feelings. Assist patient to identify coping strategies that have worked well in the past and to use them now. Assist patient to identify appropriate support persons and to enlist their aid as necessary. Refer patient to American Cancer Society, hospice, coping support groups, other support systems as necessary and appropriate.

Discharge planning and patient/family education

Discharge planning for the patient with lung cancer will depend on the severity of the illness at the time of discharge, the projected course of the disease, and the attitude and desires of the patient and family toward the disease at the time of discharge. When it seems appropriate, the patient should be referred to agencies for assistance such as the American Cancer Society, hospice care, or Meals-on-Wheels. The focus of care will be pain management and comfort measures, psychological support, nutrition, rest, exercise, and control of the noxious effects of therapy. Provide the information in Box 7-8.

Evaluation

ABGs are acceptable for patient.
Patient states that pain is relieved.
Splinting of respirations does not occur.
Sputum is thin and easily coughed up.
Patient has no adventitious breath sounds.
Patient has minimal or reduced dyspnea.
Respiratory secretions are thin, clear, and odorless.
Temperature remains within normal range.
Caloric intake is appropriate (specify) for patient. Intake includes an appropriate nutrient variety.
Patient will discuss feelings that are present.
Patient will utilize appropriate support systems, support persons, and coping strategies.

Box 7-8.

Patient Education

Lung Cancer

Take your medications exactly as ordered. If you seem to need more of any medication, notify your physician.

Notify your physician of any change in your condition.

Notify your physician of any signs of infection such as fever, change in the color and character of sputum, or redness or drainage at surgical incision sites.

Talk with your physician or nurse when you feel that you need more help or care at home than you and your family can comfortably manage. They can refer you to agencies that can provide the help you need.

Continue to drink plenty of fluids each day (usually at least 2 to 3 quarts).

Try to eat a nutritious diet. Use the antinausea drugs that have been ordered regularly before meals to help you eat.

Good mouth care before meals will also help improve your appetite.

Plan your day so that you get rest at frequent intervals. Also try to get some exercise each day. This will give you some energy and improve your feeling of well-being.

Try to carry on as many normal activities as possible even if you have to shorten the intensity or duration of these activities from your usual pattern.

As much as possible, avoid persons or situations that upset or depress you.

Be sure to keep your appointments for treatment and checkups.

Talk with your doctor about influenza and pneumonia vaccinations.

Add individual instructions for patient/family to take home if desired:

TUBERCULOSIS

Tuberculosis is an infection that is caused by the *Mycobacterium tuberculosis*. Tuberculosis occurs in richly oxygenated tissues, especially the lungs. It may also occur in the kidneys and meninges and in the growing bones of children (Madsen, 1990). Tuberculosis usually results from reactivation of the microorganism after a previous exposure. Although this disease had been on the decline, there has been an upswing since 1985 (Madsen, 1990). Those who are at greatest risk are people who have lived in geographic areas where the disease is endemic and/or medical care is scarce. In the United States, about two thirds of the active cases of TB are among Hispanics, native Americans, blacks, and Asians. The homeless are also at high risk, as are the immunosuppressed: those with HIV infection, diabetes, or chronic renal failure; those who are malnourished, on chemotherapy, or steroid dependent; or older individuals. Persons with lungs damaged by silicosis are also at special risk (Madsen, 1990).

► PATHOPHYSIOLOGY, SIGNS, AND SYMPTOMS

Tuberculosis is generally transmitted as airborne droplet nuclei. The patient is most infectious prior to diagnosis. By the time treatment has continued for a week, the patient is usually noninfectious.

When the nuclei are inhaled, the larger ones are trapped by the respiratory mucus and are coughed out. The smaller ones may find their way to the alveoli, where they can multiply unhindered as a minute tuberculosis pneumonia. At this stage the person is not infectious and is asymptomatic. During this period the organisms can be transmitted to the blood and lymph in persons who lack a normal immune response. When the immune system is normal, multiplication of the organisms is eventually suppressed and the area is sealed off by a granuloma. This process may take up to 10 weeks, during which antibodies to the organism are also being developed.

Prior to the formation of the granuloma, the person is said to have primary tuberculosis, which is not an active disease. The granuloma may eventually calcify and may never break down and become an active disease, or it may break down at a later time when the person becomes debilitated or immunosuppressed. This is called postprimary tuberculosis. If the body defenses at the time of the initial exposure are suppressed, the incubation period for the disease is about 6 months.

► DIAGNOSTIC PROCEDURES

Skin testing—Skin testing is valuable, but not without its problems. A positive skin test does not mean active disease, but only that the initial, primary infection has occurred and the immune system has responded to it. False positives may occur if the person has had another mycobacterial disease or has received BCG vaccine. False negatives may occur if insufficient time has elapsed between exposure and the skin test, if the immune system is depressed, or if the patient is taking steroids or has had a recent immunization or a viral disease. False negatives and positives may also result from improper reading of the skin test. In older adults, false readings may occur because the initial exposure and immune response were many years ago. Sensitivity to the skin test diminishes with time.

Chest x-ray—A positive skin test should be followed up with x-ray. The calcified granuloma or the active disease will show on the x-ray.

Sputum smear—A quick way to test for organisms is the sputum smear. Unfortunately, other organisms also stain acid-fast, so this must be followed up with sputum cultures. Failure to identify the mycobacterium in the sputum does not rule out tuberculosis (Madsen, 1990).

Sputum culture—For this test, three sputum specimens are usually cultured for 6 weeks. It takes the organism this long to grow and give a positive diagnosis. Meanwhile, drug therapy is begun. Sputum cultures are also used as follow-up tests to determine when the patient is negative for TB and noninfectious.

Bronchoscopy—If hemoptysis occurs for no apparent reason, this test should be included in the pulmonary workup.

► MEDICAL MANAGEMENT

Treat the infection:

Usually, drug therapy with a combination of three or more drugs is begun on initial diagnosis (clinical signs and symptoms, chest x-ray, sputum smear) so as to be sure drugs to which the organism is sensitive are included (Madsen, 1990).

Once therapy is begun, the patient is usually noninfectious within a week.

Schedule regular monitoring for adverse effects of drugs and evaluation of the progress of the disease.

Promote immune response and optimal general health by emphasizing the importance of plenty of rest and fluids, a nutritious high-carbohydrate diet, and a regular exercise program. The patient should avoid exposure to infections.

Manage symptoms by identifying and treating any particular medical problems that are present.

Drug therapy

Drug therapy for tuberculosis usually continues for 6 months after the person's sputum is negative for the organism, which makes a total treatment period of about 9 months. Treatment is usually with a combination of two drugs, isoniazid and rifampin being the two most common. These are further described in Table 7-2.

▶ **PROGNOSIS**

If the patient complies with the treatment plan, the prognosis for a successful outcome without complications is very good.

Table 7-2. Treatment of tuberculosis

Drug	Information about administration and adverse effects
Primary drugs	
Isoniazid (INH)	Dose: 10-20 mg/kg up to 300 mg po or IM daily or 5 mg/kg po (*usually* 900 mg) or IM twice weekly.
	Adverse effects: Peripheral neuritis, seizures, optic neuritis with atrophy, muscle twitching, dizziness, ataxia, toxic encephalopathy, hypersensitivity. The major risk factor is hepatitis with alcohol consumption as a co–risk factor. Hepatitis is also dose and age related and not usually seen in patients under 20 years old. INH increases Dilatin toxicity. Resistance occurs easily.
	Tests for adverse effects: SGPT/SGOT, especially in early months of therapy.
	Treatment of adverse effects: Prompt withdrawl of INH for symptoms of hepatitis/liver toxicity. Pyridoxine 10 mg as prophylaxis for neuritis; 50-100 mg for treatment. Vitamin B_{12} concurrently to reduce liver toxicity. Give with food.
	Can be given without altering dose in moderately advanced renal failure.
Rifampin	Dose: 10-20 mg/kg up to 600 mg po daily or 600 mg po twice weekly.
	Adverse effects: Orange urine, tears, sweat; hepatitis, febrile reactions, purpura (rare), flulike syndrome, gastrointestinal upset, rash, thrombocytopenia, leukopenia, hemolytic anemia, hepatorenal failure. Alters actions of other drugs, especially contraceptives.
	Tests for adverse effects: SGOT/SGPT, BUN/creatinine. Transient rise in serum transaminase during first week of therapy is common. This will resolve itself without interrupting drug therapy.
	Can be given for renal failure but dose must be modified in the presence of hepatic toxicity. Hepatic toxicity can be worsened by INH.
	Absorption is inhibited if given along with food or salicylic acid.
	Rifampin interacts with the actions of many other drugs.
Pyrazinamide	Dose: 15-30 mg/kg up to 2 g po daily or 2.5-3 g twice weekly.
	Adverse effects: Hyperuricemia, hepatotoxicity, gastrointestinal irritation, hypersensitivity.
	Tests for adverse effects: Uric acid, SGOT/SGPT.
	Nursing implications: Have patient drink 2 quarts of fluid/day; give with food.
	Dose adjustments necessary with either liver or renal dysfunction.
	INH and rifampin do not increase the incidence of hepatotoxicity.
Secondary drugs	
Ethambutol	Dose: 15-25 mg/kg po daily or 50 mg/kg po twice weekly.
	Adverse effects: Optic neuritis (reversible with discontinuation of drug; very rare at 15 mg/kg), skin rash, headache, hyperuricemia, gastrointestinal upset, hypersensitivity.
	Tests for adverse effects: Red-green color discrimination and visual acuity.
	Caution: Renal disease or when eye testing not feasible.
Streptomycin	Used as part of multidrug therapy for resistant organisms.
	Dose: 20-40 mg/kg up to 1 g IM daily or 1.5 g twice weekly.
	Adverse effects: Eighth cranial nerve damage, nephrotoxicity, neuromuscular blockade, hypersensitivity.
	Tests for adverse effects: Vestibular function, audiogram, BUN, creatinine.
	Cautions: Older patients; those with renal disease.
	May alter the action of various drugs.
Ethionamide	Used only when primary drugs have failed; used in a multidrug combination.
	Dose: 15-30 mg/kg up to 1 g po daily
	Adverse effects: Gastrointestinal disturbance, metallic taste in mouth, hepatotoxicity, neurotoxicity, difficulty in controlling blood sugar, hypersensitivity.
	Tests for adverse effects: SGOT/SGPT.
	Nursing implications: Divided dose may lessen gastrointestinal effects.

Continued.

Table 7-2. Treatment of tuberculosis—cont'd

Drug	Information about administration and adverse effects
Tertiary drugs	
Capreomycin	Used in multidrug therapy only. Dose: 15-30 mg/kg up to 1 g IM daily. Adverse effects: Eighth cranial nerve damage, nephrotoxicity, hypokalemia, hypersensitivity. Tests for adverse effects: Vestibular function, audiogram, BUN, creatinine. Cautions: Elderly patients, use of other neuromuscular blocking agents. Rarely used with renal disease.
Kanamycin	Dose: 15-30 mg/kg up to 1 g IM or IV daily. Adverse effects: Auditory toxicity, nephrotoxicity, vestibular toxicity (rare). Tests for adverse effects: Vestibular function, audiograms, BUN, creatinine. Cautions: Elderly patients; rarely used with renal disease.
Para-aminosali-cylic acid (PAS)	Used only when other drugs have failed and used in a multidrug combination. Dose: 150 mg/kg up to 12 g po daily. Adverse effects frequent: Gastrointestinal disturbance (can be severe), hematologic disorders, hypersensitivity, hepatotoxicity, increased sodium retention. Tests for adverse effects: SGOT/SGPT. Nursing implications: Gastrointestinal effects very frequent, making adherence to dosage schedule difficult. Do not give salicylates with this drug. Inhibits absorption of rifampin and vitamin B_{12}.
Cycloserine	Dose: 10-20 mg/kg up to 1 g po Adverse effects: Psychosis, personality changes, headache, somnolence, tremors, vertigo, convulsions, rash. Tests for adverse effects: Psychologic testing. Blocking of adverse effects may be achieved with pyridoxine, ataractic agents, or anticonvulsants. CNS toxicity may increase when given with INH.

Data compiled from the Madsen and Stephenson sources in the reference list and from Amin NM (1990). Let's stop the comeback of tuberculosis, Postgrad Med, November 1, pp 107-120; and Farer, LS (1982). Tuberculosis: what the physician should know, New York, American Lung Association and American Thoracic Society, p 11.

▶ NURSING MANAGEMENT—NURSING CARE PLAN
Tuberculosis

Assessment

SUBJECTIVE DATA

The most common sign of tuberculosis is a chronic cough.

Other signs include fatigue, indigestion, anorexia, late afternoon and evening fever, night sweats, and amenorrhea.

OBJECTIVE DATA

Hemoptysis is a major sign of tuberculosis. When it occurs for no apparent reason, the patient should always have a bronchoscopy and workup because the two most common reasons for this are lung cancer and tuberculosis.

<table>
<tr><td rowspan="20" style="writing-mode: vertical-lr">N U R S I N G   C A R E   P L A N</td><td>Nursing diagnoses</td><td>Expected outcomes</td><td>Nursing interventions (rationale)</td></tr>
<tr><td>Actual infection due to disease process</td><td>The sputum will remain noninfectious.</td><td>Administer drugs as ordered. (See COPD discussion for rationales not listed here.)</td></tr>
<tr><td></td><td>No adverse drug reactions will occur.</td><td>Teach patient about the drugs, why they are used, why they must be taken for the full time ordered, and their possible adverse effects. (Hepatotoxicity is a particular hazard of isoniazid.)</td></tr>
<tr><td></td><td>Respiratory secretions will be thin, clear, and odorless.</td><td>Encourage fluids as indicated.</td></tr>
<tr><td></td><td>Temperature will remain within normal range.</td><td>Monitor temperature at least every 4 hours.
Administer antipyretics and other measures as needed. (Temperature is often high; monitoring keeps the health care team informed and enables prompt treatment. Fever increases the body's metabolism, thus increasing body oxygen need.)</td></tr>
<tr><td></td><td>Potential for spread of infection will be minimized.</td><td>Respiratory isolation is necessary only for the first week of hospital treatment. The door to the room should be closed. Staff and visitors should wear masks. Patient should wear mask when out of room. Room should have nonrecirculating air. Take proper care of sputum and tissues. (Proper technique can reduce the spread of infection and the transmission of new organisms to the already ill patient.)
When patient is at home, no particular precautions should be taken, except that babies and toddlers should not visit and family members and close contacts should be tested for the disease.</td></tr>
<tr><td>Potential for altered compliance related to feeling well and not understanding chronic nature of disease</td><td>Patient will adhere to drug treatment and follow-up schedules.</td><td>Discuss the chronic nature of the disease with the patient and family.
Emphasize the importance of adhering to the drug treatment schedule.</td></tr>
</table>

Continued.

Nursing Care Plan—Tuberculosis—cont'd

Nursing diagnoses	Expected outcomes	Nursing interventions (rationale)
Potential for altered compliance related to feeling well and not understanding chronic nature of disease—cont'd		Emphasize the importance of keeping follow-up appointments and of regular monitoring of disease progress and adverse effects of drugs.
Potential altered ability to fight disease	Patient will maintain optimal (specify) nutrition and other health habits.	Instruct patient on nutritious, high-carbohydrate, varied diet and on obtaining assistance as necessary—social services, Meals-on-Wheels.
		Assist patient as necessary to plan a daily schedule that includes adequate rest as well as an appropriate level of exercise.
		Emphasize oral care prior to meals. (Cough and sputum depress appetite.)

Discharge planning and patient/family education

Discharge planning for patients with tuberculosis focuses on assisting them to maintain an optimal lifestyle, while emphasizing rest, exercise, and nutrition, and adhering to the ordered medication schedule. They must understand the importance of not stopping the medications too soon and of keeping appointments for follow-up and monitoring for adverse drug reactions. Provide patients with information in Box 7-9.

Evaluation

Sputum cultures remain noninfectious.

No adverse drug reactions occur.

Patient adheres to the drug and follow-up schedules.

Respiratory secretions are thin, clear, and odorless.

Temperature remains within normal range.

Patient maintains optimal (specify) nutrition and other health habits.

Potential for infection is minimized by adhering to techniques for preventing spread of the disease or contraction of new infections.

Box 7-9.

Patient Education

Tuberculosis

Having tuberculosis does not have to change your life drastically. However, the following instructions should be followed:

Take your medicines exactly as ordered. *Do not stop taking them for any reason.*

Keep your appointments for follow-up and for monitoring of progress of your disease and the effects of your medicines.

Eat a varied, well-balanced diet each day.

Drink 2 to 3 quarts of fluid, excluding milk, each day.

Report any changes in your symptoms to your physician.

Do not allow yourself to be exposed to persons who have infections.

Do not allow babies and toddlers to visit you until this is approved by your physician.

Get some exercise each day, but avoid becoming overtired.

Get extra rest each day. Do not allow yourself to become too tired before you rest.

Do not drink alcohol while you are taking isoniazid.

Talk with your doctor about influenza and pneumonia immunizations.

REFERENCES

Bullock BL and Rosendahl PP (1988). Pathophysiology: Adaptations and alterations in function, ed 2, Glenview, Ill, Scott, Foresman.

Esberger KK and Hughes ST, editors (1989). Nursing care of the aged, Norwalk, Conn, Appleton & Lange.

Farer LS (1982). Tuberculosis: What the physician should know, New York: American Lung Association and American Thoracic Society.

Futrell M, Brovendu S, McKinnon-Mullet E, and Browder HT (1980). Primary heatlh care of the older adult, North Scituate, Mass, Doxbury Press.

Govoni LE and Hayes JE (1988). Drugs and nursing implications, Norwalk, Conn, Appleton & Lange.

Lewis SM and Coller IC (1987). Medical-surgical nursing: Assessment and management of clinical problems, ed 2, New York, McGraw-Hill.

Madsen L (1990). Tuberculosis today, RN 53(3):44-51.

Patrick ML, Woods SL, Craven RF, et al (1986). Medical-surgical nursing: Pathophysiological concepts, Philadelphia, JB Lippincott Co.

Steffl BM (1984). Handbook of gerontological nursing, New York, Van Nostrand Reinhold.

Stephenson C (1989). Respiratory changes. In Esberger KK and Hughes ST, editors: Nursing care of the aged, Norwalk, Conn, Appleton & Lange.

West JB (1987). Pulmonary pathophysiology—the essentials, ed 3, Baltimore: Williams & Wilkins.

West JB (1990). Nurse review, vol. 1, Springhouse, Pa, Intermed.

BIBLIOGRAPHY

Glassroth J (1981). Tuberculosis: A review for clinicians, Clin Notes Resp Dis 20(2):5-13.

Iseman MD, Albert R, Locks M, et al (1980). Guidelines for short-course tuberculosis chemotherapy, Am Rev Resp Dis 121(3):611-613.

Tucker SM, Canobbio MM, Paquette EV, and Wells MF (1988). Patient care standards: Nursing process, diagnosis, and outcome, ed 4, St Louis, Mosby–Year Book, Inc.

CHAPTER 8

Musculoskeletal System

Danna Strength

Disorders and trauma of the musculoskeletal system are a common cause of debilitation, dependency, and hospitalization in older adults. These problems are characterized by chronicity and pain, quite often resulting in dramatic changes in lifestyle. The common chronic disorders of the musculoskeletal system that occur in older adults predispose them to injury through falls caused by muscle weakness, poor balance, and/or pathologic fractures.

FRACTURES

Fractures are a common result of trauma to the musculoskeletal system in the older population. Specific types or classifications of fractures are presented in Table 8-1. Fractures of the bone result in associated trauma to blood vessels, nerves, tendons, and surrounding soft tissues.

▶ PATHOPHYSIOLOGY, SIGNS, AND SYMPTOMS

Following a fracture, bone healing occurs at various rates of speed depending on the type of bone (flat bones heal more rapidly than long bones), the age of the patient (healing occurs more slowly in the aged), and the general overall condition of the patient. Fracture healing begins at the time of fracture and proceeds through the following phases (Figure 8-1):

A. *Inflammatory or hematoma formation phase—Bleeding occurs and a fracture hematoma is formed at the site. The hematoma is essential to healing because the bone ends are devitalized. Macrophages invade the area and begin the debridement process that leads to resolution of the inflammatory phase.*

B. *Cellular proliferation—Thrombocytes and fibroblasts form a fibrin network within the hematoma. Adjacent tissue grows into the clot, and revascularization begins.*

Table 8-1. Types of fractures

Type	Description
Complete	Bone separates completely, producing two fragments.
Incomplete	Bone breaks partially without separation.
Simple or closed	Bone is broken; skin is intact.
Compound or open	Fracture parts extend through the skin.
Pathologic	Fracture occurs in an area of diseased bone (osteoporosis, Paget's disease).
Compression	Bone is collapsed (vertebral fractures).
Comminuted	Bone has broken into several fragments.
Impacted (telescoped)	One bone fragment is forcibly driven into another.
Transverse	Break is across the bone.
Oblique	Line of fracture is at an oblique angle to the bone shaft.
Spiral	Line of fracture encircles the bone.

Modified from Long BC and Phipps WJ (1989). Essentials of medical-surgical nursing: A nursing process approach, ed 2, St Louis, Mosby–Year Book; and Phipps WJ, Long BC, Woods NF, and Cassmeyer VL (1991). Clinical manual of medical-surgical nursing, ed 2, St Louis, Mosby–Year Book.

C. *Osteoblastic invasion—After several days osteoblasts enter the area, collagen strands are lengthened, and calcium deposits begin to strengthen the gap between bony ends.*

D. *Callus formation—Osteoblasts build up new bone as old bone is destroyed by osteoclastic activity. The*

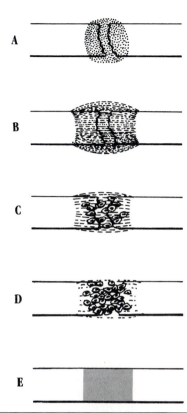

Figure 8-1. Bone healing (schematic representation). **A,** Bleeding at broken ends of the bone with subsequent hematoma formation. **B,** Organization of hematoma into fibrous network. **C,** Invasion of osteoblasts, lengthening of collagen strands, and deposition of calcium. **D,** Callus formation: new bone is built up as osteoclasts destroy dead bone. **E,** Remodeling is accomplished as excess callus is reabsorbed and trabecular bone is laid down. (From Phipps WJ, Long BC, Woods NF, and Cassmeyer VL [1991]. Medical-surgical nursing: Concepts and clinical practice, ed 4, St Louis, Mosby–Year Book, Inc, p. 1987.)

callus is formed and converted into rigid bone. The fracture ends knit together, and true bone healing has occurred.

E. *Remodeling—The osseous callus is remodeled, and bone returns to its normal prefracture state.*

These five phases of healing occur at a slower rate in the older adult, and the period of immobility and incapacitation is prolonged. Fractures are common in this age group, and the complications of immobility are a major concern. Falls of older individuals are precipitated by many factors. Among these are poor vision, generalized weakness and muscle atrophy, limitations of mobility caused by chronic medical conditions, postural instability, dizziness, tinnitus, confusion caused by cerebral ischemia, transient ischemic attacks, and pathologic fractures.

The upper extremities—especially the clavicle, acromioclavicular joint, humerus, elbow, forearm, and wrist—are common sites of fractures in older adults. These fractures are caused by direct trauma to the bone/joint in falls or by indirect trauma caused by the outstretched hands exerting force on another bone such as the clavicle. Several fractures of the upper extremities selected from this group are given more detailed discussion. The most common fracture in older adults, however, is fracture of the hip. This type of fracture is also the most life-threatening and requires a longer period of rehabilitation than do fractures of the upper extremities.

▶ DIAGNOSTIC PROCEDURES

Diagnosis of fractures is based on the history, signs, symptoms, and x-rays. Signs and symptoms include pain, muscle spasms, edema, ecchymosis, crepitation, loss of function, and shortening of the extremity in the long bones. Radiographic examination is used to determine the presence or absence of a fracture.

▶ PROGNOSIS

Recovery to a prefracture state is dependent on several factors, including overall health of the older adult and prevention of the complications of immobility. Attitudes toward recovery are not necessarily indicators for successful rehabilitation in the older adult (King, 1988). Of those older patients who require hospitalization secondary to a fall, half die within a year (King, 1988). Falls and the sequelae of falls are major health problems in those past age 65.

COLLES' FRACTURE

Colles' fracture is the classic fracture of the wrist and is caused by a fall directly onto the wrist or by breaking a fall with the outstretched hand. This fracture is one of the most common fractures of the older adult.

▶ PATHOPHYSIOLOGY, SIGNS, AND SYMPTOMS

The far end of the radius is broken off, and backward displacement occurs. The presenting symptoms are pain, swelling, limited range of motion in the fingers, and radial deviation of the wrist. Complications that frequently occur in conjunction with this fracture are shortening of the radius, fracture of the styloid process, and posterior facing of the joint. Although it will cause inconveniences, a Colles' fracture should not cause a disability or a disruption in the older person's lifestyle.

▶ MEDICAL MANAGEMENT

Reduction is maintained through casting or splinting in simple fractures. Traction with casting is used in comminuted fractures. The latter is accomplished by passing a Kirschner wire through the olecranon and one through the metacarpal bones. The wires are incorporated into the cast.

CLAVICULAR AND ACROMIOCLAVICULAR JOINT FRACTURES

Fractures of the clavicle and acromioclavicular joint are caused by direct blows or by breaking the fall with an outstretched hand. Fractures in the middle or inner two thirds of the clavicle account for 80% of these fractures (Liddel, 1988).

▶ PATHOPHYSIOLOGY, SIGNS, AND SYMPTOMS

In a displaced fracture of the clavicle, the pectoral muscle and weight of the arm pull the shoulder downward, forward, and inward, giving a slumping appearance to the affected shoulder. Fracture-dislocation of the shoulder is very common in the older patient. The undisplaced fracture may not be detected. Pain and limitation of movement are the chief symptoms in these injuries.

▶ MEDICAL MANAGEMENT

In both undisplaced and fracture-dislocation injuries, the shoulder must be kept upward and backward during healing. This is most frequently accomplished by use of the figure-of-eight or the Velpeau dressing. When alignment cannot be achieved through conservative management, open reduction is necessary. Reduction is maintained by use of wiring (Kirschner wire) in both instances or by nail fixation in fractures of the acromioclavicular joint.

FRACTURES OF THE NECK OF THE HUMERUS

Fracture of the neck of the humerus is generally caused by a fall directly onto the shoulder with the arm against the chest or in abduction rather than in extension to break the fall. Impacted fractures of the surgical neck occur frequently in older women.

▶ PATHOPHYSIOLOGY, SIGNS, AND SYMPTOMS

The pull of the pectoral muscles causes the distal fragment to be pulled inward and forward. The deltoid muscle exerts an upward pull on the fragment. Signs and symptoms include pain and limitation of motion. The affected arm hangs limply at the side.

▶ MEDICAL MANAGEMENT

Treatment consists of casting from the axilla to the wrist. Traction can be incorporated into the cast by the addition of a lead weight at the elbow. A neck-wrist strap is used to attain anterior flexion of the shoulder.

FRACTURES OF THE HIP

Fracture of the hip is the most common fracture among older adults, especially white women of small stature.

Contributory factors are osteoporosis, muscle weakness, and overall fragility related to age and lack of physical activity.

▶ PATHOPHYSIOLOGY, SIGNS, AND SYMPTOMS

There are two types of hip fracture: (1) intracapsular in which the femur is broken inside the joint or in the neck of the femur, and (2) extracapsular in which the femur is broken outside the joint or in the trochanteric region (Figure 8-2).

Clinical manifestations include severe pain, shortening and adduction, and external rotation of the affected extremity. Other manifestations include muscle spasms and hematomas, especially in extracapsular fractures. Older adults who live alone may also present with shock due to blood loss and dehydration if they were unable to summon medical assistance immediately following the injury.

▶ DIAGNOSTIC PROCEDURES

The diagnosis is made on the basis of presenting signs and symptoms and x-ray. It is important to obtain a detailed history and perform a thorough physical in order to determine associated medical problems, such as cardiovascular and respiratory illnesses, which are common in the older age group. Laboratory work includes a complete blood count, blood chemistries, blood sugar, blood urea nitrogen, and urinalysis. A chest x-ray and electrocardiogram are included in the presurgical workup.

▶ MEDICAL MANAGEMENT

Buck's extension traction is used in the period preceding surgery to decrease pain and muscle spasm, and to immobilize the affected extremity. Reduction and internal fixation are done as soon as possible to prevent avascular necrosis in intracapsular fractures and to promote early mobility, thereby avoiding the complications of immobility. Conservative management by traction is generally not used in older adults because of the lengthy immobilization involved. Intravenous therapy is ordered to reverse shock but must be carefully monitored in patients with limited cardiac reserve. Internal fixation is accomplished through the use of a variety of nails and combinations of nails and plates. In instances where satisfactory reduction and fixation or avascular necrosis is a concern, a femoral head prosthesis is selected. The blood supply to the head of the femur is depicted in Figure 8-3. The choice of the fixation method is based on the fracture site and the surgeon's preference for treatment.

▶ PROGNOSIS

Fractures of the hip are life-threatening in the older patient. The prognosis depends on early mobilization, prevention of complications, and successful management of associated medical conditions.

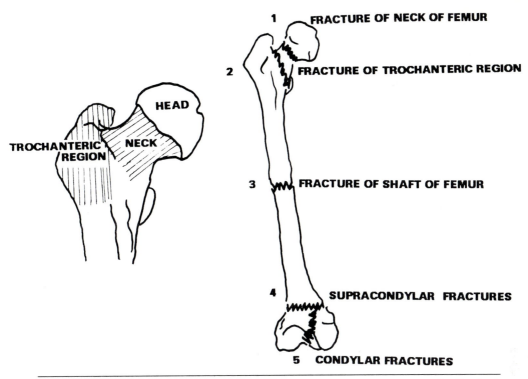

Figure 8-2. Sites of fracture of the femur. (From Brunner LS and Suddarth DS [1988]. Textbook of medical-surgical nursing, Philadelphia, JB Lippincott Co. Reprinted with permission.)

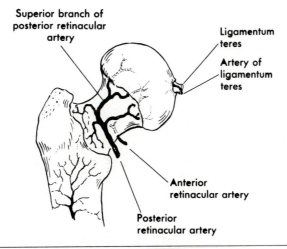

Figure 8-3. Posterior view of blood supply to head of femur. (From Phipps WJ, Long BC, Woods NF, and Cassmeyer VL [1991]. Medical-surgical nursing: Concepts and clinical practice, ed 4, St Louis, Mosby–Year Book, Inc, p. 2035.)

▶ **NURSING MANAGEMENT—NURSING CARE PLAN**
Fractured Hip: Preoperative and Postoperative

Nursing care will vary with the individual, and specific interventions and their priorities must be based on the assessment data. The nursing care plans presented here *are representative of those needed in caring for patients with fractures of the hip.*

Assessment: preoperative

SUBJECTIVE DATA
Circumstances surrounding injury
Concurrent medical problems and medications
Degree of pain
OBJECTIVE DATA
Grimacing

Vital signs
Intake and output
Presence of muscle spasms
Mental status
Condition of skin
Overall muscle strength

Nursing diagnoses	Expected outcomes	Nursing interventions (rationale)
Alteration in comfort: Acute pain related to injury/muscle spasm	Patient will verbalize a decrease in level of pain.	Assess and document level of pain. (Autonomic response to pain may be absent in older adults.) Assess and document nonverbal behaviors related to pain. (Pain sensation is decreased in older adults.) Administer analgesics and/or muscle relaxants as ordered or needed and monitor effectiveness, or instruct in use of patient-controlled analgesia (PCA) pump. (Decreased metabolism and clearance of drugs in older patients cause prolonged effects of analgesics.) Utilize proper technique in positioning. Turn every 1-2 hr using turn sheet (avoids shearing force leading to skin breakdown).
	Patient will verbalize a decrease in frequency and severity of muscle spasms.	Assess and document frequency and duration of muscle spasms. Position with pillows (reduces skeletal muscle tension). Teach relaxation techniques.
Impaired physical mobility related to fractures and treatment modality	Patient will verbalize acceptance of limitations imposed by fracture and traction.	Explain limitations of mobility imposed by fracture and Buck's extension traction. Monitor acceptance of limitations through verbalization and compliance.
	Patient will remain free of complications of immobility prior to surgery.	Observe for and prevent complications of immobility. *Respiratory* (pneumonia, chronic bronchitis, and emphysema more common in older adults). Use incentive spirometer 10 times every 2 hr. Have patient turn, cough, and deep breathe every 2 hr.

Nursing Care Plan—Fractured Hip: Preoperative—cont'd		
Nursing Diagnoses	**Expected outcomes**	**Nursing interventions (rationale)**
		Auscultate breath sounds every 2 hr. (Older adults are especially prone to respiratory complications—altered chest movement and decreased depth of respirations due to decreased elasticity of muscles and rigidity of rib cage.)
		Cardiovascular (circulatory overload, thromboemboli, fat emboli)
		Monitor vital signs every hour (take longer to stabilize in older adult).
		Monitor intravenous rate every hour. (Decreased cardiac function leads to circulatory overload if fluid is infused too rapidly.)
		Monitor intake and output every hour. (Renal blood flow and glomerular filtration rate are decreased in this age group.)
		Apply TED (thromboembolic disease) hose. (Incidence of thrombophlebitis increases with age.)
		Assess Homan's sign every 2 hr. (Initial dehydration predisposes to thrombus formation.)
		Assess for chest pain every 2 hr. (Pulmonary emboli incidence is increased in older adults, particularly after thrombophlebitis. Fat emboli are common with fractured hips.)
		Assess mental acuity every 2 hr.
		Avoid Valsalva maneuver. (Cardiac output is compromised in older adults, and maneuver decreases venous return, leading to more compromise in cardiac output.)
		Urinary
		Avoid use of indwelling catheter.
		Place on fracture pan every 2 hr if no indwelling catheter is used. (Bladder capacity is decreased in older adults.)
		Increase fluid intake to 3 L/24 hr (if within limits of cardiovascular tolerance).
		Assess for urinary retention. (Likelihood of prostatic hypertrophy is increased in older men.)
		Skin
		Assess condition of skin when turning/positioning.

Continued.

Nursing Care Plan—Fractured Hip: Preoperative—cont'd

Nursing Diagnoses	Expected outcomes	Nursing interventions (rationale)
Impaired physical mobility related to fractures and treatment modality—cont'd		Encourage patient to move freely within confines of limitations every 1-2 hr. Use trapeze for turning/movement (strengthens upper extremities and prevents shearing force). Use elbow and heel protectors.
	Patient will perform return demonstration of preoperative teaching exercise.	Teach postoperative care designed to prevent complications and encourage ambulation. Supervise return demonstration.
Altered thought processes related to pain, shock, environment, or underlying medical conditions	Patient will be oriented to person, place, and time.	Assess orientation to person, place, and time every 2 hr. (Arrhythmias, conduction defects, or other cardiovascular conditions can lead to decreased cerebral perfusion.) Reinforce orientation every 2 hr as needed. Validate patient's statements with family if possible. State expectations/instructions slowly and clearly. Allow additional time for processing of thought in all communication. (Time needed for processing responses is increased in older adults.) Encourage visits from friends, chaplain, volunteers. (Social isolation is to be avoided.)

Discharge planning and patient/family education
Rehabilitation begins on admission.
Prevention of complications leads to earlier discharge.
Teach the following:
   Use of side rails and trapeze bar to move and turn
   Use of incentive spirometer
   Coughing and deep breathing
   Dorsal and plantar flexion of unaffected extremity
   Relaxation techniques for pain and muscle spasms
Remember: Nurse will need to reinforce teaching frequently because of possible alteration in thought process.

Evaluation
Patient verbalizes minimal pain.
Patient verbalizes no muscle spasms.
Patient accepts physical limitations.
No signs and symptoms of complications are present.
Patient performs postoperative exercises.
Patient is oriented to person, place, and time and to daily events.
Patient relates daily events to family/staff.

Assessment: postoperative

SUBJECTIVE DATA

Verbalization of pain

OBJECTIVE DATA

Routine postoperative assessment, including guarding behavior, grimacing, vital signs (shock and hemorrhage), incision site, wound drainage, and intake and output

Complications, such as thrombophlebitis, fat embolism, pneumonia, urinary tract infection, and skin breakdown

Mental status

Support systems/living arrangements

	Nursing diagnoses	Expected outcomes	Nursing interventions (rationale)
N U R S I N G C A R E P L A N	Impaired physical mobility related to medically prescribed limitations	Patient accepts medically prescribed limitations such as position restrictions.	Maintain slight abduction of leg with pillows or abduction bolster (decreases stress on fixation). Maintain leg in straight alignment. Use trochanter roll (prevents external rotation). Maintain extension of knee in bed. Keep head of bed low (avoids hip flexion contracture and increases cerebral perfusion). Place pillow between legs when turning patient (generally turning to unoperative side).
		Patient will recognize own physical limitations.	Assist to stand on unaffected extremity to transfer or to use partial weight bearing (if arthroplasty).
		Patient will accept assistance in some aspects of rehabilitation.	Teach use of walker. (Crutch walking is seldom taught to frail older adults.) Encourage quadricep and gluteal setting 10 times/hr. Perform range of motion (ROM) exercises four times a day. Maintain strength in upper extremities through flexion and extension and use of trapeze bar. (Increased upper extremity strength is needed when using assistive devices.)
		Patient will remain free of postoperative complications.	Continue assessment for complications (see preoperative sections and Table 8-2). Perform neurovascular assessment. Compare pedal pulses (may be decreased in older adults as a result of underlying circulatory changes rather than neurovascular compromise). Compare color and temperature of extremities. Assess capillary refill. Assess ability to move extremity.

Continued.

Nursing Care Plan—Fractured Hip: Postoperative—cont'd

Nursing Diagnoses	Expected outcomes	Nursing interventions (rational)
Self-care deficit: bathing/hygiene/grooming, related to decreased strength and endurance	Patient will participate in self-care activities pertaining to personal hygiene.	Instruct patient to ask for assistance when needed or when becoming tired. Plan care around rest periods. (Frail older adults tire more quickly and require longer rest periods.) Provide equipment for morning care. (Minimize unnecessary activity when encouraging self-care.)
	Patient will demonstrate increased strength and endurance in performance of activities of daily living.	Reduce assistance—increase amount of self-care daily. Supervise exercises designed to maintain or increase strength.
Knowledge deficit related to limited exposure to therapeutic regimen/discharge planning	Patient will identify need for additional information regarding medical and nursing interventions.	Assess understanding of prescribed treatment plan. Assess ability and readiness to learn. Teach at patient's level of understanding. Allow time for feedback. (Response time is slower in older adults.)
	Patient will cooperate with regimen of progressive ambulation.	Teach muscle-strengthening exercises. Follow through with physical therapy regimen.
	Patient will demonstrate correct use of assistive devices—walker, cane.	Teach use of assistive devices, e.g., walker (Box 8-1), cane. Observe return demonstration.
	Patient will verbalize knowledge of home care treatment program.	Assess home situation for safety. (Older adults who have fallen are prone to subsequent falls.) Plan for discharge with family and multidisciplinary team, utilizing community resources. Give specific written discharge instructions (should be simply stated and in large print).

Discharge planning and patient/family education
Begins immediately after fracture fixation
Multidisciplinary approach to rehabilitation:
  Nursing and medical staff
  Occupational and physical therapy
  Social services
Focus of multidisciplinary team:
  Prevention of complications
  Ambulation, transfer technique, use of assistive de-
vices (see Box 8-1 for patient education in correct use of walker)
  Discharge to home
Assessment of safety of home environment essential:
  Grab bars by commode and tub/shower
  No loose throw rugs
  No electrical cords in walkways
  Elevated toilet seats

Table 8-2. Complications of immobility

System involved	Mechanism	Potential complication	Intervention
Cardiovascular	Failure of vessels in legs to assume or maintain a state of vasoconstriction, resulting in pooling of venous blood	Deep-vein thrombosis Pulmonary embolism Increased workload on heart Diminished cardiac output Decreased ability to adapt to erect posture	Active and passive range of motion (ROM) Frequent turning Slow mobilization Positioning to avoid pressure over major vessels
Respiratory	Decreased movement Decreased stimulus to cough Decreased depth of ventilation	Pooling of secretions in bronchi, bronchioles Hypostatic pneumonia	Active and passive ROM Stimulation to take maximal sustained inhalations and cough Frequent turning
Skin	Pressure or shearing forces (two or more tissue layers sliding on each other or tissue sliding on another surface) disrupting or decreasing circulation to an area	Skin breakdown (abrasion or pressure ulcer)	Early identification of areas at risk Turning Pressure-relieving pads, mattresses, flotation devices, special beds
Gastrointestinal	Decreased bowel motility Change in dietary habits Disadvantageous positioning to defecate	Constipation Impaction	Increased fluid intake More roughage in diet Encouragement to use bedside commode or toilet when possible
Musculoskeletal			
Muscles	Disuse	Atrophy Weakness	Active ROM Exercise
Joints	Limited motion leading to muscle and tendon shortening	Contracture Fibrosis or bony ankylosis around joints	Active and passive ROM Exercise Encouragement to perform own activities of daily living (ADL) as possible
Bones	Disruption of balance of osteoblastic/osteoclastic activity with destruction of bone matrix and release of calcium	Osteoporosis	Isometric and active exercise to tolerance
Urinary	Increased urinary pH, increased citric acid Poor bladder emptying	Renal stones Urinary stasis	Increased fluid intake Decreased calcium intake Improved position for bladder emptying (that is, bedside commode or toilet when possible)
Neurologic	Loss of normal stimuli	Confusion, restlessness, forgetfulness	Provision of stimulation and diversionary material

From Phipps WJ, Long BC, and Woods NF [1991]. Medical-surgical nursing: Concepts and clinical practice, ed 4, St Louis, Mosby–Year Book.

Box 8-1.

Patient Education

Correct Use of Walker

Walker should always rest on all four legs—never on two.

Maintain correct body position:
Erect posture
Elbows slightly bent
Wrists extended
Shoulders relaxed

Wear hard-soled, laced shoes.

In standard walker, move walker and weaker leg together.

After taking step, you should be centered in the walker.

Be alert for possible hazards—wet floors, cracks in sidewalks.

Additional instructions for the individual patient and/or family:

Living areas well lighted
Chairs with arms
Knowledge of community agencies:
Meals-on-Wheels
Home health services
Evaluation
Patient complies with medically prescribed regimen.
Patient seeks help when needed to comply with therapeutic regimen.

No signs and symptoms of complications are present.
Patient performs self-care activities pertaining to hygiene and ADL unassisted without tiring.
Patient asks questions and seeks additional information about treatment plan.
Patient maintains schedule of progressive ambulation.
Patient uses assistive devices correctly.
Patient describes specifics of home treatment program.

PATIENTS WITH A FRACTURE IN TRACTION OR CASTS

Medical management and nursing care vary and are dependent on the extent, location, and selected treatment for the injury, as well as on the patient's age, general health, and response to the injury. Older adults are seldom treated with traction because it increases the time of immobility. Casts are used frequently in the management of fractures of the upper and lower extremities. Boxes 8-2 and 8-3 describe the purposes, types, advantages, and disadvantages of traction and casts. See Boxes 8-4 and 8-5 for nursing care of patients who are in traction and casts.

Box 8-2.

Traction

Purposes of traction

Release contractures
Correct deformities
Reduce pain and muscle spasm
Reduce a fracture
Immobilize and maintain alignment

Types of traction

Manual—applied at time of injury; use steady firm pull
Skin—applied to skin and soft tissue, for example, Buck's extension for hip fracture
Skeletal—applied by placing Steinmann pin or Kirschner wire through the bone and attaching traction to wire or pin

Advantages

More weight can be applied with skeletal traction than with skin traction.
Skin is visible for inspection.

Disadvantages

Pin alters skin integrity, predisposing to infection.
Traction increases time of immobilization and likelihood of complications (seldom used in older people for this reason).

Box 8-3.

Casts

Purposes of casts

Maintain correct alignment
Immobilize for healing

Types of casts

Varied, but include the following:
    Short or long arm casts
    Short or long leg casts—either may incorporate a walking heel
    Body casts
    Hip spica—single or double

Advantages

Cast decreases time of immobilization (unless large cast, e.g., hip spica).
Cast decreases likelihood of complications of immobility.
Synthetic casts (fiberglass) are light, strong, and water resistant.

Disadvantages

Incision site is not visible for inspection.
Pressure points are not visible for inspection.

Box 8-4.

Nursing care of patients in traction

Place patient on an orthopedic bed—bed boards, Balkan frame, trapeze bar.

Ensure that weights and pulley ropes hang freely.

Prevent rope knots from catching in pulleys.

Perform neurovascular checks once an hour.

Avoid pressure on the popliteal space.

Avoid pressure on bony prominences, such as malleoli, soft tissue, and achilles tendon.

Keep patient in proper body alignment.

Teach patient to move within the confines of traction.

Prevent complications of immobility.

Monitor for signs and symptoms of fat emboli.

Provide pin care for skeletal traction.

Perform active/passive exercise on unaffected joints four times a day.

Never remove traction without a physician's order.

Box 8-5.

Nursing care of patients with casts

Drying the cast

Expose to circulating air—may be suspended from Balkan frame or elevated on pillow. Turn patient every 2 hours.

Do not use a heat lamp or hair dryer.

Use palms of hands in lifting or moving casts. Fingertips may dent the cast, causing pressure on the skin.

Large casts may take up to 72 hours to dry.

Protecting the skin

Examine edges of cast for roughness or loose plaster.

Petal edges of cast with moleskin or adhesive tape if not covered with stockinette.

Remove all loose plaster.

Wash skin around cast thoroughly without dampening cast. Synthetic cast is water resistant.

Apply alcohol to the skin around cast edges to toughen the skin. (Lotions soften and increase likelihood of skin breakdown.)

Support entire length of casted extremity on pillows to avoid pressure from edge of cast to skin.

Instruct patient to *never* insert any object under the cast.

Prevention of other complications

Evaluate neurovascular status every ½ to 1 hour for first 12 hours—compare with opposite extremity.

Check for five Ps: pain
pallor
pulselessness
paresthesia
paralysis

Prevent edema by elevating the casted area.

Outline the perimeter of drainage—include date, time, and initials.

Assess the cast for odor and "hot" spots.

Assess patient for pain and systemic signs of infection.

Assess for cast syndrome, which may occur in patients with large body casts because of obstruction of duodenum. Remain alert for prolonged nausea/vomiting, abdominal distension, pain, acid-base imbalance.

Care of the cast

Clean with damp cloth and dry cleaner.

Avoid getting cast damp—unless it is synthetic.

Remember

Notify the physician immediately of any abnormality.

▶ **NURSING MANAGEMENT—NURSING CARE PLAN**
  Traction or Cast

Assessment

SUBJECTIVE DATA	*Draining wound/odor*
Itching sensation	*Neurovascular data*
Expressions of loss/powerlessness	*Bladder or bowel incontinence*
OBJECTIVE DATA	*Motor or sensory deficits*
General skin condition/bony prominences	*Level of mobility*
Nutritional and hydration status	*Sense of power*
Presence of edema or discoloration	*Mental status*

	Nursing diagnoses	Expected outcomes	Nursing interventions (rationale)
N U R S I N G C A R E P L A N	Comfort, altered: Acute pain related to fracture and muscle spasm	See the preoperative nursing care plan for patient with a hip fracture.	
	Impaired physical mobility related to either cast or traction	See the preoperative nursing care plan for patient with a hip fracture.	
	Altered thought processes related to injury, aging, or social isolation of hospital environment	See the preoperative nursing care plan for patient with a hip fracture.	
	Impaired skin integrity or potential impaired skin integrity related to injury, cast, traction, or immobility	Skin will remain intact.	Place patient on an orthopedic bed—boards, Balkan frame, trapeze bar. Assess and document skin condition/turgor every 2 hr. (Well-hydrated skin is less prone to breakdown. Condition of tongue is a better indicator of hydration than pinching of skin because of reduced skin turgor in the older adult.) Turn patient every 2 hr. Perform ROM every 2 hr (stimulates circulation, promotes skin integrity). Use protective devices—elbow and heel protectors, alternating pressure mattress. Keep cast clean and dry. Keep bed free of crumbs, loose plaster. Keep linens clean and dry. Cleanse perianal area thoroughly with water and nondrying soap (superfatted) after each voiding/bowel movement. Remove TED hose, bathe and dry legs thoroughly every 24 hr. (Using superfatted soap during bath reduces dryness and pruritus due to decreased production of sebum in older adults.) Increase protein and carbohydrate intake. Maintain fluid intake at 3 L/24 hr if not contraindicated. (Well-hydrated skin is less likely to break down.)

Continued.

Nursing Care Plan—Traction or Cast Cont'd

Nursing Diagnoses	Expected outcomes	Nursing interventions (rationale)
Impaired skin integrity—cont'd		Avoid friction/shearing forces when turning or lifting patient in bed. (Skin is easily broken because of thinning of the epidermis in older adults. Healing is frequently slowed because of circulatory impairment.)
	Pin site will remain free of infection.	Assess pin sites every shift. Perform pin care as ordered or according to unit policy as needed.
Powerlessness related to loss of control or hospitalization	Patient will verbalize feelings of powerlessness.	Assist patient in identification of factors contributing to feelings. Assist patient to express feelings regarding powerlessness.
	Patient will identify factors within own control.	Assess patient's locus of control. Consider locus of control when planning care. Allow control of activities and schedule when possible (helps patient to increase sense of power and maintain independence).
	Patient will participate in making decisions regarding care.	Engage patient in decision-making process. (Individuals who have an internal locus of control are affected more by the loss of decision-making ability than those with an external locus of control.)
	Patient will seek active involvement in aspects of personal care.	Reinforce right to ask questions regarding medical and nursing management. (Assertive skills and behavior lead to increased feelings of control.) Reinforce positive feelings about self and involvement in care and exercise program.

Discharge planning and patient/family education
Instruct the patient in traction to do the following:
  Perform inspection of skin, particularly over bony prominences.
  Move properly within confines of traction.
  Use side rails/trapeze bar in moving and turning.
  Perform range of motion exercises on unaffected joints.
  Avoid modifying pulleys, ropes, knots, weights.
  Report any unusual sensations or increase in pain.
Instructions for the patient with a cast are presented in Box 8-6.

Evaluation
No skin breakdown occurs.
Vital signs are normal—no infection at pin site.
Patient discusses feelings in an open, honest manner.
Patient discusses factors that can be self-controlled.
Patient demonstrates problem-solving/decision-making behavior.
Patient participates actively in self-care.

Box 8-6.

Patient Education

Care of a Cast

Keep the cast dry unless it is a synthetic cast.

Do not insert any instrument or utensil (back scratcher, spoon) under the edge of the cast to scratch.

Report to your physician any breaks or cracks in the cast.

If lower extremity cast, elevate the casted extremity when sitting. This will reduce or prevent swelling.

Do not bear weight on a casted lower extremity unless a walking heel has been incorporated into the cast.

Soiled cast may be cleaned with *slightly* dampened cloth.

If cast becomes wet, do not dry with a hair dryer. You may use an oscillating fan.

Be alert for circulatory problems. Danger signs to watch for include coldness, numbness, pain, blueness or paleness of fingernails or toenails, and swelling or tightness.

Call your physician if circulatory problems above occur.

Ask your physician about performing isometric exercises.

Physician's telephone number _____.

Additional instructions for the individual patient and/or family:

OSTEOPOROSIS

Osteoporosis is a relatively common disorder of bone metabolism in which bone mass is reduced. Causative factors include a decrease in regular exercise as the person grows older, prolonged immobility, estrogen deficiencies in the postmenopausal woman, large doses of corticosteroids in long-term administration, calcium deficiency or an age-related decrease in calcium absorption, and disturbances in protein metabolism. The incidence of osteoporosis is greater in fair, white women of small stature who are over 50 years of age. Men and black women do not develop osteoporosis as frequently or as early because of their greater bone mass. The incidence in women over age 75 is 90% (Liddel, 1988). Osteoporosis affects an estimated 15 to 20 million Americans.

▶ PATHOPHYSIOLOGY, SIGNS, AND SYMPTOMS

Osteoporosis results when bone resorption occurs at a faster rate than bone formation, leading to brittle, fragile, and porous bone. The peak bone mass is achieved in the adult at approximately 35 years of age. After that age, normal bone remodeling decreases and age-related loss of bone occurs. The causative factors vary, but the basic pathology is the reduction of mineral and protein matrix components with a loss of bone mass.

Back pain and fatigue are common complaints of patients with osteoporosis. Since the skeleton is weakened, the work of supporting the body in an upright position is shifted to the muscle mass, which is reduced in older people. This leads to back pain and fatigue. Pain may also be due to compression fractures of the vertebrae. Loss of height is another common feature of osteoporosis. This is attributable to collapse of the vertebrae and resultant development of kyphosis (dowager's hump).

▶ **DIAGNOSTIC PROCEDURES**

Osteoporosis can be diagnosed by x-ray and nuclear scans. It is diagnosed on x-ray when 25% to 40% demineralization has occurred. The bones have a "washed-out" appearance as a result of demineralization. Computerized axial tomography is used to monitor bone mass of the hip and spine.

Laboratory studies such as complete blood counts, serum calcium, serum phosphate, alkaline phosphatase, and urine calcium excretion may rule out other medical conditions that lead to bone loss. The serum and urinary calcium, serum phosphate, and phosphatase are normal in osteoporosis.

▶ **MEDICAL MANAGEMENT**

The management of osteoporosis in those already diagnosed is directed toward arresting or slowing the progression of the disease and relieving pain. The ideal management is directed toward prevention and is begun much earlier in life.

The average recommended daily dose of calcium is 800 mg/day. Since the absorption of dietary calcium is less efficient in older adults, the recommended daily dosage is increased to 1500 mg/day. Inadequate amounts of dietary vitamin D and lack of sunshine resulting from the restricted lifestyle of many older adults are also a problem. Vitamin D up to 400 IU or 5 μg may be incorporated into the diet or may be prescribed as a supplement. Some calcium preparations contain vitamin D.

Outdoor activities or exercises such as walking are frequently suggested to increase weight bearing and to take advantage of sunlight to enhance vitamin D production. All exercise should be within limits of tolerance and should be increased in duration as strength is gained.

Estrogen replacement therapy is controversial. Estrogen decreases the rate of bone resorption but has been associated with an increase in the incidence of breast and endometrial cancer. Progesterone may be used in combination with estrogen replacement therapy to reduce the risk of endometrial cancer. Calcitonin (Calcimar) is also used in routine treatment of osteoporosis. The New England Journal of Medicine (July 12, 1990) reported a study by Watts et al (1990) which concluded that etidronate (EHDP) reverses slow bone loss and can prevent compression fractures of the vertebrae. EHDP is yet to be approved for the treatment of osteoporosis by the Food and Drug Administration.

Additional treatment is based on the symptomatology. Fractures and muscle spasms are common complications. Fractures are commonly seen in the hips, shoulders, vertebrae, and wrists of older adults with osteoporosis. Immobilization of the fracture site is achieved through bed rest, casting or braces, and corsets.

During the last 10 to 15 years increased emphasis has been placed on prevention of the disorder. Preventive therapy is based on the inclusion of adequate amounts of calcium and vitamin D in the diet to maintain bone remodeling, a weight-bearing exercise program, avoidance of agents that interfere with calcium absorption, and estrogen/progesterone replacement therapy.

▶ NURSING MANAGEMENT—NURSING CARE PLAN
Osteoporosis

Fractures related to falls and pathology are common in patients with osteoporosis. See the sections on hip frac- *tures and patients in casts and traction for information on the management of older adults with fractures.*

Assessment

SUBJECTIVE DATA
Complaints of back pain, fatigue
Exercise program
Lifestyle
OBJECTIVE DATA
Age, race, sex, stature

Age menopause occurred
Estrogen/progesterone replacement therapy
Intake of calcium and vitamin D
Laboratory results
X-ray results

	Nursing diagnoses	Expected outcomes	Nursing interventions (rationale)
N U R S I N G C A R E P L A N	Knowledge deficit related to limited exposure to health measures/home care	Patient will identify need for additional information.	Assess and document patient's readiness to learn. Teach patient to select foods high in calcium and vitamin D. Develop and implement a suitable exercise program that includes weight bearing (walking for 20 minutes three times a week). Teach patient to avoid agents that interfere with calcium metabolism—alcohol, caffeine, nicotine. Caution patient to avoid lifting heavy objects (even small grocery sacks in advanced cases) since this leads to compression fractures of the vertebrae.
		Patient will demonstrate ability to follow controlling measures.	Administer postteaching quiz.
	Potential for injury related to falls	Patient will increase home safety.	Plan with patient/family for environmental safety at home—removal of small rugs, careful placement of electrical cords, lights in hallways and staircases. (Falls resulting in fractures are the most frequent accidents in older adults.) Have grab bars installed by commode and tub. Assess outside exercise area for obstacles—broken sidewalks, rocks, holes in ground, walks, or streets, unleashed dogs.
		Patient will increase postural stability.	Teach patient to avoid hyperextension of neck. Teach patient to rise slowly from bed or chair and to avoid any sudden movement (prevents dizziness and postural instability).

Discharge planning and patient/family education
Instruct the patient to do the following:
  Place a bed board under a firm, nonsagging mattress.
  Use proper body mechanics in sitting, standing, and sleeping.
  Walk and maintain a regular exercise program.
  Select a diet high in calcium, protein, and vitamin D.
  Avoid bending and lifting.
  Rest at least a couple of times a day.
Nurse and/or social worker should assess the home for safety prior to discharge.

Provide patient education on measures to manage osteoporosis (Box 8-7).
Evaluation
Patient seeks additional information regarding management of disorder.
Patient complies with weight-bearing exercise program.
Patient complies with dietary suggestions.
Small rugs are removed from home environment.
Overall home safety factors are improved.
Patient avoids situations leading to postural instability.

Box 8-7.

Patient Education

Measures to Manage Osteoporosis

Maintain a healthy lifestyle by doing the following:
  Eats three balanced meals every day.
  Eat foods high in calcium and vitamin D—these include low-fat milk, cottage cheese, and yogurt.
  Take vitamin supplements—total daily intake should be 1500 mg of calcium and 400 IU of vitamin D after age 35.
  Maintain a sustained program of regular weight-bearing exercise. Walk for at least 20 minutes three times a week, preferably in the sunshine.

Limit caffeine intake to one source per day if unable to stop usage.* Foods high in caffeine are coffee, tea, chocolate, and cola beverages.
Limit alcohol intake to one source per day if unable to stop usage.*
Avoid use of nicotine.*

Talk with physician about hormone replacement in early menopause.

---

*Alcohol, caffeine, and nicotine interfere with calcium metabolism.

Additional instructions for the individual patient and/or family:

DEGENERATIVE JOINT DISEASE (OSTEOARTHRITIS)

Degenerative joint disease is a noninflammatory, non-systemic, slowly progressive disorder of the joints. There are two types: (1) primary osteoarthritis, which begins without any known causative factors, and (2) secondary osteoarthritis, which is due primarily to excessive joint use with resultant wear and tear on the joint. Other causative factors of secondary osteoarthritis include congenital skeletal defects, joint trauma, and inflammatory arthritis. Aging, genetic difference, and obesity are also contributing factors in the development of osteoarthritis (Luckmann and Sorensen, 1987). Degenerative joint disease is a disorder of the aging process. It is generally thought to occur earlier and more frequently in women (Graves, 1988). Radiographic evidence supports a universal prevalence by the age of 80.

▶ PATHOPHYSIOLOGY, SIGNS, AND SYMPTOMS

In degenerative joint disease two processes occur: (1) a deterioration of the joint cartilage and (2) the development of new bone, osteophytes, at the marginal aspects of the joint. It is theorized that cartilage deterioration is caused by a release of lysosomal enzymes that promote the digestion or breakdown of protein polysaccharides, resulting in damage to the cartilage. Another theory suggests that inadequate nutrition leads to deterioration of cartilage. Older adults, particularly those living alone, frequently have inadequate nutritional intake. Inadequate nutrients to the synovial fluid, which provides nutrients to the cartilage, could lead to degeneration of the articular cartilage and decreased ability to repair the cartilage. Osteophytes that develop as a result of the loss of matrix components from the cartilage cause erosion of the cartilage with a proliferative response at joint margins.

Osteoarthritic changes occur not only in the articular cartilages and joints but also in the soft tissues surrounding joints. Degenerative joint disease is characterized by aching pain in the joints, surrounding muscles, and soft tissues. A distinguishing feature is pain on use; however, muscle spasm may cause pain even when the joint is at rest. Night pain and morning stiffness are characteristic of the disease, particularly as it progresses. The joints most frequently affected are the weight-bearing joints and the distal interphalangeal joints. Crepitation and limitation of motion are frequently noted on mobility. The distal interphalangeal joints are affected with Heberden's nodes. Involvement of the proximal interphalangeal joints is less frequent. Nodes occurring on these joints are called Bouchard's nodes. As the disease progresses there may be loss of mobility and development of contractures.

▶ DIAGNOSTIC PROCEDURES

A complete history and physical are of primary importance (Table 8-3). The history should include information pertaining to the description, duration, and location of the pain as well as mention of activities that precipitate pain. Radiographic examination may reveal narrowing of the joint spaces, osteophytes, and in some instances bony sclerosis. Changes seen on x-ray do not necessarily correlate with the degree of pain experienced. Laboratory tests and diagnostic procedures include the erythrocyte sedimentation rate (ESR) and synovial fluid analysis. The ESR is normal in most instances, but exceptions may occur in cases of erosive osteoarthritis. The synovial fluid may be increased in amount but shows little or no sign of inflammation.

▶ MEDICAL MANAGEMENT

Medical management is symptomatic. The primary aim of treatment is control of pain because there is no treatment modality that prohibits the progression of joint destruction. Pain control is achieved primarily through use of analgesics and nonsteroidal antiinflammatory drugs (NSAIDs). The most common analgesic prescribed in the treatment of degenerative joint disease is aspirin; however, in older patients acetaminophen is preferred to salicylates even though acetaminophen has no antiinflammatory properties. Effective pain management can be achieved with acetaminophen without risking gastric irritation and potential gastric hemorrhage, which could result from therapeutic levels of salicylates. This complication is a greater threat in older patients because of shrinking of the gastric mucosa and a decrease in gastric mucus production. NSAIDs have both analgesic and antiinflammatory properties. A common side effect of all

Table 8-3. Diagnostic studies—degenerative joint disease

Procedure	Result

History and physical	Positive signs and symptoms:
	    Aching pain
	    Muscle spasms
	    Morning stiffness
	    Crepitation
	    Limitation of motion
	    Heberden's or Bouchard's
	      nodes

Radiographic examination	Narrowing of joint spaces Osteophytes Bony sclerosis
Laboratory tests	ESR—normal Synovial fluid—increased in amount Signs of inflammation—negative

these drugs is gastrointestinal irritation. Ibuprofen (Motrin, Rufen) is a common drug in this classification. Muscle relaxants may be ordered to control muscle spasms but are not usually used in very old patients (those past 75 years of age).

Nonpharmacological methods of pain management include the use of moist heat to relieve pain, spasm, and stiffness; orthotic devices, such as braces and splints, to support inflamed joints; weight reduction when obesity is a factor; and behavior modification programs. Conservative methods of pain control also include occupational and physical therapy, which are very effective in the older patient. When conservative management fails, reconstructive surgery may be recommended.

▶ PROGNOSIS

The prognosis for osteoarthritis of the hands is good in terms of functional abilities and pain control. When the larger weight-bearing joints are involved, prognosis is more guarded.

▶ NURSING MANAGEMENT

Nursing management of osteoarthritis is presented at the conclusion of the sections on arthritis.

RHEUMATOID ARTHRITIS

Rheumatoid arthritis is a chronic, systemic disease in which inflammatory changes occur throughout the body's connective tissue. The disease is progressive, produces deformity, and is characterized by remissions and exacerbations. Remissions occur most frequently in the early stages of the disease. The exact etiology is unknown. Suggested etiologies include the following: (1) infectious pathogens, particularly viruses; (2) autoimmunity; (3) metabolic abnormalities; and (4) genetic factors. Psychosocial factors such as stress may have an etiologic role, but this theory is less accepted.

Rheumatoid arthritis occurs at any age, but it occurs most frequently in females between 20 and 40 (Luckmann and Sorensen, 1987). The sex ratio is 3:1, female to male. The incidence is about the same in the United States and Canada. Rheumatoid arthritis rarely occurs in tropical climates.

▶ PATHOPHYSIOLOGY, SIGNS, AND SYMPTOMS

If unarrested, rheumatoid arthritis passes through four stages (Figure 8-4):
1. *Synovitis—Joint inflammation, or synovitis, develops and becomes chronic, leading to an increase in the production of synovial fluid and an increase in the thickness of the synovial membrane.*
2. *Pannus formation—Pannus, or granulation inflammatory tissue, is formed. It is derived from the synovial membrane and extends over the articular cartilage, destroying it in the process. As the disease progresses, the joint capsule and subchondral bone are destroyed.*

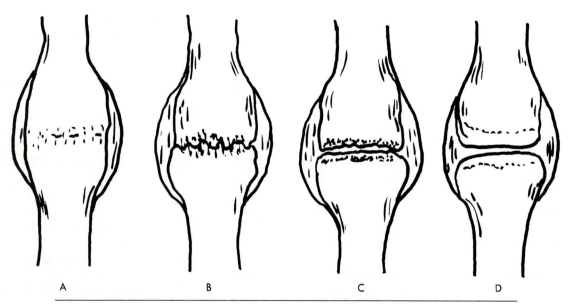

A   B   C   D

Figure 8-4. Pathologic changes of the joint in rheumatoid arthritis. **A,** Joint capsule synovial inflammation with synovitis. **B,** Inflammation progression to pannus formation. **C,** Fibrous ankylosis. Inflammation subsided. **D,** Bony ankylosis. (From Luckmann J and Sorensen KC [1987]. Medical-surgical nursing: A psychophysiologic approach, Philadelphia, WB Saunders Co. Reprinted with permission.)

3. *Fibrous ankylosis—Pannus is replaced by tough fibrous tissue, which occludes the joint space. This leads to decreased motion in the joint and deformity.*
4. *Bony ankylosis—The fibrous tissue calcifies and changes into osseous tissue. This may result in total immobilization of the joint.*

▶ DIAGNOSTIC PROCEDURES

A thorough history will most likely reveal an insidious onset with early nonspecific complaints of fatigue, general malaise, weakness, and weight loss (Table 8-4). The presenting symptoms generally are erythema, swelling, stiffness, and warmth as well as tenderness and pain over the affected joint(s). Physical examination may reveal enlarged lymph nodes, fever, and subcutaneous nodules over bony prominences, bursae, and tendon sheaths. Joint involvement frequently includes the small joints of the hands and wrists but may also include the larger joints of the ankle, cervical spine, elbow, hip, knee, and shoulder, and the sternoclavicular and temporomandib-

Table 8-4. Diagnostic studies—rheumatoid arthritis

Procedure	Result

History and physical	Positive history of:
	  Joint pain and swelling
	  Morning stiffness
	  Muscle spasms
	  Erythema
	  Edema
	Positive physical signs:
	  Enlarged lymph nodes
	  Subcutaneous nodules
	    over bony promi-
	    nences, bursae, tendon
	    sheaths
	  Ulnar deviation

Radiographic examination	Bony cysts Cartilage erosion Narrowing of joint spaces Osteoporosis Soft tissue swelling
Laboratory tests	
Complete blood count	Decreased RBC Increased WBC
C-reactive protein	Increased
Erythrocyte sedimentation rate	Increased
Rheumatoid factor	Hemagglutination inhibition titer—positive
Synovial fluid analysis	Inflammatory, increased volume, decreased viscosity
Serum protein electrophoresis	Increased α- and γ-globulin Decreased albumins

ular joints. Involvement of the temporomandibular joint further complicates problems with chewing in older adults, particularly those with dentures. As the disease progresses, muscle atrophy and tendon destruction occur around the joint. This causes subluxation to occur and produces ulnar deviation, "swan neck," and boutonniere deformities. The systemic nature of the disease manifests itself in extraarticular complications such as vasculitis, peripheral edema, neuropathy, myopathy, and cardiopulmonary disorders.

Radiographic examination may reveal bony cysts, erosion of cartilage, narrowing of joint spaces, osteoporosis, and soft tissue swelling. Laboratory studies include a complete blood count, C-reactive protein, rheumatoid factor, erythrocyte sedimentation rate, synovial fluid analysis, and serum electrophoresis.

▶ MEDICAL MANAGEMENT

The major goals of treatment are to relieve pain and symptoms, maintain mobility and power of joints, and prevent crippling deformities. A variety of regulatory technologies are used in an attempt to achieve these goals.

Pharmacological management may include five stages of treatment (Table 8-5). The drug of choice to reduce inflammation, pain, and temperature is one of the salicylates.

In conjunction with the pharmacological management, a balanced diet, alternating moist heat and cold, rest and joint protection, and orthotic devices such as braces and splints are frequently prescribed in the first stage of treatment. In the second stage the nonsteroidal antiinflammatory drugs (NSAIDs) are used for their analgesic and antiinflammatory actions. All of the agents in this category produce some degree of gastric irritation and should be taken with meals. These drugs are being used with increasing frequency in the management of rheumatoid arthritis in older adults (Graves, 1988). The supportive treatment modalities begun in the first phase are continued throughout the remainder of the stages of treatment, with the addition of occupational and physical therapy. Remissive drugs such as gold are given in the third stage. In the fourth stage, adrenocorticosteroids are introduced. The patient may be hospitalized at this point for reconstructive surgery. Immunosuppressive drugs are ordered in the fifth level of treatment. Informed consent is required for patients receiving immunosuppressive therapy.

In the most severe cases, treatment may progress to a sixth stage in which cytotoxic therapy is introduced. Patients are required to sign an informed consent when these drugs are used.

▶ NURSING MANAGEMENT

Nursing management of rheumatoid arthritis is presented at the conclusion of the sections on arthritis.

Table 8-5. Medications prescribed in the five stages of treatment of rheumatoid arthritis

Medication	Action	Side effects/toxic effects	Precautions
First stage—salicylates			
Acetylsalicylic acid, choline salicylates	Analgesic, antipyretic, antiinflammatory	Gastric irritation; dose-related salicylism; skin rash; hypersensitivity	Take with food, milk, or antacid; space every 4-6 hr to maintain antiinflammatory effect.
Second stage—nonsteroidal antiinflammatory drugs (NSAIDs)			
Indomethacin (Indocin)	Analgesic, antiinflammatory	Headache; dizziness; insomnia; confusion; gastrointestinal (GI) irritation	Take with food, milk or antacid; if central nervous system symptoms develop, discontinue and notify physician.
Ibuprofen (Motrin)	Same as indomethacin	Same as indomethacin, but believed to be less irritating to GI tract; fluid retention	Absorption is delayed if taken with food.
Tolmetin (Tolectin)	Same as ibuprofen	Same as ibuprofen	Take with food or milk.
Naproxen (Naprosyn)	Same as ibuprofen	Same as ibuprofen; also drowsiness	Take with food, milk, or antacid; avoid driving until dosage effect is established.
Fenoprofen (Nalfon)	Same as ibuprofen	Same as naproxen	Absorption is delayed if taken with food; avoid driving until dosage effect is established.
Sulindac (Clinoril)	Same as ibuprofen	Same as ibuprofen; also skin rash	Take with food, milk, or antacid; do not use with acetylsalicylic acid.
Piroxicam (Feldene)	Analgesic; antiinflammatory	Gastric irritation; anemia; skin rash; fluid retention; dizziness; headache	Take with food or antacid.
Third stage—remissive drugs			
Gold salts: IM gold sodium thiomalate (Myochrysine)	Antiinflammatory; effect not noted for 3-6 months after beginning therapy	Renal and hepatic damage; corneal deposits; dermatitis; ulcerations in mouth, hematologic changes	Have a urinalysis and complete blood count (CBC) before injection; report dermatitis, metallic taste in mouth, or lesions in mouth to physician.
Gold thioglucose (Solganal) Gold—oral: auranofin (Ridaura)			Oral gold may produce fewer side effects than injectable, but periodic laboratory tests are required.

Adapted from Phipps WJ, Long BC, and Woods NF [1991]. Medical-surgical nursing: Concepts and clinical practice, ed 4, St Louis, Mosby–Year Book, Inc.

Table 8-5. Medications prescribed in the five stages of treatment of rheumatoid arthritis—cont'd

Medication	Action	Side effects/toxic effects	Precautions
Penicillamine (Cuprimine)	Antiinflammatory (mechanism unclear); effect not expected to be noted until several months after beginning treatment	Fever; skin rash; nephrotic syndrome; hematologic changes; GI irritation; lupuslike syndromes; allergic reactions (33% probability if allergic to penicillin); retarded wound healing	Have a urinalysis, CBC, and differential, hemoglobin, and platelet count at least weekly for 3 months, then monthly; report skin rash, fever to physician; food interferes with absorption—take on empty stomach between meals.
Antimalarials: hydroxychloroquine (Plaquenil)	Antiinflammatory (mechanism unknown); effect not expected to be noted for 6-12 months after beginning therapy	GI disturbances; retinal edema that may result in blindness	Have an eye examination before beginning therapy and every 6 months thereafter
Fourth stage—corticosteroids (oral and intraarticular)			
Adrenocorticosteroids: prednisone (Deltasone), prednisolone (Delta-Cortef)	Interfere with body's normal inflammatory response	Fluid retention; sodium retention, potassium depletion; hypertension; decreased healing potential; increased susceptibility to infection; GI irritation; hirsutism; osteoporosis; fat deposits; diabetes mellitus; myopathy; adrenal insufficiency or adrenal crisis if abruptly withdrawn	Take with food, milk, or antacid; dosage not to be increased or decreased without physician's supervision; take in morning if taken on a once a day basis.
Fifth stage—immunosuppressive drugs			
Azathioprine (Imuran)	Interferes with body's normal inflammatory response; suppresses immune system	Skin rashes; GI ulcerations, bone marrow depression, decreased resistance to infection	Avoid use during pregnancy; have frequent CBCs; informed consent is required.

GOUT (GOUTY ARTHRITIS)

Primary gout is an inborn disease of purine metabolism manifested by hyperuricemia and joint inflammation. Secondary gout is an acquired disease. Acquired hyperuricemia occurs in certain hematologic conditions (leukemia and multiple myeloma), in chronic renal disease (glomerulonephritis), in hypertensive cardiovascular disease, and with prolonged use of thiazides.

Gout usually occurs in the middle years (45 to 64), and there is a male/female ratio of 7:1.

▶ **PATHOPHYSIOLOGY, SIGNS, AND SYMPTOMS**

Hyperuricemia is caused by the overproduction and/or undersecretion of uric acid. Both overproduction and undersecretion of uric acid may occur in the same individual. Joint inflammation results from the deposition of uric acid crystals in connective tissue and joints, especially on the great toe, knuckles, and ears. Uric acid tends to precipitate and form deposits in cartilaginous tissue, epiphyseal bone, and periarticular structures. These deposits are called tophi (Figure 8-5).

The onset is sudden and begins with an attack of acute pain, generally in fewer than four of the peripheral joints. Pain is accompanied by signs of inflammation at the involved joint(s) and sometimes by chills and fever. Untreated attacks generally subside in 1 week. In chronic gouty arthritis, there is bone destruction and deformity in the involved joint(s). Renal disease is another complication. There is an increased incidence of nephrolithiasis and albuminuria on an intermittent basis. Cardiovascular complications include hypercholesterolemia and hypertriglyceridemia.

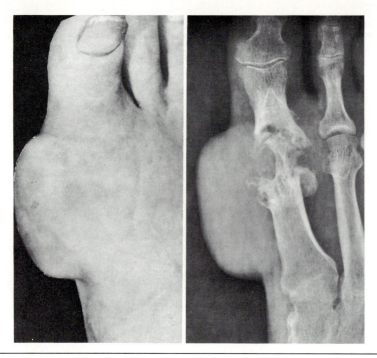

Figure 8-5. Gout of long duration. The mass is associated with extensive urate deposits. (From Brashear HR and Raney RB [1986]. Handbook of orthopaedic surgery, St Louis, Mosby–Year Book, Inc.)

Table 8-6. Diagnostic studies—gouty arthritis

Procedure	Findings
History	Family history of the disorder
	Acute, severe joint pain
	Renal stones
Physical	Inflamed joints
X-ray	Presence of tophi
	Bone destruction
Laboratory tests	Increased serum uric acid
	Decreased WBC in acute attacks
	Increased ESR in acute attacks
	Synovial fluid—sodium urate crystals

▶ **DIAGNOSTIC PROCEDURES**

A family history of primary gout and a history of acute, severe joint pain or renal stones are important diagnostic findings (Table 8-6). A differential diagnosis from other forms of arthritis such as osteoarthritis and rheumatoid arthritis must be made. The physical examination will reveal an inflamed joint(s) and possibly the presence of tophi. X-rays are taken of the affected joint(s) and an intravenous pyelogram is performed to determine the presence of renal stones and to determine renal function.

Laboratory findings reveal elevated serum uric acid levels. During acute attacks the white blood cell count is elevated, as is the erythrocyte sedimentation rate. Microscopic examination of synovial fluid aspirated from a joint or tophus reveals sodium urate crystals.

▶ **MEDICAL MANAGEMENT**

The management of gouty arthritis is directed toward (1) termination of the acute attack, (2) prevention of recurrent attacks, and (3) prevention of complications such as tophi and renal stones. Drug therapy consists of colchicine, probenecid, and allopurinol. Colchicine is effective in the relief of pain. It is of definite differential diagnostic value because it has no effect on nongouty arthritis or on uric acid metabolism. Probenecid (Benemid) is a uricosuric medication that inhibits tubular reabsorption of urate, thereby increasing urinary excretion of uric acid and decreasing the level of serum urate. It also aids in the prevention of uric acid stone formation. Allopurinol (Zyloprim) acts by regulating the production of uric acid and has no effect on the urinary excretion of uric acid.

Supportive therapy includes the use of analgesics, immobilization of the joint and bed rest, applications of heat and cold, and possibly intraarticular injections of corticosteroids.

▶ **NURSING MANAGEMENT—NURSING CARE PLAN**
  Degenerative Joint Disease, Rheumatoid Arthritis, Gouty Arthritis

When properly managed, patients with gouty arthritis rarely develop deformities; however, there may be extensive joint destruction in advanced stages of gout. This *requires the same nursing management as rheumatoid arthritis and degenerative joint disease, and the following material applies to all three diseases.*

Assessment

SUBJECTIVE DATA
History of disorder
History of medical treatment and self-management
Complaints of joint involvement—pain, stiffness
Limitation of activities

OBJECTIVE DATA
General health status
Presence of signs and symptoms
  Systemic in rheumatoid arthritis—fever, anemia, inflamed joints

Local in degenerative joint disease—Heberden's and/or Bouchard's nodes
Systemic in gouty arthritis—chills and fever, inflamed joints
Deformities—seldom seen in gouty arthritis
Ability for self-care in activities of daily living—range of motion, strength, ambulation
Diagnostic studies—x-rays, laboratory work

N U R S I N G C A R E P L A N	Nursing diagnoses	Expected outcomes	Nursing interventions (rationale)
	Comfort, altered: chronic pain related to inflammatory process and joint degeneration	Patient will identify activities that increase or decrease pain.	Assess duration, intensity, location, and type of pain. Assist patient in identifying acceptable level of pain. (Pain is especially difficult for the older person. Pain represents another loss to older adults who have already experienced many losses.) Identify and document activities that precipitate, increase, or decrease pain. Help patient identify effective mechanisms for coping with chronic pain. Establish rest-activity-rest program. (Periods of activity need to be shorter in older adults because of decreased muscle mass and underlying medical conditions that cause fatigue. Heart cannot meet demands of vigorous/prolonged activity because of decreased functional capacity in the older adult.)
		Patient will verbalize increased comfort after administration of analgesics/antiinflammatory agents.	Administer prescribed analgesics/ antiinflammatory agents. (Physicians are prescribing nonsteroidal antiinflammatory agents [NSAIDs] to older adults with increasing frequency.) Instruct patient in rationale for drug therapy and necessary precautions. (Caution patient to observe for darkened stools or blood in vomitus and to take medication with food. Older persons have a decrease in gastric mucus production and an increased tendency for gastrointestinal bleeds.)

Continued.

Nursing Care Plan—Degenerative Joint Disease, Rheumatoid Arthritis, Gouty Arthritis—cont'd

Nursing diagnoses	Expected outcomes	Nursing interventions (rationale)

Impaired physical mobility related to pain, joint degeneration, and muscle atrophy	Patient will maintain range of motion in affected joints.
	
	Patient will increase muscle strength through exercise.
		Assess level of mobility.
		Instruct patient in transfer techniques—bed to chair, commode to bed.
		Check range of motion every 4 hr.
		Develop a plan for maintaining/ increasing mobility and strength:
		  Isometric exercises
		  Use of trapeze bar
		Instruct patient in use of supportive devices (for correct use of walker see Box 8-1).
		Instruct patient in correct body alignment—lying, sitting, standing. (Encourage patient to stand straight at all times because stooped posture increases instability in older adults.)
		Teach patient to rest and protect joints through use of splints/ braces.
		Assess need for outpatient physical therapy or visits by a home health agency.

Potential impaired skin integrity related to decreased activity, nutritional state, and aging	Patient will identify measures to promote skin integrity.	Assess condition of skin over bony prominences and affected joints every 2 hr. (Skin over involved joints is shiny, and in older adults there is a decrease in subcutaneous tissue and thinning of skin that predisposes to skin breakdown.) Instruct patient in methods of skin assessment. Turn and reposition once an hour. Keep skin clean and dry—especially perianal area. Use protective measures—foam protectors, sheepskin protectors, alternating-pressure mattresses. Establish a skin care routine and implement it every 2 hr. Avoid friction and shearing forces in moving, transferring, or turning patient. (Thin skin of older adults is easily injured.) Promote intake of well-balanced diet (at least three meals/day). Maintain fluid intake at 3 L/24 hr—unless contraindicated by underlying medical conditions. (There is decreased pain and decreased likelihood of skin breakdown in well-hydrated patients.)

Nursing Care Plan—Degenerative Joint Disease, Rheumatoid Arthritis, Gouty Arthritis—cont'd		
Nursing diagnoses	**Expected outcomes**	**Nursing interventions (rationale)**
Self-care deficit: bathing/hygiene, dressing/grooming, feeding, toileting, related to fatigue or pain	Patient will perform self-care activities at optimal level of independence.	Assess functional level of self-care. Offer rest/pain medication prior to self-care. (Give lowest effective dose because of slower excretion and metabolism and less protein to bind drugs in older adults.) Encourage independence in performance of activities of daily living. (Independence increases feelings of self-esteem and self-worth, which are frequently decreased in older adults.) Instruct patient in use of assistive devices—long-handled reachers (Figure 8-6).
Low self-esteem related to body image disturbance or altered role performance	Patient will demonstrate appropriate assertive behaviors.	Help patient identify personal strengths. Increase patient's understanding of nature of disease process—permanence, progressivity, periodicity. Help patient identify community resources for home assistance/care.
	Patient will demonstrate adjustment to lifestyle changes.	Explore feelings regarding loss—mobility, independence, body image, role. (Low self-esteem and loss increase susceptibility to depression, which is common in older adults.) Encourage decision making and participation in plan of care. (Decreased social interactions and decreased control over self and environment in older persons produce a decrease in self-esteem.) Encourage daily grooming activities. (Improved appearance [body image] increases self-esteem.) Discuss impact on patient/family of change in role performance. Acknowledge patient's accomplishments. (Self-esteem is increased through positive appraisals by others.)
Potential for trauma related to impaired mobility and environmental factors	Patient will identify factors posing threat.	Assess home for needed adaptations. (Electrical outlets at waist level eliminate need for stooping—with resultant dizziness—to plug/unplug appliances.) Assess ability to protect self. (Increased incidence of falls in older adults is secondary to poor vision, postural instability, dizziness/vertigo associated with medical conditions.) Assess knowledge of home caregiver(s).

Continued.

Nursing Care Plan—Degenerative Joint Disease, Rheumatoid Arthritis, Gouty Arthritis—cont'd		
Nursing diagnoses	**Expected outcomes**	**Nursing interventions (rationale)**
Potential for trauma related to impaired mobility and environmental factors—cont'd		Assess ability to apply and use assistive/supportive devices. Plan with client/family for removal of environmental hazards—mats, rugs, electrical cords. Plan with client/family for purchase and installation of safety devices—grab bars in bathroom, elevated toilet seats, long-handled reaching device. Arrange for home health visit to assess functioning in home.

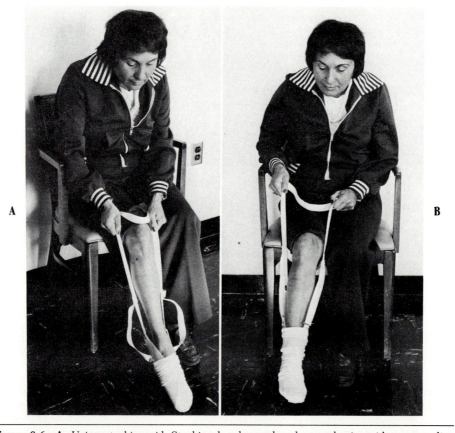

Figure 8-6. A, Using stocking aid. Stocking has been placed over plastic guide; garter clips at end of strap have been attached to top of stocking. Woman then places her foot into stocking. **B,** Straps are used to pull stocking over foot and up leg; when top of stocking is at knee, patient can release garters. This apparatus is useful for persons who cannot bend over to reach feet. (From Phipps WJ, Long BC, Woods NF, and Cassmeyer VL [1991]. Medical-surgical nursing: Concepts and clinical practice, ed 4, St Louis, Mosby–Year Book, Inc, p. 2050.)

Patient Education

Rheumatoid Arthritis, Degenerative Joint Disease, Gouty Arthritis

Avoid fad diets, "miracle cures and drugs"—these are expensive forms of quackery.

Take only those medications prescribed by your physician.

Take medication on prescribed schedule in prescribed amounts.

Do not "double up" on medication when discomfort increases unless directed by your physician. Again: take only prescribed amounts.

Be alert for signs of gastric irritation.
  Nausea/vomiting
  Burning or hurting in stomach
  Indigestion
  Blood in vomitus or stools

Avoid obesity. Additional weight increases strain on weight-bearing joints.

Maintain good posture to avoid additional strain on joints and muscles.

Perform prescribed exercises on a regular schedule.

Avoid lifting. If you need to move an object, pull it toward you.

Avoid fatigue. Rest at least twice a day.

Simplify activities.

Pace yourself and avoid rushing when performing activities.

Patient Education

Specifics for Gouty Arthritis

Avoid crash diets and fasting—both increase the serum uric acid level.

Maintain a fluid intake level of 3 L/24 hr unless physician orders a restriction of fluids.

Avoid aspirin—it interferes with excretion of uric acid.

Avoid drinking alcoholic beverages.

Eat foods that have a high alkaline-ash content. Examples are citrus fruit, milk, and potatoes.

Avoid foods with a high purine content. Examples are anchovies, brains, liver, sardines, and shellfish.

Additional instructions for the individual patient and/or family:

Discharge planning and patient/family education
Essentials of discharge planning include instructing the patient to do the following:
   Protect joints
   Conserve energy
   Maintain medication schedule
   Avoid "miracle cures and drugs"
Box 8-8 gives instructions needed by patients with rheumatoid arthritis, degenerative joint disease, or gouty arthritis. Additional specifics that apply only to gouty arthritis are presented in Box 8-9. Provide the patient with printed information on arthritis and its treatment (see Box 8-12).
Evaluation
Patient discusses activities that alter pain perception.

Patient exhibits increased comfort after compliance with medical program.
Range of motion in affected joints is improved.
Muscle strength is increased.
Patient assesses own skin.
Skin remains intact.
Patient increases participation in self-care activities without fatigue or pain.
Patient directs caregivers when unable to perform aspects of care.
Patient discusses positive feelings about self.
Patient makes alterations in lifestyle without hostility.
Patient modifies factors in self and environment posing threat of injury.

JOINT REPLACEMENT ARTHROPLASTY

Arthroplasty may involve the reconstruction of a joint or the partial or total replacement of the joint. The aims of arthroplasty are to relieve pain, improve mobility, restore function, and correct deformity. Arthroplasty is not a panacea for all joint problems, but it is an effective procedure for patients in whom joint degeneration or deformity has occurred and for those in whom the vascular supply to the bone has been compromised.

Total hip and knee replacements are generally performed in patients over the age of 60 who have unrelenting pain and joint destruction that has led to loss of function and mobility. Hip arthroplasty is also performed in older adults who have experienced a fractured hip.

Over the last three decades total joint replacement arthroplasty has become a common orthopedic procedure. The hip was the first joint for which total replacement was attempted. Total hip arthroplasty (Figure 8-7) is the most common joint replacement in the older patient, followed in frequency by total knee replacement (Figure 8-8). Joint replacements are also performed on the shoulder and metacarpophalangeal joints as well as the elbow, wrist, and ankle. The last three are more complex joints and are replaced less frequently.

Prostheses are secured in place with methyl methacrylate, a pliable polymer that hardens, or through the use of self-adhering replacements. The latter method is the newer one and is gaining widespread usage. Self-adhering prostheses are composed of ceramic and metallic components, and bone particles are used as the natural interfacing material. Rehabilitation is longer with this method because the bone particles must granulate and ossify in order to hold the prosthesis firmly in place; however, there is less likelihood of loosening when this method is used.

In total knee replacements the patient is placed on a continuous passive motion (CPM) device in the postanesthesia room. This device increases circulation and movement of the joint. Initially, 10 degrees of extension and 50 degrees of flexion are prescribed, with progression to 90 degrees of flexion by the time of discharge (Liddel, 1988). Bilateral total knee replacements are being performed simultaneously with increasing frequency.

▶ MEDICAL MANAGEMENT

Drugs frequently ordered in the postoperative period include antiinfective agents, narcotic analgesic agents, antiemetic agents, anticoagulants, sedatives, and antipyretic agents. Oxygen therapy at 2 to 3 liters per nasal cannula for 24 hours and intermittent positive pressure breathing treatments are ordered through respiratory therapy. An incentive spirometer is kept at the patient's bedside for use every hour. Ambulation orders are based on the type of surgery performed (cement or noncement) and the physician's preference. However, patients are generally out of bed within 24 to 72 hours with no weight bearing. Drains are placed in the wounds and connected to suction devices. The drains may be removed as early as the second postoperative day.

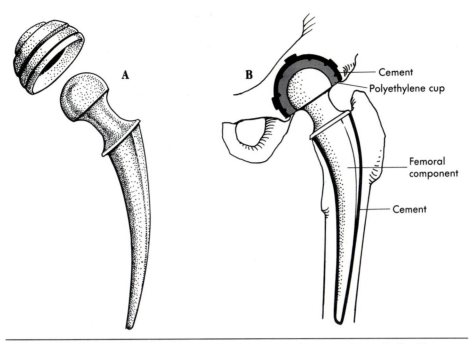

Figure 8-7. A, Acetabular and femoral components of total hip prosthesis. **B,** Total hip prosthesis in place. (From Phipps WJ, Long BC, Woods NF, and Cassmeyer VL [1991]. Medical-surgical nursing: Concepts and clinical practice, ed 4, St Louis, Mosby–Year Book, Inc, p. 2074.)

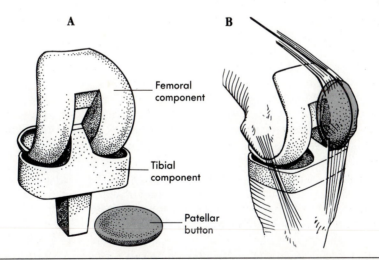

Figure 8-8. A, Tibial and femoral components of total knee prosthesis. Patellar button, made of polyethylene, protects posterior surface of patella from friction against femoral component when knee is moved through flexion and extension. **B,** Total knee prosthesis in place. (From Phipps WJ, Long BC, Woods NF, and Cassmeyer VL [1991]. Medical-surgical nursing: Concepts and clinical practice, ed 4, St Louis, Mosby–Year Book Inc, p. 2074.)

▶ **NURSING MANAGEMENT—NURSING CARE PLAN**
Joint Replacement Arthroplasty

Assessment: Preoperative

SUBJECTIVE DATA
History and management of disorder
Concurrent medical problems and medications
*Verbalizations regarding readiness for surgery and re-
habilitation program*

OBJECTIVE DATA
Vital signs
Mental status
Level of functional ability
Overall muscle strength

	Nursing diagnoses	Expected outcomes	Nursing interventions (rationale)
N U R S I N G C A R E P L A N	Potential for infection related to alteration in skin integrity	Patient will be free of signs and symptoms of infection.	*Preoperative/Intraoperative* Administer intravenous antibiotic as ordered. Clean and close operating room suite the night before surgery. Control traffic in operating room suite—inside and outside circulating nurses. *Postoperative* Monitor vital signs every 2 hr. (Ability to regulate temperature is diminished in the aged. Heat loss is difficult because of decreased ability to perspire and dilate peripheral vessels. Normal laboratory values are better indicators of infection than vital signs.) Assess dressing for drainage every 2 hr. (Hemostasis is more likely to be a problem in older adults.) Measure drainage from suction device every shift. Change dressing using aseptic technique. (Signs of infection may be masked because of depressed or delayed inflammatory reaction and immune response.) Assess incision (after dressing removal) for wound edge approximation, color, and temperature every 4 hr. (Healing occurs at a slower pace in older people.)
	Impaired physical mobility related to prescribed bed rest	Patient will increase activity, with partial weight bearing (PWB) progressing to full weight bearing (FWB) as tolerated.	Maintain slight abduction/limited flexion of operative leg (hip arthroplasty). Assist in position changes/transfer technique, changing from PWB to FWB. (Caution—Patients with confusion or dementia may try FWB before it has been ordered.) Instruct in proper use of cane and walker (see Box 8-1 for walker).

Nursing Care Plan—Joint Replacement Arthroplasty—cont'd		
Nursing diagnoses	**Expected outcomes**	**Nursing interventions (rationale)**
		Supervise in hip ROM and strengthening exercises—no active abduction (avoids dislocation of prosthesis). (Muscle atrophy and weakness normally present in the older adult are compounded by immobility.)
		Maintain proper functioning of continuous passive motion (CPM) device in knee arthroplasty.
		Assist in arranging for postdischarge physical therapy.
Comfort, altered: acute pain related to total joint replacement (hip or knee)	Patient will verbalize decrease in pain.	Assess pain—duration, intensity, location, type. (Older adults are more tolerant of pain, have a higher pain threshold. Do not allow to endure pain without relief.)
		Instruct in use of patient-controlled analgesia (PCA) pump, or administer analgesics as ordered/needed or prior to activity. (Lowest effective dose is ordered because of decreased circulation and increased likelihood of adverse effects in older adults.)
		Change position within therapeutic guidelines every 2 hr. (Total hip—Some physicians allow patients to turn to *operative* side only, whereas others allow to turn to *unoperative* side only.)
		Assess extremities for numbness, tingling. (Sensations are decreased in older adults who may have difficulty in describing sensations accurately.)
Altered tissue perfusion related to interruption of arterial flow, venous pooling, or potential hemorrhage	Patient will remain free of circulatory/neurovascular complications.	Assess vital signs every 2 hr. (Vital signs take longer to stabilize in the older adult and need to be taken more frequently.)
		Assess surgical dressing every 2 hr. (Older adults are more susceptible to hemorrhage and shock since blood vessels have decreased ability to constrict and older patients have decreased clotting factors.)
		Monitor hemoglobin/hematocrit every day. (See rationale for assessing surgical dressing.)
		Measure output of suction device.

Continued.

Nursing Care Plan—Joint Replacement Arthroplasty—cont'd

Nursing diagnoses	Expected outcomes	Nursing interventions (rationale)
Altered tissue perfusion related to interruption of arterial flow, venous pooling, or potential hemorrhage—cont'd		Apply TED hose—remove once every 24 hr and reapply (decreases venous pooling and thrombus formation in older adults, who are more prone to complications). Monitor functioning of pneumatic stockings (lessens venous pooling and thrombus formation). Perform neurovascular checks once an hour—edema, deep pain, paresthesia, paralysis, capillary refill. Test Homan's sign every 2 hr. Assess pulses distal to operative site. (Compare with pulses before surgery. Pedal pulse may have been absent because of vascular disease.) Avoid pressure on popliteal area. Assess for pulmonary emboli. (Older people are more susceptible following thrombophlebitis.) Compare skin color and temperature with opposite extremity.
Knowledge deficit related to discharge planning/home maintenance	Patient will comply with planned home management program.	Assess knowledge level. Assess home environment. Involve multidisciplinary team in discharge planning. Instruct patient in specifics of home care (see Boxes 8-10 and 8-11).

Assessment: Postoperative

SUBJECTIVE DATA

Verbalization of pain, nausea

OBJECTIVE DATA

Assessment of incision, including color, drainage/suction apparatus, and dressing

Peripheral pulses

TED (thromboembolic disease) hose or pneumatic sequential compression stockings

Hemoglobin and hematocrit

Vital signs

Intake and output

Complications—wound infection, respiratory, urinary, thrombophlebitis

Discharge planning and patient/family education

Essentials of discharge planning for patients with total hip and knee arthroplasty include instructing the patient/family to do the following:

Maintain outpatient physical therapy program.

Continue prescribed exercise program at home.

Contact physician regarding prophylactic antibiotic therapy if dental work or surgery, such as cystoscopy, is indicated.

Continue use of assistive devices as needed, particularly when in crowds.

Provide instructions for home care after total hip replacement (Box 8-10) or total knee replacement (Box 8-11), and give patient the arthritis advice in Box 8-12.

Evaluation

Vital signs are within normal postoperative parameters.

No cardinal signs of infection are noted.

The following are normal: hemoglobin and hematocrit, RBC, WBC and differential, protein, serum osmolarity, and coagulation studies.

Activity is advancing from partial weight bearing with walker to full weight bearing.

Pain is decreasing with less need for analgesics.

There is no evidence of circulatory/neurovascular complications.

There is no evidence of prosthesis dislocation.

Box 8-10.

Patient Education

Tips for Home Care After Total Hip Replacement

Call physician when questions arise. Doctor's telephone number: _____.

Keep legs uncrossed at all times.

Keep hips in neutral straight position at all times. Use rolled towels from hip to knee on both sides when in bed.

Keep firm pillow between legs when turning to unoperative side in bed.

Sit in high chair with arm rest to push up and out.

Sit with both feet on floor in neutral straight position.

Use an elevated toilet seat with arm rests.* Do *not* bend forward to rest elbows on knees. Seat may be purchased from Medical Supply.

Flex hip no more than 90 degrees when sitting (a right angle—L).

Use long-handled reacher to pick up objects from floor.

Use long-handled stocking aid to assist in putting on hose or socks.

Use a tub or shower chair when bathing.*

These tips help to avoid flexion greater than a right angle and avoid internal or external rotation of hips.

*If ordered by a physician, Medicare pays 80% of the cost of any special equipment.

Additional instructions for the individual patient and/or family:

Box 8-11.

Patient Education

Total Knee Replacement

Call physician when questions arise. Doctor's telephone number: _____.

Use stationary bicycle for 10 minutes four times a day, to improve range of motion and strengthen muscles.

Continue quadricep setting exercises 10 times per hour during waking hours.

Avoid placing stress on joint. Do not engage in excessive bending or twisting.

Avoid obesity. Obesity places additional stress on weight-bearing joints.

Use a tub or shower chair when bathing.

Sit in high chair with arm rest to push up and out.

Use grab bars by commode and tub or shower.

Box 8-12.

Arthritis advice

Arthritis means inflammation of a joint. The disease categories commonly known as arthritis—which is also known as "rheumatic disease"—include over 100 different conditions. They vary in symptoms and probably in cause. Some forms are better understood than others, but the causes of most of them are not yet known. Many effective treatments are used today to control arthritis symptoms, but *there are few cures.*

Most forms of arthritis are usually chronic, lasting for years. The more serious forms involve inflammation—swelling, warmth, redness, and pain. In older people, the two most common forms of arthritis are rheumatoid arthritis and osteoarthritis.

Rheumatoid arthritis

Rheumatoid arthritis (RA) is an inflammation of the joint membrane. It varies in severity and can cause severe crippling. RA afflicts three times more women than men, and it usually appears in the middle years, although it can begin at any age.

RA can affect many body systems but most frequently appears in the joints—fingers, wrists, elbows, hips, knees, and ankles. Persistent swelling and pain in joints on *both* sides of the body are typical symptoms. Morning stiffness is especially common.

RA should be treated as soon as it is discovered because uncontrolled inflammation of joint membranes can damage the joints.

Osteoarthritis

Osteoarthritis (OA) is often a mild condition, causing no symptoms in many people and only occasional joint pain and stiffness in others. Still, some people experience considerable pain and disability.

OA is also called degenerative joint disease, a more accurate name since "osteoarthritis" implies that inflammation is a part of the disease, which is not usually the case. While wear and tear on the inside surface of the joint is probably a cause of some cases, heredity and being overweight may be other possible factors.

Although OA is almost always present in older people, the condition can occur at any age, especially after a joint injury. Joint stiffness in OA can be brief, is often relieved by activity, and may recur upon rest. The large weight-bearing joints of the body—knees, hips and spine—are most often affected.

Treatment

The aim in treating arthritis is to relieve pain and stiffness, stop joint destruction from inflammation, and maintain mobility.

MEDICATIONS

Aspirin is the medicine most often used to treat arthritis. It relieves pain and reduces joint inflammation. But aspirin should be taken for arthritis only under medical supervision since large doses are required to reduce

U.S. Department of Health and Human Services, Public Health Service, National Institutes of Health.

Box 8-12.

Arthritis advice—cont'd

inflammation. In some patients, long-term use of aspirin can cause stomach irritation or other side effects, and may interfere with blood clotting.

Acetaminophen—a common aspirin substitute—does not reduce inflammation, although it can relieve aches and pains. "Arthritis-strength" aspirins are plain aspirin with small amounts of caffeine or antacids.

Newer prescription medicines used in place of aspirin are nonsteroidal antiinflammatory drugs (NSAIDs). These include ibuprofen, naproxen, fenoprofen, tolmetin, and sulindac. They are similar to aspirin in their ability to reduce inflammation and may have fewer side effects. Indomethacin, oxyphenbutazone, and phenylbutazone are other NSAIDs that provide relief for patients with arthritis but they may have more side effects. At this time, one of the newest NSAIDs, piroxicam, offers the advantage of a once-daily dosage.

Other stronger or nonaspirin drugs available by prescription include antimalarial drugs (such as hydroxychloroquine), gold salts, steroids (including prednisone and cortisone), and penicillamine (not the same as penicillin). These drugs can have more serious side effects than aspirin.

PHYSICAL THERAPY

Physical therapy is fundamental to treatment. People with arthritis tend not to move around very much, and while rest can reduce inflammation, too much rest stiffens joints. So rest and exercise must be balanced.

Daily exercise like walking or swimming can help maintain joint mobility. Good posture and proper eating (to prevent overweight) can help relieve joint strain.

SURGERY

Surgery is sometimes used in patients with RA or OA when joints are severely damaged and the more conservative forms of treatment have failed to control pain. Hip and knee joints are replaced most often. The purpose of surgery is to relieve pain and restore function for patients for whom other forms of treatment have not been successful.

Unproven and "quack" cures

Arthritis symptoms, especially in RA, may go away by themselves but then reappear weeks, months, or years later. This sudden disappearance of symptoms makes arthritis an ideal target for quack products or gimmicks. Some of the more common unproven or unsafe remedies are described here.

DMSO (DIMETHYL SULFOXIDE)

Currently, this drug is approved *only* for the treatment of interstitial cystitis, a bladder disorder. Studies are now being conducted to determine the safety and effectiveness of DMSO for the treatment of certain illnesses, but as yet there is no evidence that it is useful for arthritis.

SPECIAL DIETS

Diet is not a factor in the cause or treatment of arthritis. Any ads promoting certain foods, vitamins, or diets as "cures" are false.

MEDICAL DEVICES

Magnetic bandages, vibrators, or other gadgets are of no use in treating arthritis. Be wary of ads that use words such as "cure" or "miracle treatment."

Warning signs of arthritis

Any recurring joint symptoms (lasting longer than 6 weeks) should be checked with a doctor, no matter how mild or "temporary." A physical examination, x-ray studies, and specific laboratory tests can distinguish arthritis from other ailments and can identify the specific type of arthritis.

Important arthritis warning signs are as follows:
- Pain, tenderness, or swelling in one or more joints
- Pain and stiffness in the morning
- Recurring or persistent pain and stiffness in the neck, lower back, or knees
- Symptoms such as these that go away for a week or a month but return

Resources

The Independence Factory (PO Box C, Middletown, OH 45042) sells practical aids (zipper pulls, enlarged-handle toothbrushes, etc.) for those with hand and limb limitations.

For more information, write to the Arthritis Foundation (3400 Peachtree Rd, NE, Rm 1101, Atlanta, GA 30326) or the National Institute of Arthritis, Diabetes, and Digestive and Kidney Diseases (NIH, Bldg 31, Rm 9A04, Bethesda, MD 20205).

PAGET'S DISEASE

Paget's disease (osteitis deformans) is an inflammatory disorder of the bone that is characterized by a proliferation of osteoclasts and osteoblasts. Rates of bone formation and bone resorption may not always proceed at the same speed. The etiology of Paget's disease is unknown, but recent experimental evidence supports a slow virus infection of osteoclasts as the cause (Mirra, 1987). Paget's disease occurs primarily in men over 40, and the incidence increases with age. There is a familial tendency (Mirra, 1987).

▶ PATHOPHYSIOLOGY, SIGNS, AND SYMPTOMS

Increased activity of the osteoclasts leads to increased bone resorption, resulting in a compensatory increase in bone formation to repair the resorbed bone. This abnormal remodeling produces bones that are deformed and enlarged. These bones also have an abnormal increase in vascularity, which produces an increase in the warmth of the skin over involved bones. Bones affected by Paget's disease are structurally weak and easily fractured. Pathologic fractures are the most common complications of Paget's disease.

The onset is insidious, and bone pain and fatigue are frequently the earliest symptoms. Pain may vary in intensity from mild to severe and may be dull, aching pain or sharp, knifelike pain. Skeletal deformities include bowing of the femur and tibia, barreling of the chest, kyphosis, and enlargement of the skull. Skeletal deformities lead to systemic complications as the disease progresses. Kyphosis and bowing of the legs produce a marked reduction in height. The stooping posture of the older adult is increased by kyphosis, with a resultant increase in postural instability. The most frequently involved bones are those of the pelvis followed by the femur, skull, tibia, and spine.

▶ DIAGNOSTIC PROCEDURES

Radiographic examination reveals areas of increased bone density adjacent to areas of decreased bone density. X-rays demonstrate bony enlargement, opacity, radiolucency, and a widened cortex. Affected bones are prone to linear fractures. Serum alkaline phosphatase, serum acid phosphatase, and levels of urinary hydroxyproline are usually increased and are diagnostic of Paget's disease (Table 8-7). It is important to remember that some patients with symptoms of Paget's disease will have normal serum alkaline phosphatase and urinary hydroxyproline levels.

▶ MEDICAL MANAGEMENT

Medical management is directed toward control of pain and progression of the disease. Acetylsalicylic acid and nonsteroidal antiinflammatory drugs are useful in con-

Table 8-7. Diagnostic studies—Paget's disease

Test	Laboratory value
Serum alkaline phosphatase	Increased
Serum acid phosphatase	Increased
Urinary hydroxyproline	Increased

trolling pain. Corticosteroids in high dosages will suppress the disease, but high doses are not recommended because they are not well tolerated. In the older patient the increased likelihood of gastrointestinal bleeding is intensified. Calcitonin (Calcimar) produces marked pain relief and a decrease in serum alkaline phosphatase levels and urinary hydroxyproline excretion levels. Cytotoxic drugs such as mithramycin (Mithracin) and actinomycin (Dactinomycin) have been used effectively in the relief of pain and in the reduction of the laboratory values previously discussed. These drugs may decrease new bone formation by decreasing osteoblastic activity. Pain relief has also been achieved through the use of diphosphonates such as disodium etidronate (EHDP). Although this drug relieves pain more slowly, it is effective in reducing indices of bone resorption. EHDP reduces alkaline phosphatase values to normal and reduces neurologic signs and symptoms.

▶ PROGNOSIS

Pathologic fracture usually occurs in the destructive phase of the disease and is a frequent complication in affected bones. In edentulous adults, bony deformity of the maxilla can lead to difficulty in mastication and improperly fitting dentures that result in deficits in nutritional requirements.

More serious complications involve the neurologic and circulatory systems. Loss of hearing is associated with involvement of the temporal bone. Overgrowth of bone at the base of the skull can lead to brain stem compression. Spinal cord lesions with resultant paralysis have been noted and are attributable to compression of the spinal cord related to bony overgrowth or to pathological fractures of the vertebrae. In widespread involvement, the increased blood flow to the vascular bones is associated with a high cardiac output. In rare instances, high cardiac output failure has resulted. Cardiac output is already compromised in the older adult and cannot compensate for this increased blood flow.

Sarcoma is one of the most rare and dreaded complications of Paget's disease. Sarcomas originate most frequently in the long bones, skull, face, and pelvis. Treatment is symptomatic, and the prognosis of patients with sarcoma associated with Paget's disease is poor.

▶ NURSING MANAGEMENT

The multiple complications challenge nurses providing care to patients with Paget's disease. The most common complication is pathologic fracture. The nursing management of patients with fracture(s) is covered earlier in this chapter in the section on patients with a fracture in traction or casts.

REFERENCES

Graves M (1988). Physiologic changes. In Hogstel MO, editor: Nursing care of the older adult, New York, John Wiley & Sons, Inc, pp 63-89.

King PA (1988). Mobility and activity. In Burnside I, editor: Nursing and the aged: A self-care approach, New York, McGraw-Hill, pp 383-447.

Liddel DE (1988). Musculoskeletal and locomotion problems. In Brunner LS, Suddarth DS, Bare BG, et al, editors: Textbook of medical-surgical nursing, Philadelphia, JB Lippincott Co, pp 1534-1636.

Long BC and Phipps WJ (1989). Essentials of medical-surgical nursing: A nursing process approach, ed 2, St Louis, The CV Mosby Co.

Luckmann J and Sorensen KC (1987). Medical-surgical nursing: A psychophysiologic approach, Philadelphia, WB Saunders Co.

Mirra JM (1987). Pathogenesis of Paget's disease based on viral etiology, Clin Orthop 217(April):162-170.

Phipps WJ, Long BC, Woods NF, and Cassmeyer VL (1991). Clinical manual of medical-surgical nursing, ed 2, St Louis, Mosby–Year Book, Inc.

Watts NB et al (1990). Intermittent cyclical etidronate treatment of postmenopausal osteoporosis, N Engl J Med 323(2):73-79.

BIBLIOGRAPHY

Bahr RT Sr (1989). Musculoskeletal system. In Burggraf V and Stanley M, editors: Nursing the elderly: A care plan approach, Philadelphia, JB Lippincott Co, pp 150-181.

Boyer MJ (1988). Management of patients with rheumatic disorders. In Brunner LS, Suddarth DS, Bare BG, et al, editors: Textbook of medical-surgical nursing, Philadelphia, JB Lippincott Co, pp 1217-1241.

Buergin P (1990). Interventions for the person with motor problems. In Phipps WJ, Long BC, and Woods NF, editors: Medical-surgical nursing: Concepts and clinical practice, ed 4, St Louis, Mosby–Year Book, Inc.

Buergin P (1990). Problems of the musculoskeletal system. In Phipps WJ, Long BC, and Woods NF, editors: Medical-surgical nursing: Concepts and clinical practice, ed 4, St Louis, Mosby–Year Book, Inc.

Buergin P (1990). Interventions for persons with trauma to the musculoskeletal system. In Phipps WJ, Long BC, and Woods NF, editors: Medical-surgical nursing: Concepts and clinical practice, ed 4, St Louis, Mosby–Year Book, Inc.

Buergin P (1990). Interventions for the person with degenerative disorders of the musculoskeletal system. In Beare PG and Myers JL, editors: Principles and practice of adult health nursing, St Louis, The CV Mosby Co.

Carpenito LJ (1989). Nursing diagnosis: Application to clinical practice, ed 3, Philadelphia, JB Lippincott Co.

Christ MA and Hohloch FJ (1988). Gerontologic nursing, Springhouse, Pa, Springhouse.

Corbett JV (1987). Laboratory tests and diagnostic procedures with nursing diagnoses, ed 2, Norwalk, Conn, Appleton & Lange.

Corbett RW (1990). Nursing management of adults with specific musculoskeletal disorders. In Beare PG and Myers JL, editors: Principles and practice of adult health nursing, St Louis, The CV Mosby Co, pp 1353-1380.

Epstein C (1977). Learning to care for the aged, Reston, Va, Reston.

Evans RA (1990). Calcium and osteoporosis, Med J Aust 152(8):431-433.

Graffam S (1989). Pain in the elderly. In Burggraf V and Stanley M, editors: Nursing the elderly: A care plan approach, Philadelphia, JB Lippincott Co, pp 356-368.

Hamilton GP (1988). Health care of the older adult. In Brunner LS, Suddarth DS, Bare BG, et al, editors: Textbook of medical-surgical nursing, Philadelphia, JB Lippincott Co, pp 141-168.

Hogstel MO and Taylor-Martof M (1988). Perioperative care. In Hogstel MO, editor: Nursing care of the older adult, New York, John Wiley & Sons, Inc, pp 335-353.

Kanis JA and Gray RES (1987). Long-term follow-up observations on treatment in Paget's disease of bone, Clin Orthop Related Res 217(April):99-124.

Kim MJ, McFarland GK, and McLane A (1991). Pocket guide to nursing diagnoses, ed 4, St Louis, The CV Mosby Co.

Klinger JL, editor (1974). Self-help manual of arthritis patients, New York, The Arthritis Foundation, Allied Health Professions Section.

Lane PL (1990). Nursing interventions common to musculoskeletal problems. In Beare PG and Myers JL, editors: Principles and practice of adult health nursing, St Louis, The CV Mosby Co, pp 1333-1352.

Lederer JR, Marculescu GL, Mocnik B, and Seaby N (1991). Care planning pocket guide: A nursing diagnosis approach, ed 4, Redwood City, Calif, Addison-Wesley Nursing.

Lubkin IM (1986). Chronic illness: Impact and interventions, Boston, Jones & Bartlett.

Morand EF and Littejohn GO (1990). Medical problems in joint replacement patients: A retrospective study of 243 total hip arthroplasties, Med J Aust 152(8):408-413.

Mourad LA (1989). Musculoskeletal systems. In Thompson JM, McFarland GK, Hirsch JE, et al, editors: Mosby's manual of clinical nursing, ed 2, St Louis, The CV Mosby Co, pp 375-475.

Nade S (1990). Infection after joint replacement—What would Lister think? Med J Aust 152(8):394-397.

Nichols LW (1986). Drugs used for inflammatory disorders: Anti-inflammatory and related agents. In Spencer RT, Nichols LW, Lipkin GB, et al, editors: Clinical pharmacology and nursing management, Philadelphia, JB Lippincott Co, pp 346-366.

U.S. Department of Health and Human Services, Public Health Service, National Institutes of Health, National Institute on Aging (1982). Age page: Arthritis advice.

CHAPTER 9

Endocrine and Hematologic Systems

Laura Talbot

DIABETES MELLITUS
(NON–INSULIN-DEPENDENT DIABETES)

Non–insulin-dependent diabetes mellitus (NIDDM or type II) is a non–ketosis-prone class of diabetes. The National Institutes of Health subdivides this class of diabetes into two kinds, obese NIDDM and nonobese NIDDM. NIDDM is of insidious onset and usually occurs in those over 40 years of age. It is estimated that 90% of those affected are obese and have a high hereditary predispositon.

▶ PATHOPHYSIOLOGY, SIGNS, AND SYMPTOMS

Non–insulin-dependent diabetes mellitus occurs because of a need for insulin. Many theories have been proposed to explain the occurrence of NIDDM. One theory of aging regards immunodeficiency as the possible origin of the disease. Some type of stress, such as a virus, initiates an insidious decline in the immunologic system. Another theory suggests that a decline in the efficiency of the immune system resulting from the aging process makes the individual succeptible to a virus. The beta cell destruction that occurs causes an insulin deficiency.

In type II diabetes the pancreas produces insulin, but the amount produced is not adequate to metabolize the food eaten. Hyperglycemia occurs, often times without ketosis. The pancreatic production of insulin is enough to prevent ketosis but is not sufficient for metabolism. As the blood glucose level rises, glucose spills into the urine, resulting in glycosuria. Polyuria is caused by the
osmotic diuretic effect of glucose, which prevents reabsorption of water in the renal tubules. Because of this diuretic effect, polydipsia (excess thirst) and polyphagia (excess hunger) ensue.

A serious complication is hyperglycemic, hyperosmolar, nonketotic coma (HHNK), which results from the high serum glucose and nonketotic state of the type II diabetic.

Atherosclerosis due to hyperlipemia is commonly seen in the diabetic. A high incidence of peripheral vascular disease results from this coupling of hyperlipemia and hyperglycemia. The vascular degeneration that occurs affects multiple organs, including the kidneys, eyes, heart, and peripheral limbs. With impaired circulation and high blood glucose, infections are common and the healing process is slowed.

▶ DIAGNOSTIC PROCEDURES

The following results of blood tests are diagnostic for diabetes mellitus:

Fasting blood sugar (FBS)	>140 mg/dl
Postprandial blood sugar	>200 mg/dl
Oral glucose tolerance test (GTT)	>200 mg/dl

▶ MEDICAL MANAGEMENT

Because of the high incidence of obesity in patients with NIDDM, weight reduction through diet and exercise is the primary medical focus. Oral hypoglycemics are recommended only if weight reduction fails to decrease the hyperglycemia and the older adult is incapable of administering or receiving insulin, possibly as a result of vision loss or arthritis. If the individual is having symptoms, insulin is recommended.

The present medical management of the older adult with asymptomatic fasting hyperglycemia or an impaired glucose tolerance avoids drug therapy. There is a high risk of inducing hypoglycemia in this population.

▶ PROGNOSIS

There is no cure for diabetes, only management through diet, exercise, and/or medication. Weight reduction is the goal of the obese patient with NIDDM. Many times control of the disease can be obtained through weight loss, diet, and exercise. However, oral hypoglycemic agents are prescribed if diet and exercise do not achieve the desired control

▶ NURSING MANAGEMENT—NURSING CARE PLAN
Diabetes

Assessment

SUBJECTIVE DATA
Polydipsia (thirst)
Polyphagia (hunger)
Fatigue

OBJECTIVE DATA
Polyuria (excessive urination)
Obesity
Frequent infections
Blurred vision

	Nursing diagnoses	Expected outcomes	Nursing interventions (rationale)
N U R S I N G C A R E P L A N	Knowledge deficit related to management of the disease process, i.e., diet, exercise, and/or medication	Patient will verbalize an understanding of the disease process of diabetes that will include a demonstration and interactive discussion on diet, exercise, and/or medication.	Assess individual learning needs, ability to learn, and factors that would influence learning. (Many older individuals have had limited formal education. In addition, many older adults have arthritis, which may affect their ability to give self-injections or operate a glucometer.) Teach the basic concepts of the disease process at the level of the patient. (This will provide a common ground for discussion.) Discuss the purpose of diet and exercise as it relates to diabetes. Explain how insulin and oral hypoglycemics interplay in the disease process. Explain the purpose of testing the urine and/or blood for glucose. Teach the patient how to test urine and/or blood glucose levels.
	Sensory/perceptual alterations (visual and/or auditory) related to the aging process	Patient will demonstrate the use of methods designed for the individual with visual and auditory impairment.	Assess the patient's status. (Visual acuity, depth perception, peripheral vision, and visual field may all be altered by the diabetes and the aging process.) Provide instructions in large-print black letters on a white background or on audio tape, depending on the patient's ability to see and hear. Assess the patient's color perception. (The aging process causes a distortion of color in the blue-green spectrum.)

Continued.

Nursing Care Plan—Diabetes—cont'd

Nursing diagnoses	Expected outcomes	Nursing interventions (rationale)
Sensory/perceptual alterations (visual and/or auditory) related to the aging process—cont'd		Be sure the patient can see the different color gradients when testing the urine and blood. Obtain the book *Materials and Aids for the Visually Impaired Diabetic* from the National Diabetes Information Clearinghouse, Box NDIC, Bethesda, MD 20892—(301) 468-2162.
Altered nutrition: more than body requirements, related to NIDDM in the obese	Patient will attain and maintain ideal body weight through a nutritional regimen.	Assess causative factors that attribute to obesity, i.e., stress, sedentary lifestyle, and/or inadequate nutritional knowledge. Have patient follow the American Diabetes Association (ADA) diet to assist weight reduction and minimize catabolism of lean body tissue. Instruct patient in keeping a diet diary to see pattern of eating. Encourage the patient to weigh weekly and record weight to keep track of the weight loss to date. Discuss an exercise routine to promote weight reduction and better utilization of carbohydrates.
Altered peripheral tissue perfusion related to atherosclerosis	Patient will demonstrate how to examine skin, legs, and feet.	Examine skin, legs, and feet for any breakdown, lesions, or reddened areas. Assess the patient's vision. If visually impaired, teach foot care and the importance of manually checking for changes, including warm spots, cracks, new blisters, and nail changes. Evaluate neurovascular status of the legs and feet. Note any loss of sensation in the lower extremities.
	Patient will maintain the integrity of the skin, legs, and feet.	Teach skin, leg, and foot care using the patient education guide (Box 9-1).
Potential for injury: hypoglycemia, related to oral hypoglycemic medication, diet, and/or exercise	Patient will describe the signs and symptoms of hypoglycemia and methods to avoid their occurrence.	Assess the patient's current knowledge of hypoglycemia and hyperglycemia to obtain a knowledge base from which to start teaching. Encourage the patient to wear a Medic Alert tag in case of an emergency in which the patient is unconscious. Teach action, dosage, side effects, and toxic effects of oral hypoglycemic medications. Be sure the patient understands not to take over-the-counter medications without consulting the physician. (Medications that interact with sulfonylureas are

Nursing Care Plan—Diabetes—cont'd		
Nursing diagnoses	Expected outcomes	Nursing interventions (rationale)
		chloramphenicol [Chloromycetin], salicylates, clofibrate [Atromid-S], and phenylbutazone.) Alcohol should be avoided because it lowers blood sugar.
		Teach the patient to consume 4 ounces of unsweetened orange juice or 1 tablespoon of honey, syrup, or molasses if the signs and symptoms of hypoglycemia occur. If the attack does not subside after 15 minutes, the patient should test the blood sugar and consult the physician.
		Encourage the patient to carry a glucagon emergency kit in case he or she is unable to eat or becomes unconscious. In addition, teach a family member how to use the kit.

Box 9-1.

Patient Education

Skin, Leg, and Foot Care

Examine your feet daily. Look for any breaks in the skin, lesions, calluses, corns, or ingrown toenails.

Have your physician check any injury to your legs, feet, or toes.

A magnifying glass may assist in your examination of your feet.

If unable to bend over to examine your feet, try using a small mirror to examine the bottom of each foot.

Wash your feet regularly. Be sure to dry thoroughly between the toes. Apply lanolin lotions for dry skin.

Toenails should be kept trimmed straight across. See a podiatrist for calluses, corns, ingrown toenail.

Shoes should fit properly. Look for reddened areas, blisters, or chafing, which indicate a poorly fitting shoe. Break new shoes in slowly.

Use a thermometer to ensure the right temperature of your bath water. This will avoid unintentional water burn on your legs and feet.

Discharge planning and patient/family education

The primary cause of hypoglycemia is decreased food intake, excessive exercise, or too high a dose of an oral hypoglycemic agent or other drugs. Table 9-1 illustrates the difference between high blood sugar (hyperglycemia) and low blood sugar (hypoglycemia).

Teach the patient and significant others the signs and symptoms of hypoglycemia.

Teach the patient and significant others the route, dosage, side effects, and intervening factors related to oral hypoglycemic medications (Box 9-2).

Involve the family and significant others in the teaching.

Have patient perform a return demonstration on all teaching.

Refer the patient to the American Diabetes Association for additional information and community support.

Consult a discharge planner or social worker to evaluate the home environment for safety.

A home health nurse may be needed to evaluate prior teaching and assist in its integration in the home setting (Box 9-3).

Consult with the dietitian in planning a diet that fits the individual's lifestyle.

Many organizations have been established to assist the individual with diabetes. An excellent organization to belong to is the American Diabetes Association. It provides support, booklets, and educational materials. There are also local chapters to assist the diabetic. For more information write or call the Association.

American Diabetes Association
1970 Chain Bridge Road
McLean, VA 22109
(800) ADA-DISC

Eli Lilly & Company provides a free booklet on diet, exercise, insulin, and oral hypoglycemic medications.

Eli Lilly & Company
Indianapolis, IN 46285
(317) 276-2000

For patients using blood glucose testing to assess their diabetes, Becton Dickinson offers free booklets on blood glucose testing.

Becton Dickinson
Consumer Products
Franklin Lakes, NJ 07417
(800) 627-1579

Evaluation

Patient understands the basic concepts of diabetes mellitus type II and how it relates to diet, exercise, and medication.

Patient or significant others demonstrate the use of aids and materials for the visually impaired.

Patient attains and maintains ideal body weight through exercise and a nutritional regimen.

Patient's skin, legs, and feet maintain their integrity.

Skin remains supple and intact.

Legs and feet maintain sensation, are free of lesions, and are infection-free.

Hypoglycemic reactions are recognized and treated promptly. Preventive measures related to medication, diet, and/or exercise are implemented.

Table 9-1. Comparison of hypoglycemia and hyperglycemia

Hypoglycemia	Hyperglycemia
Low blood glucose	High blood glucose
Sweating	Thirsty
Pale skin	Dry flushed skin
Faintness	Nausea/vomiting
Awareness of heart beating	Diarrhea
	Dry mouth
Personality changes	Hunger
Hunger	Fast heart beat
Fast heart beat	Increased urination
Tremors/shakes	Fever
Light-headedness	Confusion
Headache	
Double vision	

Box 9-2.

Patient Education

Oral Hypoglycemic Medications

Remember to do the following while taking oral hypoglycemic medications:
- Follow your diet.
- Test your urine or blood daily.
- Take medication as directed.
- Do not take over-the-counter medications (even aspirin) without first consulting your doctor.
- Take medication prior to a meal.

Report the following side effects to your physician:
- Upset stomach
- Ringing in the ears
- Weakness
- Numbness
- Headache
- Rash
- Yellowing of the skin
- Hypoglycemic reaction

Additional instructions for the individual patient and/ or family:

Box 9-3.

Patient Education

Exercise, Rest, and Diet

Exercise on a regular basis. Walking is one exercise that costs little, requires no skill, and can be done anywhere.

Exercise only to tolerance. Do not overdo it. Build your strength and tolerance up slowly.

Follow the diet prescribed by your doctor.

It may help to join a support group to assist you in following your diet (e.g., Weight Watchers or Overeaters Anonymous).

Weigh yourself weekly and keep a record of your weight.

Additional instructions for the individual patient and/ or family:

HYPOTHYROIDISM (MYXEDEMA)

Hypothyroidism (myxedema) is a deficiency of thyroid hormones in the adult. It predominantly occurs in women in their 60s. Current research suggests that there is a large older population who have unrecognized hypothyroidism.

Primary hypothyroidism, the most common type, is believed to be the result of an autoimmune disease. It frequently occurs following Hashimoto's thyroiditis, or it may be an iatrogenic reaction to hyperthyroidism therapy.

Secondary hypothyroidism is a failure of the pituitary gland to secrete thyroid-stimulating hormone (TSH) or an insufficient secretion of thyrotropin-releasing hormone (TRH) from the hypothalamus.

▶ PATHOPHYSIOLOGY, SIGNS, AND SYMPTOMS

With an inadequate secretion of thyroid hormone, the body's metabolism, as well as mental and physical function, are slowed. The degree of severity of the disease ranges from mild myxedema with minimal symptoms to severe myxedema with life-threatening complications.

The physical appearance of the individual changes. The hair becomes dry and sparse; the face is masklike and puffy, with periorbital edema; the skin is dry and coarse and has a yellowish cast; and there is an increase in weight. Common complaints are memory loss, lethargy, fatigue, menorrhagia or amenorrhea, an inability to tolerate cold temperatures, and constipation. An acceleration of atherosclerosis and coronary artery disease is a major complication of myxedema, and acute organic psychosis (myxedema madness) may also occur.

▶ DIAGNOSTIC PROCEDURES

Laboratory tests are performed to determine levels of thyroxine (T_3), triiodothyronine (T_4), TSH, and cholesterol (Table 9-2).

▶ MEDICAL MANAGEMENT

The treatment for hypothyroidism is replacement of the thyroid hormone through therapy. Levothyroxine sodium, thyroglobulin, and liotrix are commonly available replacements.

▶ PROGNOSIS

Myxedema coma is a life-threatening complication of hypothyroidism that is commonly seen in the older person who has gone without treatment. It occurs in areas with a cold climate but rarely in warm climates. Coma is accompanied by severe hypothermia, which is followed by seizures, hypotension, respiratory depression, carbon dioxide retention, and cardiovascular collapse. If left untreated, death will ensue.

Table 9-2. Test results in hypothyroidism

Test	Primary hypothyroidism	Secondary hypothyroidism
T_3 and T_4	Decreased	Decreased
TSH	High	Low
Serum cholesterol	Increased	Low

▶ **NURSING MANAGEMENT—NURSING CARE PLAN**
  Hypothyroidism

Assessment

SUBJECTIVE DATA
Fatigue
Memory loss
Slowing of thought processes

OBJECTIVE DATA
Bradycardia
Hypotension
Arrhythmias
Weight gain
Hypothermia

	Nursing diagnoses	Expected outcomes	Nursing interventions (rationale)
N U R S I N G C A R E P L A N	Knowledge deficit regarding replacement therapy and disease process	Patient will verbalize an understanding of the disease process of hypothyroidism that will include a demonstration and interactive discussion on replacement therapy, activity level, and management of environmental stresses.	Assess the patient's knowledge of the disease process to obtain a baseline for teaching. Explain the disease process to the patient at his or her level. Teach the patient about the thyroid hormone medication. Include the name, purpose, dosage, time and route of administration, and side effects. Assist in planning an exercise program tailored to the patient's present level of fitness. Assist the patient in planning alternatives for environmental stresses such as a cold climate and/or stressful situations.
	Potential alteration in cardiac output related to coronary artery disease, decreased metabolic rate, atherosclerosis	Patient will maintain present level of cardiac output.	Assess the patient's pulse, blood pressure, and temperature to determine his or her present cardiovascular level. Monitor level of consciousness and orientation. Be alert to changes and reorient as necessary. Measure intake and output plus daily weight to evaluate fluid status. Obtain a baseline electrocardiogram to note any existing arrhythmias and to be alert to future changes. Assess respiratory status. Be alert to adventitious sounds, rapid, labored respirations, the development of an S_3 gallop, or distended neck veins.

Continued.

Nursing Care Plan—Hypothyroidism—cont'd

Nursing diagnoses	Expected outcomes	Nursing interventions (rationale)
Constipation related to decreased activity, slowed metabolic rate, and/or decreased peristalsis	Patient will be able to describe an appropriate bowel regimen, including diet, exercise, and appropriate fluid intake.	Assess elimination pattern, diet, and fluid intake to obtain a baseline of present patterns. Encourage the patient to drink at least 2 liters of fluid per day if not contraindicated by a preexisting condition. Assist patient in establishing a daily bowel routine. Provide a high-fiber, low-fat, low-calorie diet. Assess present activity level. Discuss alternating periods of rest with increasing levels of exercise to increase muscle tone and promote peristalsis. Assess for laxative abuse by questioning the patient on the frequency of use and the type and amount of laxative used.

Discharge planning and patient/family education

Arrange for outpatient follow-up by physician and/or visiting nurse.

Provide written instructions for taking medication (Box 9-4).

Tell patient to consult the doctor if any of the following occur:

Becomes out of breath on mild exertion

Feels heart beating or skipping at rest

Has large, unexplained weight gain

Experiences pain or tightness in the chest

Arrange a home health nurse referral to ensure follow through on the teaching and to assist if an impaction occurs.

Constipation is a frequent concern of individuals with hypothyroidism. Prevention is the best method of addressing this problem. Box 9-5 lists preventive methods that should be followed.

Evaluation

Patient verbalizes an understanding of the disease process of hypothyroidism.

Preventive measures related to replacement therapy, activity level, and/or environment are implemented.

Patient remains oriented to person, place, and time.

Lungs remain clear without adventitious sounds.

Heart rate and rhythm are appropriate.

Preventive measures related to constipation are implemented.

Bowel movements are regular without signs or symptoms of constipation reoccurrence.

Box 9-4.

Instructions for taking medications

The name of your medication is ——————————————————. It should be taken —————————— times a day
at the prescribed dosage of ———————————. Remember:
   Take your medication at the same time each day.
   Medication must never be discontinued without first consulting with your doctor.
   Never take an over-the-counter medication without first consulting with your doctor.

Box 9-5.

Patient Education

Preventing Constipation

Drink at least eight glasses of water a day.

Be sure you are eating enough fiber in your diet. Include fresh fruits and vegetables and whole grain breads and cereal.

Set aside a regular time during the day to go to the toilet to defecate without interruptions.

Try drinking a warm liquid to stimulate your bowels.

Plan an exercise program, for this too will stimulate your bowels.

Avoid laxatives. You can become dependent on them.

Additional instructions for the individual patient and/or family:

BREAST DISEASE

Little is known of the etiology of breast disease, but there are specific factors that indicate an increased risk to certain groups. Diseases of the breast occur predominantly in women. Heredity plays a major part, and women with a family history are at greater risk. In addition, the endocrine system influences breast lesions, as evidenced by the decreased incidence of benign breast lesions after menopause versus a sudden increase in breast cancer after menopause.

Carcinoma of the breast is a malignancy most frequently seen in the upper outer quadrant and tail of Spence. Staging of the cancer is based on lymph node involvement, metastases, and the extent of the primary lesion.

▶ PATHOPHYSIOLOGY, SIGNS, AND SYMPTOMS

A painless, palpable mass is usually the first sign of cancer of the breast. It is usually hard, nonmobile, slow growing, and irregular in shape. Other signs are nipple retraction, enlarged lymph nodes, discharge from the nipple, breast edema, change in contour, and an orange-peel appearance of the breast.

▶ DIAGNOSTIC PROCEDURES

A conclusive diagnosis can be made only by microscopic examination of the involved tissue obtained by biopsy. Breast self-examination, mammography, and thermography assist in identifying the lesion.

▶ MEDICAL MANAGEMENT

Radiotherapy—can be used for local control and also as a palliative treatment for recurrent cancer.
Hormonal manipulation—may be used in combination with radiotherapy and/or surgery; also used in palliative treatment and in delaying advancement of the cancer
Cytotoxic chemotherapy—used as a prophylactic measure after surgery for those at risk for recurrent cancer; also used with those having recurrence of the breast cancer
Surgical interventions are as follows:
Partial mastectomy (lumpectomy)—removal of the tumor and approximately 1 inch of tissue surrounding the lesion; performed when lesion is small and peripherally located
Simple mastectomy (total mastectomy)—removal if lesion is confined to the breast without lymph node involvement
Modified radical mastectomy—removal of the breast and pectoralis minor muscle, with axillary dissection; performed when the lesion is localized
Conventional radical mastectomy—removal of the breast, pectoral muscle, and adjacent tissue, with axillary dissection; performed when lesion has significant infiltrate
Extended radical mastectomy—removal of the breast and pectoral muscles, axillary dissection, and removal of the upper internal mammary lymph node chain; performed when lesion is in an area where it will spread to the upper internal mammary lymph node chain, such as in the medial quadrant

▶ PROGNOSIS

The prognosis is dependent on the cancer staging. Without lymph node involvement, survival time is lengthened by surgical intervention. With lymph node involvement and/or systemic spread, the treatment is palliative.

▶ **NURSING MANAGEMENT—NURSING CARE PLAN**
Breast Disease

Assessment
SUBJECTIVE DATA
A nontender mass
OBJECTIVE DATA
A palpable lump

Nipple discharge
Enlarged lymph nodes
Distorted contour of the breast

	Nursing diagnoses	Expected outcomes	Nursing interventions (rationale)
N U R S I N G C A R E P L A N	Knowledge deficit related to screening and management of breast disease	Patient will verbalize an understanding of breast disease that will include a demonstration and interactive discussion on breast self-examination and the importance of routine mammography.	Assess the patient's ability and willingness to learn breast self-examination. (A patient with severe arthritis may not be able to perform self-examination because of limited dexterity. In this case discuss alternatives, e.g., significant others.) Teach how to perform a breast self-examination and what a mass feels like. Discuss the American Cancer Society recommendations for frequency of breast self-examination. Discuss the American Cancer Society recommendations for frequency of mammography.
	Body image disturbance related to mastectomy	Patient will verbalize the importance of breasts to her sexual image and describe ways to enhance her appearance, such as a prosthesis, clothing, and reconstructive surgery.	Explore with patient the significance of her breasts to her sexual image. Discuss fears she may have in relation to her significant other. Discuss the different types of prostheses available, where they can be purchased, and the price. Provide pictures of clothing that would be comfortable and attractive, yet provide a natural look. Explore the possibility of reconstructive surgery with the patient, including her thoughts and feelings on the surgery.

Discharge planning and patient/family education
Arrange for outpatient follow-up examination by physician.
Patient should have an annual mammography after age 50.
Patient should perform monthly breast self-examination (Box 9-6).
Refer the patient to Reach to Recovery, a program sponsored by the American Cancer Society. It provides a *support network and resources for the individual with breast cancer.*

Evaluation
Patient states the overall concepts of breast disease.
Patient performs breast self-examination monthly.
Patient has mammography annually.
Patient discusses the sexual importance of her breasts, and ways to improve her physical appearance are implemented.

Box 9-6.

Patient Education

Breast Self-Examination

Select a day that is easy to remember when the examination can be performed. It is recommended that breast self-examination be performed once a month. If you are still having periods, the recommended time is 1 week after your period begins.

Use a mirror in which you have full view of both breasts.

First examine your breasts in four positions:
    Arms at your side
    Hands on hips with muscle flexion
    Arms above the head
    Leaning over at the waist

Look for any skin changes, dimpling, size and contour differences in your breasts.

Next palpate your breasts one at a time with the arm on the palpated side placed over your head. In a circular motion, start from the outer portion under the arm and rotate inward, noting any lumps.

Palpate the nipple and try to express any fluid.

Additional instructions for the individual patient and/or family:

ANEMIA

Anemia is a symptom of multiple diseases that is demonstrated by laboratory findings of decreased red blood cells (RBCs), hemoglobin (Hb), and/or hematocrit (Hct). Anemias are classified by their mean corpuscular volume (MCV) and mean corpuscular hemoglobin (MCH). Microcytic anemia is an MCV of <80, normocytic is an MCV between 80 and 94, and macrocytic is an MCV of >94. Hypochromic anemia is an MCH of <27, normochromic is an MCH between 27 and 32, and hyperchromic is an MCH of >32. Iron-deficiency anemia is a hypochromic microcytic anemia, hypoplastic (aplastic) anemia is a normochromic normocytic anemia, and vitamin B_{12} deficiency (pernicious anemia) is a megaloblastic anemia. The etiology of these three anemias is as follows:

Iron-deficiency anemia is the result of a need for iron, usually due to chronic blood loss.

Aplastic (hypoplastic) anemia is a panhypoplasia of the bone marrow that is commonly idiopathic but can be the result of a chemical agent, radiation, or drugs.

Pernicious anemia is the result of a vitamin B_{12} deficiency due the atropic gastric mucosa not secreting intrinsic factor.

▶ PATHOPHYSIOLOGY, SIGNS, AND SYMPTOMS

The signs and symptoms associated with anemia are the result of hypoxia to the tissues and are identical regardless of the type of anemia involved. The cardiovascular and pulmonary systems try to compensate for the hypoxia. As a result the following symptoms appear: fatigue, headache, pallor, dyspnea, tinnitus, irritability, and unusual or bizarre behavior.

▶ DIAGNOSTIC PROCEDURES

Diagnosis is made on the basis of laboratory findings. The following are laboratory changes associated with each classification of the anemia:

Iron-deficiency anemia—Hct is low; Hgb is low; MCH, MCH concentration, and MCV are all reduced; serum iron is low; iron binding capacity is elevated; serum ferritin is low; erythrocyte count is reduced.

Aplastic anemia (hypoplastic)—MCV is borderline high; platelets are decreased; reticulocytes are decreased; serum iron is increased; erythrocyte count is less than 1 million/mm^3; leukocyte count is low (less than 2000/mm^3).

Pernicious anemia—Serum iron is increased; MCV is >100; Schilling test shows inappropriate urine excretion of B_{12}, indicating an intrinsic factor deficit; radioisotopic assay is <150 pg/ml; erythrocyte count is less than 3 million/mm^3; bone marrow biopsy shows an increase of megaloblasts; serum bilirubin is increased; there is a positive response to a therapeutic trial of vitamin B_{12}.

▶ MEDICAL MANAGEMENT

Iron-deficiency anemia—ferrous sulfate or ferrous gluconate, 300 mg orally; parenteral iron therapy if oral therapy is unsuccessful

Aplastic (hypoplastic) anemia—bone marrow transplant

Pernicious anemia—monthly intramuscular injections of vitamin B_{12}

▶ PROGNOSIS

The prognosis varies according to the type of anemia involved. For iron-deficiency anemia, the outcome depends on the identification and correction of the underlying cause. Pernicious anemia requires monthly injections of B_{12} for the rest of the patient's life. Aplastic anemia has a high mortality rate with serious complications of hemorrhage and infection.

▶ **NURSING MANAGEMENT—NURSING CARE PLAN**
Anemia

Assessment

SUBJECTIVE DATA
Fatigue
Headache
Dizziness
Behavior change
Irritability

OBJECTIVE DATA
Decrease in RBCs
Decrease in Hct and Hgb

	Nursing diagnoses	Expected outcomes	Nursing interventions (rationale)
N U R S I N G C A R E P L A N	Knowledge deficit related to the disease process of anemia and therapy required	Patient will verbalize an understanding of the disease process of anemia that will include an interactive discussion on therapy required to correct the anemia.	Assess the patient's knowledge level and ability to learn. Discuss the major concepts of the disease process of anemia. Teach the patient about the specific medication needed for the particular type of anemia. If the patient has pernicious anemia, emphasize that vitamin B_{12} must be taken for life. Discuss the signs and symptoms that indicate medical intervention is necessary.
	Altered nutrition: less than body requirements, related to fatigue and anorexia	Patient will maintain weight through eating a nutritional diet.	Monitor intake to ensure that patient is eating a well-balanced diet. Provide small, frequent meals to avoid overdistension of the stomach. Check weight daily to ensure that patient is maintaining weight and obtaining sufficient calories. Assist patient with oral hygiene to improve food taste. Provide for a pleasant environment to increase food desire.
	Activity intolerance related to tissue hypoxia	Patient will be able to perform desired activities.	Assess present activity level and response to it. Evaluate vital signs at rest and immediately after activity to assess response to the activity. Alternate rest periods with periods of activity. Assist with activities of daily living to conserve energy. Take safety precautions by having patient sit at edge of the bed before standing and walking so as to prevent falls. Gradually increase the activity to the patient's tolerance level.

Discharge planning and patient/family education
See leukemia care plan.

Evaluation
See leukemia care plan.

LEUKEMIA

Leukemia is a neoplastic disease characterized by a proliferation of leukocytes and their precursors. There are several types of leukemia, but chronic lymphocytic leukemia (CLL) is the leukemia seen late in life, usually after 50 years of age. It occurs more commonly in men than in women.

▶ PATHOPHYSIOLOGY, SIGNS, AND SYMPTOMS

Chronic lymphocytic leukemia is specifically characterized by an accumulation of mature lymphocytes in the circulating blood and lymphoid tissues, including the lymph nodes, bone marrow, liver, and spleen. It has an insidious onset, and the individual is often asymptomatic for years. Many times the disease is detected on routine blood work. Early symptoms are fatigue with exercise intolerance, anorexia, and weight loss. Early signs are lymph node enlargement and bone marrow infiltration with progression to lymphocytes in the blood. Anemia and thrombocytopenia result from the bone marrow involvement. Splenomegaly and hepatomegaly occur as a result of the accumulation of white blood cells in the liver and spleen. Hypogammaglobulinemia is seen late in the disease, accompanied by a decreased resistance to infection.

▶ DIAGNOSTIC PROCEDURES

Diagnosis is based on the following findings:
   Leukocyte count—elevated

Differential WBC count—small lymphocytes
Platelets—low
Bone marrow biopsy—hypercellular with lymphocytes predominating
Blood smear—many blast cells
RBC count—low
Other—hemolytic anemia, hypogammaglobulinemia

▶ MEDICAL MANAGEMENT

Medical management of chronic lymphocytic leukemia is palliative. Intervention does not begin until active progression of the disease is present. The agents used in chemotherapy of chronic lymphocytic leukemia are chlorambucil, cyclophosphamide, triethylenemelamine, and prednisone. Radiation therapy provides symptomatic relief of splenomegaly, hepatomegaly, and lymphadenopathy. Blood components are used to temporarily correct anemia.

▶ PROGNOSIS

The course of the disease is progressive in nature. Remissions following therapy will increase survival time. The prognosis is worse for those in the later stages of the disease, with secondary infection being the usual cause of death.

▶ **NURSING MANAGEMENT—NURSING CARE PLAN**
Leukemia

Assessment

SUBJECTIVE DATA
Fatigue
Weight loss
Exercise intolerance

OBJECTIVE DATA
Anemia
Splenomegaly
Hepatomegaly
Lymphadenopathy

	Nursing diagnoses	Expected outcomes	Nursing interventions (rationale)
N U R S I N G C A R E P L A N	Knowledge deficit related to the disease process and indicators signifying progression of the disease, especially in the asymptomatic person	Patient will verbalize an understanding of the disease process of leukemia that will include an interactive discussion on indicators of disease progression and a need for health care evaluation.	Assess individual's learning needs, ability to learn, and factors that would influence learning. Teach the importance of regular periodic examinations by a health care professional. Integrate examining the patient and teaching self-examination. Be sure to do the following: Inspect the skin and mucous membranes for bleeding, petechiae, ecchymosis, hematoma formation, purpura, signs and symptoms of a skin infection. Palpate the lymph nodes for lymphadenopathy. Palpate the liver and spleen for enlargement. Palpate bones and joints for pain, tenderness, and/or swelling.
	Potential for infection related to hypogammaglobulinemia	Patient will describe signs and symptoms of respiratory infection, skin infection, urinary tract infection, and preventive measures.	Check the blood work. Consult with physician about prophylactic doses of γ-globulin for patients with low γ-globulin levels. Administer appropriate antibiotics on the basis of culture and sensitivity. Emphasize oral and personal hygiene to avoid infection. Place patient in reverse isolation during times of susceptibility. Examine patient for signs of infection. Administer blood transfusions as ordered when replacement is needed. Evaluate vital signs for evidence of infection. Teach patient the signs and symptoms of respiratory infection, skin infection, and urinary tract infection.

Nursing Care Plan—Leukemia—cont'd		
Nursing diagnoses	**Expected outcomes**	**Nursing interventions (rationale)**
Potential for injury related to bleeding and hemolytic anemia from thrombocytopenia	Injury will be avoided and preventive measures will be implemented.	Assess patient for areas of bleeding. Check all body orifices, mucous membranes, and skin. Monitor and evaluate blood work. Note especially a low platelet count, which indicates greater susceptibility to bleeding. Check catheter and IV sites frequently for bleeding. Administer blood transfusion as needed for replacement of blood components. Instruct patient on safety precautions such as using a soft toothbrush, avoiding falls, and using an electric razor.

Discharge planning and patient/family education

Arrange for outpatient follow-up by physician and/or visiting nurse.

Teach patient about iron therapy (Box 9-7).

Consult with dietitian to ensure addressing patient's food preferences as well as obtaining a balanced diet.

It is important for the patient to eat a diet with foods high in iron, vitamins, and protein and to monitor weight to ensure intake of the appropriate number of calories.

Help patient set up an activity schedule so that activities and rest periods can be planned.

The patient should be prepared to adjust his or her schedule so that energy can be conserved.

Tell the patient to sit on the side of the bed for a few minutes before rising if dizziness is experienced.

If overly tired, patient should take a few minutes to rest and not overexert.

Have patient contact the doctor if any of the following changes are noticed:

General—fatigue, out of breath, awareness of heart beating, fainting spells, headache, loss of appetite, fever, flulike symptoms

Skin—small purplish spots, nose bleed, blood in the stool or urine, bleeding gums, bruising

Pain in the bones or joints

Instruct patient on the importance of taking antibiotic as directed.

Teach self-examination of the skin.

Review methods of avoiding infection (Box 9-8).

Emphasize the importance of periodic examination and blood work by a health care professional.

Evaluation

Patient verbalizes an understanding of the disease process of anemia and the therapy required to correct the problem.

Patient's weight is maintained.

Patient performs desired activities without dyspnea, fatigue, or tachycardia.

Patient understands the basic concepts of chronic lymphocytic leukemia and states the indicators of disease progression that warrant health care evaluation.

Patient describes signs and symptoms of infection and methods of prevention.

No injury has occurred. Preventive measures are implemented.

Box 9-7.

Patient Education

Iron Therapy

Iron is best absorbed on an empty stomach. Take it between meals. If you get an upset stomach, take it with food.

The iron medication will change the color of your stool to a dark-green or black color.

Even though you start to feel better, continue to take your iron medication until told to stop.

Certain items decrease the absorption of iron. Avoid taking milk, tea, coffee, eggs, and antacids at the same time as your iron (wait at least 1 hour).

Ascorbic acid enhances the absorption of iron. Try eating an orange with your iron.

Additional instructions for the individual patient and/or family:

Box 9-8.

Patient Education

Avoiding Infection

Avoid situations where you are likely to be exposed to disease or infection, such as crowds or visits by grandchildren with colds.

Eat a well-balanced diet.

Contact your doctor at the first signs of any type of infection—urinary tract infection, respiratory infection, skin infection, etc.

As a preventive measure, be sure to obtain a yearly flu vaccination.

Do not overexert yourself. Alternate periods of activity with rest periods.

Arrange furniture for easy maneuverability.

Additional instructions for the individual patient and/or family:

BIBLIOGRAPHY

Ebersol P and Hess P (1985). Toward healthy aging: Human needs and nursing response. St Louis, The CV Mosby Co.

Herget M and Williams A (1989). New aids for low-vision diabetics, Am J Nurs. 89(10):1319-1322.

Hull M (1989). How to set up a diabetes education program, RN 52(11):61-64.

Huzar J (1989). Diabetes now: Preventing acute complications, RN 52(8):34-40.

Robertson C (1989). Coping with chronic complications, RN 52(9):34-38, 40, 42-43.

Thompson J, McFarland G, Hirsch J, et al (1989). Mosby's manual of clinical nursing, ed 2, St Louis, The CV Mosby Co.

CHAPTER 10

Gastrointestinal System

Mildred O. Hogstel

Older adults have many chronic conditions that affect the gastrointestinal system. Some of them, constipation for example, are more bothersome than dangerous. Others, like periodontal disease, can be prevented if proper dental and mouth care is consistent. Even cancers of the gastrointestinal tract, if diagnosed and treated early, often have a good prognosis. The gastrointestinal problems that are most common in older adults are listed in Table 10-1.

PERIODONTAL DISEASE

Although there are some people in their late 90s and early 100s who still have all of their teeth, the majority of persons over the age of 65 have lost teeth as a result of periodontal or gum disease (commonly called pyorrhea). Most of these older people did not have the advantage of proper care when they were children and young adults, so it was an expectation that they would need dentures in later life. However, original teeth are meant to last a lifetime. People should never have to lose their teeth if

proper care is maintained throughout life (for example, brushing, flossing, seeing a dentist regularly, and using fluoridated water). Functioning teeth are essential to adequate nutrition, which is so important in maintaining good health in old age, and to a positive self-concept related to appearance.

▶ PATHOPHYSIOLOGY, SIGNS, AND SYMPTOMS

Inadequate cleansing of the teeth causes the accumulation of plaque, which is a greater problem as a person ages. Bacteria in the plaque irritate the gums. Without treatment, infection forms between the teeth and gums. The gums recede and the infection spreads to the roots of the teeth, which become loose and fall out or have to be extracted. The most common signs and symptoms of periodontal disease are the following:

    Bleeding gums
    Swollen gums
    Inflamed (red) gums
    Pus between gums and teeth
    Sensitive gums
    Painful gums
    Receding gum line (gum pulling away from bottom of tooth)
    Loose teeth
    Lost teeth

▶ DIAGNOSTIC PROCEDURES

A careful examination and assessment of the mouth, teeth, and gums by a qualified dentist will determine the presence and degree of periodontal disease.

▶ MEDICAL MANAGEMENT

The primary goal is to prevent periodontal disease through the following:

Table 10-1. Common gastrointestinal problems of older adults

System affected	Condition
Upper gastrointestinal tract	Periodontal disease
	Oral cancer
	Hiatal hernia
	Cancer of the stomach
Lower gastrointestinal tract	Cancer of the colon
	Diverticulosis
	Constipation
	Fecal incontinence

Brushing the teeth at least two times a day
Flossing well at least every 24 hours
Having the teeth professionally cleaned at least every
   6 months
Drinking fluoridated water (most water supplies con-
   tain fluoride)
Using toothpaste that contains fluoride
Using an antibacterial or antiplaque mouth rinse
If periodontal disease has progressed to involve several
of the teeth so that bleeding, infection, and receding gums
are present, a prophylactic program can still be insti-
tuted. Sometimes the pockets around the teeth in which

the bacteria collect can be eliminated by surgery. But
once the roots are involved and the teeth are loose, there
are few options except to extract the involved teeth and
replace them with a bridge, a partial plate, full dentures,
or possibly dental implants if the bone structure is sat-
isfactory. Dental implants can be used to replace only
one tooth or all of the teeth.

▶ PROGNOSIS

The prognosis is good with early treatment and a con-
sistent preventive program. If the disease is in the late
stages, the teeth will most likely be lost.

▶ NURSING MANAGEMENT—NURSING CARE PLAN
Periodontal Disease

Assessment

SUBJECTIVE DATA

"My gums are sore and bleed."
"I haven't taken care of my teeth like I should have."

OBJECTIVE DATA

Bleeding gums
Receding gums
Loose teeth

	Nursing diagnoses	Expected outcomes	Nursing interventions (rationale)
N U R S I N G C A R E P L A N	Altered nutrition: less than body requirements, related to inability to chew because of painful, loose, or missing teeth	Patient will be able to eat 100% of all three meals each day.	Assess food preferences. Provide preferred foods that are easy to chew and swallow (ground and chopped but not pureed).
		Patient will eat foods from the four major food groups and all six essential nutrients each day.	Provide foods from the four major food groups and the six essential nutrients each day. Observe, evaluate, and record the amount and type of foods eaten.
	Body image disturbance related to distortion of the mouth due to loss of teeth	Patient will see a dentist for evaluation and treatment of dental problems.	Provide the names of several dentists if the patient does not have a dentist. Arrange for transportation and financial assistance if needed.
		Patient will follow the dentist's treatment plan.	Teach patient about dental and mouth care (brushing, flossing, rinsing). Teach patient about the need for following the dentist's suggestions.
		Patient will lose no more teeth and will obtain partial dentures if needed.	Teach patient care of dentures (safety, cleansing, storing).

Discharge planning and patient/family education
Give the patient the following printed materials to take
home:
Taking Care of Your Teeth and Mouth, Age Page, Na-
   tional Institute on Aging, National Institute of Dental
   Research (Box 10-1)
Dental Outlook-Keeping a Healthy Mouth—Tips for
   Older Adults, W160 9-152/12.89R, American Dental

Association, Division of Communications, 211 East
Chicago Ave, Chicago, IL 60611
Evaluation
Patient eats an adequate nutritious diet daily.
The remaining teeth are free of gum disease (no pain,
   swelling, bleeding).
A partial plate has been fitted where teeth had been lost.
Patient smiles freely and feels good about self.

Box 10-1.

Taking care of your teeth and mouth

A healthy smile is a bonus at any age. Too often older people—especially those who wear dentures or false teeth—feel they no longer need dental checkups. Because the idea of preventive dental care dates back to the 1950s, many people over age 65 have not grown up with the idea of preventive care of the teeth.

If you haven't learned the basic elements of good oral health, it is not too late to start. And even if you have, it's a good time to be reminded.

Tooth decay (cavities)

Tooth decay is not just a disease of children; it can continue throughout life as long as natural teeth are in the mouth. Tooth decay is caused by bacteria that normally live in the mouth. The bacteria stick to teeth and form a sticky, colorless film called dental plaque. The bacteria in plaque, which live on sugars, produce decay-causing acids that dissolve minerals in the tooth surfaces. In the presence of gum disease, tooth decay can develop on the exposed roots of the teeth.

Research has shown that adding fluoride to the water supply is the best and least costly way to prevent tooth decay. Just as with children, fluoride is important for adult teeth. In addition to drinking fluoridated water, the use of fluoride toothpastes and mouth rinses can add protection. Fluoride mouth rinses are available in two different strengths, one for daily use and one for weekly use. Daily fluoride rinses can be bought without prescription. Your dentist or dental hygienist may give you regular fluoride treatments in the dental office or prescribe a fluoride gel or mouth rinse for use at home.

Periodontal (gum) disease

Periodontitis, a common cause of tooth loss after age 35, is caused by buildup of plaque. If plaque is not removed from the teeth every day it may harden into calculus (tartar)—a substance which only your dentist or dental hygienist can remove. Bacteria in plaque can irritate the gums which become inflamed and bleed easily. If left untreated, the disease gets worse as pockets of infection form between the teeth and gums, causing the gums to recede. The infection spreads toward the roots of the teeth and, eventually, teeth become loose and are lost.

To prevent gum disease it is important to remove plaque thoroughly by brushing and flossing your teeth each day. Also, by carefully checking your teeth and gums, you may find early signs such as red, swollen, or bleeding gums. Be sure to see your dentist at once if these signs are present.

Cleaning your teeth and gums

An important part of good oral health care is knowing how to brush and floss properly. Careful daily brushing removes plaque (containing disease-causing bacteria) which routinely forms on the teeth. Gently brush the teeth on all sides with a soft-bristle brush and fluoride toothpaste. Use circular and short back and forth strokes, taking special care to brush carefully along the gum line. Lightly brushing your tongue also helps to remove plaque and food debris and makes your mouth feel fresh.

In addition to toothbrushing, the use of dental floss is necessary to keep the gums healthy. Proper flossing is especially important because it removes plaque and left over food that a toothbrush cannot reach. Your dentist or dental hygienist can show you the best way to brush and floss your teeth. If toothbrushing or flossing results in bleeding, pain, or irritation, see your dentist at once.

A new antibacterial or antiplaque mouth rinse is now available. This mouth rinse is an addition to but not a substitute for a trip to the dentist's office and careful daily brushing and flossing. Your dentist may prescribe this rinse for you.

Some people with arthritis or other conditions that limit motion may find it hard to hold a toothbrush. To overcome this, the brush handle can be attached to the hand with a wide elastic band or may be enlarged by attaching it to a sponge, styrofoam ball, or similar object. Those with limited shoulder movement might find brushing easier if the handle of the brush is lengthened by attaching a long piece of wood or plastic. Electric toothbrushes are of benefit to many.

Other conditions of the mouth

Xerostomia (dry mouth), which makes you feel thirsty or feel the need to sip liquids frequently, is common in many adults. It may cause difficulty in eating, swallowing, tasting, and speaking. Dry mouth is usually caused by salivary glands failing to function properly. This is a side effect of many medications and certain medical treatments and also can accompany emotional or physical problems. Dry mouth can affect oral health by contributing to tooth decay and gum disease. If you think you have dry mouth, talk with your dentist or physician. To relieve the dryness, drink extra water and avoid sugary snacks, caffeinated beverages, tobacco, and alcohol, which can increase dryness of the mouth.

Some kinds of cancer therapies, such as radiation to the head and neck and chemotherapy, can cause tooth decay, sores, and painful gums. These problems may develop because of a decrease in saliva. It is important that you see a dentist and finish any necessary dental work before beginning radiation treatments to the head and neck region. Severe tooth decay which results from reduced saliva flow during cancer therapy can be prevented by good plaque removal practices and the daily use of a fluoride gel.

From U.S. Department of Health and Human Services, Public Health Service, National Institutes of Health.

Box 10-1.

Taking care of your teeth and mouth—cont'd

Mouth cancer often goes unnoticed in its early and curable stages. This is true in part because many older people do not visit their dentists often enough and because pain is not an early symptom of the disease. If you notice any red or white spots or sores in the mouth that bleed or do not go away within 2 weeks, be sure to have them checked by a dentist. Regular checkups not only help keep a healthy mouth, but are necessary for the early discovery of oral cancer.

Dentures

If you have dentures (false teeth), you should keep them clean and free from food deposits that can cause permanent staining, bad breath, and gum irritation. Once a day, brush all surfaces of the dentures with a denture-care product. Remove your dentures from your mouth and place them in water or a denture-cleansing liquid while you sleep. It is also helpful to rinse your mouth with a warm salt-water solution in the morning, after meals, and at bedtime.

Partial dentures should be cared for in the same way as full dentures. Because bacteria tend to collect under the clasps of partial dentures, it is especially important that this area be cleaned thoroughly.

Dentures will seem awkward at first. When learning to eat with false teeth, you should select soft, nonsticky food. Cut food into small pieces, and chew slowly using both sides of the mouth. Dentures tend to make your mouth less sensitive to hot foods and liquids and less able to detect the presence of harmful objects such as bones. If problems in eating, talking, or simply wearing dentures continue after the first few weeks, your dentist may be able to make proper adjustments.

In time, dentures need to be replaced or readjusted to the changes in the tissues of the mouth that may have occurred over time. Do not try to repair dentures at home, as this can damage the dentures and injure the tissues of the mouth.

Dental implants

Dental implants are designed to look like teeth and are surgically inserted through the gum surface to rest on or within the bone of the jaw. Implants are useful only for patients with enough bone structure. Thus, if you are considering having an implant, it is important that you select an experienced dental specialist with whom you can discuss your concerns to be sure the procedure is right for you.

Professional care

In addition to practicing good oral hygiene at home, it is important to have regular dental checkups—whether you have natural teeth or dentures. It is also important to follow through with any special treatments which may be necessary to ensure oral health care. For instance, if you have sensitive teeth caused by receding gums, your dentist may suggest that you use a special toothpaste for a few months. Teeth are meant to last a lifetime. By using the right preventive measures you can protect your teeth and gums for years to come.

Additional dental health information

Although general dentists take care of the dental needs of most older people, some dentists have a special interest in the care of geriatric patients. The American Society for Geriatric Dentistry, 1121 W Michigan St, Indianapolis, IN 46202, has the names and addresses of several hundred such dentists.

For information on dental research and general dental care write to the National Institute of Dental Research, Building 31, Room 2C-35, Bethesda, MD 20892. For information on general dental care write to the American Dental Association, 211 E Chicago Avenue, Chicago IL 60611.

The National Institute of Dental Research publications include:

Dry Mouth (Xerostomia)
Fever Blisters and Canker Sores
Fluoride to Protect the Teeth of Adults
Periodontal Disease and Diabetes
Periodontal (Gum) Disease
Rx for Sound Teeth
Tooth Decay

ORAL CANCER

The most common types of oral cancer in older adults are included in Chapter 4.

HIATAL HERNIA

Hiatal hernia, sometimes referred to as diaphragmatic hernia, is a herniation of part of the stomach up through the esophageal opening in the diaphragm. It is especially common in obese older females. There are estimates that more than 50% of women over age 65 have some degree of the condition.

▶ **PATHOPHYSIOLOGY, SIGNS, AND SYMPTOMS**

The primary cause is a structural weakness of the muscles in the diaphragm around the esophagogastric opening. Other contributing factors are "obesity, pregnancy, ascites, tumors, tight corsets, . . . heavy lifting on a con-

tinual basis . . . increased age, trauma, poor nutrition, . . . a forced recumbent position . . . congenital weakness" (Elrod, 1987, pp. 963, 965). Stress may also be a predisposing factor.

Symptoms experienced by patients with hiatal hernia may include the following:

Burning in the epigastrium, especially after eating a full meal and/or spicy foods

Heartburn when lying down or bending over after eating, drinking alcohol, or smoking

Dysphagia, painful swallowing

Regurgitation (bitter or sour taste in mouth from stomach contents)

Some patients with hiatal hernia do not have any symptoms. Others have symptoms that are similar to those experienced with gallbladder disease, peptic ulcer, or angina (Elrod, 1987, p. 965).

▶ DIAGNOSTIC PROCEDURES

Fluoroscopy or x-ray of the upper gastrointestinal tract while swallowing a barium solution is the primary method of diagnosis. Esophagoscopy may also be performed. It is important to rule out other diseases of the esophagus and stomach such as peptic ulcer and carcinoma.

▶ MEDICAL MANAGEMENT

Medical management is primarily conservative and includes having the patient do the following:

Avoid eating large meals and highly seasoned or fatty foods (five small meals a day are better than three large meals).

Avoid any foods that cause regurgitation.

Do not eat within 2 hours before going to bed. (Because the incidence of hiatal hernia is very high in older adults and often not diagnosed, no older adult should lie down for at least 1 hour after eating.)

Sleep with the head of the bed raised at least 6 inches. (An electric or mechanical bed may be purchased or blocks can be placed under the head of the bed.)

Limit alcohol intake and smoking.

Do not wear tight clothes.

Avoid lifting and straining.

If obese, lose weight.

Take medications if needed (e.g., antacids, Gaviscon)

Surgery is usually not performed but may be necessary if severe complications occur such as "stenosis, strangulation, chronic esophagitis, or bleeding" (Elrod, 1987, p. 966).

▶ PROGNOSIS

The prognosis is good if the patient follows the physician's suggestions for controlling symptoms. If surgery is necessary, the usual complications of abdominal or thoracic surgery are possible. Some dietary restrictions are necessary even after successful surgery.

▶ NURSING MANAGEMENT—NURSING CARE PLAN
Hiatal Hernia

Assessment

SUBJECTIVE DATA

"I have this burning in the pit of my stomach after I eat."

"Sometimes I have trouble swallowing."

OBJECTIVE DATA

Obese female over age 65

Patient's hand pressing on stomach

N U R S I N G C A R E P L A N	Nursing diagnoses	Expected outcomes	Nursing interventions (rationale)
	Altered nutrition: potential for more than body requirements, related to stress in life situation	Patient will maintain or obtain body weight appropriate for age, height, and build.	Assess food and fluid intake. Weigh weekly. Teach patient about weight reduction diet if needed. Help to determine reasons for stress. Recommend stress reduction methods (counseling, biofeedback).
	Health-seeking behaviors (relief from symptoms of hiatal hernia) related to present abdominal discomforts	Patient will be able to state definition, causes, and methods of relieving discomforts of hiatal hernia. Patient will follow recommendations to relieve discomforts.	Teach patient about hiatal hernia (definition, causes, treatment). Recommend methods of relieving discomfort (Box 10-2).

Discharge planning and patient/family education
Teach the patient about hiatal hernia and how to live with it (see Box 10-2).
Give the client printed information on digestive do's and don'ts (Box 10-3).
Evaluation
Patient obtains (maintains) normal weight.

Stress has been reduced.
Patient can discuss definition, causes, and treatment of hiatal hernia.
Patient experiences minimal discomfort from hiatal hernia.

Box 10-2.

Patient Education

Methods to Relieve Discomforts Caused by Hiatal Hernia

Eat five small meals a day instead of three large ones.

Eat slowly.

Avoid the following foods and fluids:

Spices	Coffee
Fat	Tea
Alcohol	Orange juice
Chocolate	Colas
Caffeine	

Lose weight if needed.

Do not lie down for 2 to 3 hours after eating.

Elevate head of bed at least 6 inches.

Do not wear tight clothes.

Do not bend over after eating.

Avoid lifting and straining.

Do not smoke.

Reduce emotional stress.

Take an antacid after meals if needed.

Additional instructions for the individual patient and/or family:

Box 10-3.

Digestive do's and don'ts

The digestive system performs the amazing task of breaking down the food you eat into the nutrients your body needs. Most of the time this system stays remarkably free of trouble. As you grow older, however, your body begins to work less efficiently in some ways and your lifestyle may change. As a result, you may occasionally have a digestive problem.

During the chemical process of digestion, food is broken down into pieces tiny enough to be taken into the blood. The blood, in turn, carries these food elements to cells in all parts of the body where they are changed into energy or used to form new structures.

Many body organs are involved in the process of digestion: the esophagus, stomach, pancreas, gallbladder, liver, small intestine, and colon. Most people have few, if any, digestive problems related to aging. Changes that may occur are usually minor and include slower action of the muscles of the digestive system and reduced acid production in some people. Both of these events can affect how fast food travels through the system, slowing down digestion. It is important to remember, however, that this usually does not lead to problems.

Changes in lifestyle can interfere with the workings of the digestive system. Such lifestyle changes include increased use of medicines, reduced exercise, and changes in eating habits.

The digestive system

Digestion begins in the mouth. As you chew your food, tiny glands give off a fluid, saliva, which lubricates food so that it can be swallowed easily. Saliva also contains an enzyme which begins to change carbohydrates—like vegetables and breads—into a form the body can absorb. Once the food is swallowed, peristaltic (wavelike) motions push it through the esophagus and into the stomach. Stomach muscles crush and mix the food with enzymes and acids, creating a mixture called chyme. The stomach allows small amounts of the chyme to enter the duodenum, the first part of the small intestine. The stomach holds the rest of the chyme until the duodenum is ready to receive it. It is in the duodenum that most digestion takes place. There, juices from the liver and pancreas break down fats, protein, and carbohydrates. As the digested food passes into the last two thirds of the small intestine, nutrients are absorbed into the blood. The remaining material is pushed into the colon, part of the large intestine. This material includes water and waste—the part of food that is not digested, such as fiber from fruits, vegetables, and grains. The lining of the colon absorbs water from the material and, when the waste is solid enough, nerves in the wall of the large intestine signal the urge for a bowel movement.

Taking care of the system

You can take the following steps to keep your digestive system working at its best:

- Eat a well-balanced diet that includes a variety of fresh fruits, vegetables, and whole grain breads, cereals, and other grain products.
- Eat slowly and, whenever possible, try to relax for 30 minutes after each meal.
- Exercise regularly.
- Drink alcohol in moderation, if at all.
- Avoid large amounts of caffeine.
- Use caution when taking over-the-counter medications and always follow your doctor's directions exactly when taking prescribed medications.

When to see a doctor

No matter how well you treat your digestive system, there are times when things go wrong. Often the problem will take care of itself. Sometimes, however, symptoms can be a signal that something more serious is wrong. Some important warning signs are the following:
- Stomach pains that are severe, last a long time, are recurring, or come with shaking, chills, and cold, clammy skin.
- Blood in vomit or recurrent vomiting.

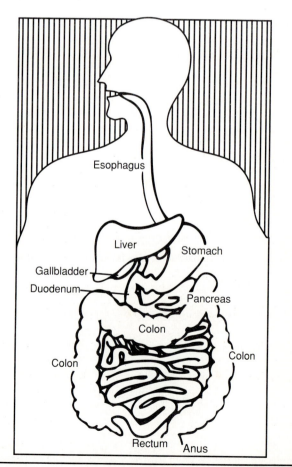

From U.S. Department of Health and Human Services, Public Health Service, National Institutes of Health.

Digestive do's and don'ts—cont'd

- A sudden change in bowel habits and consistency of stools lasting more than a few days (for example, diarrhea for more than 3 days or the sudden onset of constipation).
- Blood in stools or coal-black stools.
- Jaundice (a yellowing of the skin and the whites of the eyes) or dark, tea-colored urine.
- Pain or difficulty in swallowing food.
- Continuing loss of appetite or unexpected weight loss.
- Diarrhea that wakes you up at night.

If you have any of these symptoms, see a doctor at once.

Digestive diseases

Disorders of the digestive tract cause more hospital admissions than any other group of diseases. They occur most often in people who are middle-aged or older.

Digestive problems can result from such things as infection, defects present at birth, certain diseases, poisons, and stress. But the causes of many digestive diseases are unknown. There is evidence that diet may be involved in a few of them. For example, low intake of fiber (the part of the plant that is not digested) is thought to play a role in constipation, cancer of the colon, and diverticulosis, a condition in which small sacs form in the intestine. Alcoholism has been linked to pancreatitis (inflammation of the pancreas), but definite proof still has not been found.

Progress is being made in diagnosing and treating many digestive diseases. In addition to the upper and lower "GI series" which uses x-rays and barium to find trouble spots, doctors can use a new, flexible instrument called the endoscope to see inside the esophagus, stomach, duodenum, and colon. The endoscope can also be used to perform biopsies and some forms of mini-surgery. There are also better techniques for getting images of body organs, such as ultrasound and the CT scan (computed tomographic scan), which takes detailed, three-dimensional x-rays.

Treatment advances include new drugs for peptic ulcer, a vaccine to prevent chronic hepatitis, and a drug which can dissolve gallstones in some patients.

Some of the digestive disorders which most commonly cause problems for older people are the following:

Constipation—A decrease in the number of bowel movements, along with prolonged or hard passage of stools. Older people report this problem much more often than younger ones do. "Regularity" does not necessarily mean one bowel movement every day. Normal bowel habits can range from three movements each day to one each week. A poor diet, drinking too few liquids, inactivity, some prescription medications, or misusing laxatives can lead to constipation. Regularity is usually improved by eating foods high in fiber and staying physically active.

Diarrhea—A condition in which body wastes are discharged from the bowel more often than usual and in a more or less liquid state. There are many possible causes, but many cases are related to infection. Treatment of the underlying disorder is needed, along with replacement of lost fluids.

Diverticulosis and diverticulitis—In diverticulosis, which is common in older people, small sacs form on the wall of the large intestine. Although they usually cause no symptoms, occasionally there is pain in the lower left side of the abdomen. Treatment includes a diet high in fiber and liquids. Sometimes the sacs become inflamed, causing fever. The condition is then known as diverticulitis. Treatment consists of bed rest and antibiotics.

Functional disorders—Sometimes symptoms such as pain, diarrhea, constipation, bloating, and gas are caused by a "functional" disorder such as irritable bowel syndrome. In these disorders there are no signs of disease, and yet the intestinal tract still fails to work properly. A functional disorder may cause discomfort, but it is unlikely to lead to a serious disease. A doctor may prescribe medication to relieve symptoms. Because diet and stress are thought to trigger functional disorders, the same guidelines that help to keep your system running smoothly should help control the symptoms.

Gallbladder disease—In this disease, stones (usually composed of cholesterol) form in the gallbladder. The stones are often "silent," that is, they cause no symptoms or discomfort, but sometimes they cause problems requiring drug treatment or surgery. Severe pain in the upper abdomen may mean that a gallstone has lodged in one of the tubes leading from the gallbladder.

Gas—Some gas is normally present in the digestive tract. It is usually caused by swallowing air or eating foods such as cauliflower, brussels sprouts, brown beans, broccoli, bran, and cabbage. The body rids itself of gas by means of belching and flatulence (passing gas through the rectum). However, if it collects in some portion of the digestive tract, it can lead to pain and bloating. A change in dietary habits will often relieve extra gas.

Gastritis—An inflammation of the stomach, gastritis is a symptom, not a disorder, and can be caused by many different digestive ailments. Treatment is aimed at correcting the condition that is causing the gastritis.

Heartburn—A burning pain felt behind the breastbone occurs after meals and may last for many minutes to several hours. It is often caused by eating foods such as tomato products, chocolate, fried foods, or peppermint, and smoking cigarettes. It is relieved by a change in diet, taking an antacid, sleeping with the head of the bed raised 6 inches, or stopping cigarette smoking.

Peptic ulcer—A sore on the lining of the stomach or duodenum (the small intestine just below the stomach) occurs when the lining is unable to resist the damaging effects of acid and pepsin that are produced by the stomach to digest foods. Antacids, which neutralize acid in

Continued.

Digestive do's and don'ts—cont'd

the stomach, and drugs that decrease the production of acid or coat the ulcer are very useful in treating peptic ulcer.

Indigestion—This is a common condition involving painful, difficult, or disturbed digestion. Doctors often call it dyspepsia. The symptoms may include nausea, regurgitation, vomiting, heartburn, abdominal fullness or bloating after a meal, and stomach discomfort or pain. Overeating or eating the wrong foods can cause symptoms, but they may also be related to other digestive problems such as peptic ulcer, gallbladder disease, or gastritis. Indigestion usually can be controlled through diet or by treating the specific disorder.

Hemorrhoids—Veins in and around the rectum and anus have become weakened and enlarged. The condition is caused by pressure in the rectal veins due to constipation, pregnancy, obesity, or other conditions. The veins may become inflamed, develop blood clots, and bleed. Hemorrhoids are treated with frequent warm baths, creams, or suppositories, and if necessary, by injections or surgery.

Hiatal hernia—In this condition part of the stomach slides up through the diaphragm (a thin muscle which separates the abdominal cavity from the chest cavity) into the chest cavity. Hiatal hernias are common after middle-age and rarely cause symptoms. Contrary to popular myth, hiatal hernias do not cause heartburn, although they are sometimes associated with it. Usually, they do not need surgical or drug treatment.

Milk intolerance—The inability to digest milk and milk products properly is caused by a deficiency of lactase, the intestinal enzyme that digests the sugar found in milk. Some people develop this problem as they grow older. The symptoms, which include cramps, gas, bloating, and diarrhea, appear 15 minutes to several hours after consuming milk or a milk product. Most people can manage the problem by eating fewer dairy products, taking smaller servings more frequently, or adding a special nonprescription preparation to milk that makes it easy to digest. If fewer dairy products are eaten, other foods that have calcium (such as dark green leafy vegetables, salmon, and bean curd) should be substituted to help keep the bones strong. Many people can eat yogurt without having discomfort.

Ulcerative colitis—This is a chronic disorder that usually develops in young adults, but also appears in older people. In ulcerative colitis, parts of the large intestine become inflamed, causing abdominal cramps and often rectal bleeding. Joint pain and skin rashes may also develop. The symptoms are usually controlled with drugs, but some patients eventually need surgery. Sometimes irritable bowel syndrome (IBS) is incorrectly called "spastic colitis." However, IBS does not cause inflammation and it is not related to ulcerative colitis.

For further information about these and other digestive disorders consult your physician. You can also write to the National Digestive Diseases Education and Information Clearinghouse, 1555 Wilson Blvd, Suite 600, Rosslyn, VA 22209.

CANCER OF THE STOMACH

Fortunately the incidence of cancer of the stomach has been decreasing over the past several decades, although it is still one of the most common types of cancer in the older age group. It occurs more frequently in men than in women.

▶ PATHOPHYSIOLOGY, SIGNS, AND SYMPTOMS

There is no specific known cause for cancer of the stomach, although diet and genetic factors have been considered possible contributory factors. Persons with pernicious anemia or decreased gastric acid are at high risk for developing gastric cancer. One of the major problems is that there are few specific symptoms in the early stages. Because symptoms may be the same as for other nonmalignant gastric problems such as gastritis, peptic ulcer, or simple indigestion, the individual does not seek treatment. The symptoms may be intermittent and vague abdominal discomforts such as dyspepsia or regurgita- *tion. Bleeding may occur, but the blood in the feces will not be obvious to the individual. Other symptoms may be fullness, dysphagia, weight loss, anorexia, constipation, nausea, vomiting, and hematemesis (Deters, 1987, pp. 1039-1040).*

▶ DIAGNOSTIC PROCEDURES

A variety of procedures and tests are used to aid in the diagnosis of gastric cancer. These include the following:
   Guaiac test for occult blood
   Analysis of gastric secretions for decreased gastric acid and cytologic examination of cells
   Blood chemistry for possible anemia
   Barium x-ray of stomach
   Gastroscopy

▶ MEDICAL MANAGEMENT

Surgery is the primary method of treatment. The type of surgery depends on the condition of the patient and the site and degree of the lesion, but usually the entire stomach is removed (gastrectomy). If the lesion has gone through the stomach wall and involved adjacent organs, or if metastasis has already occurred, radiation therapy and chemotherapy are also used, although with limited success. Sometimes surgery is only palliative and is used to prevent hemorrhage and relieve pain and other immediate complications.

▶ **PROGNOSIS**

If the cancer has been confined to the stomach and has not infiltrated through the muscle wall, involved the lymph nodes, or metastasized, the prognosis is fair. "Without lymph node involvement it is estimated that 5 to 15 percent of clients will have a 5-year cure" (Deters, 1987, p. 1041).

▶ **NURSING MANAGEMENT—NURSING CARE PLAN**
Cancer of the Stomach or Colon

Assessment

SUBJECTIVE DATA	OBJECTIVE DATA
Vague abdominal complaints (e.g., fullness)	*Severe loss of weight*
Increase in constipation	*Pale color*
Feelings of fatigue	*Poor appetite*

	Nursing diagnoses	Expected outcomes	Nursing interventions (rationale)
N U R S I N G C A R E P L A N	*Preoperative* Altered nutrition: less than body requirements, related to anorexia	Patient will be able to eat 75% of each meal offered.	Assess food and fluid preferences. Provide small, attractive, appetizing meals. Provide food and fluid supplements if ordered (need to improve nutritional status prior to surgery).
	Fatigue related to loss of blood	Patient will sleep at least 7 hr each night and will take morning and afternoon rest periods in bed.	Provide desired snack at bedtime. Give backrub and make bed. Do not interrupt sleep or rest periods. Provide a quiet environment.
	Anxiety related to possible diagnosis of cancer	Patient will express fears and concerns regarding surgery and diagnosis.	Encourage patient to express fear and concerns about surgery. Listen attentively. Explain preoperative and immediate postoperative procedures (e.g., enemas, medications, skin preparation).
	Postoperative Potential for infection related to surgical incision	No signs of infection will occur (temperature will remain normal; incision site will show no edema, redness, or drainage).	Take vital signs every 4 hr after immediate postoperative period. Observe abdominal dressing every 4 hr for excess drainage, and change when ordered.
	Pain related to trauma of tissues during surgery	Pain will be relieved.	Assess patient's pain and use of patient-controlled analgesia (PCA) pump frequently. Reposition for comfort as needed.
	Altered nutrition: less than body requirements, related to change in digestive process	No vomiting will occur.	Maintain patency of nasogastric tube. Provide oral and nasal care several times a day.
		Food and fluid intake will be tolerated.	Assess bowel sounds. Monitor intravenous fluids. Provide small amounts of clear fluids (e.g., water, broth, carbonated beverages) when allowed.
		Patient will maintain weight within or gain weight to normal range for age, height, frame.	Initiate progressive diet as tolerated. Weigh patient before breakfast three times a week.

Continued.

Nursing Care Plan—Cancer of the Stomach or Colon—cont'd

Nursing diagnoses	Expected outcomes	Nursing interventions (rationale)
Knowledge deficit (postoperative care and complications) related to changes in gastrointestinal tract	Patient will progressively and safely ambulate without fear.	Teach patient how to get out of bed without discomfort.
		Teach patient safety factors in ambulating soon after surgery.
	Patient will be able to state essentials of care needed at home after discharge.	Teach patient and family about dietary restrictions (e.g., small meals), dumping syndrome (if gastrectomy), colostomy care (if removal of sigmoid colon/rectum), weighing weekly, wound management, prevention of complications, and activities allowed.
		Demonstrate and teach about the use of medications (analgesics and chemotherapy) and care of colostomy, if needed.
		Refer patient to a home health agency for follow-up home care if needed.
Hopelessness (potential) related to questionable prognosis	Patient will adapt to the fact of living with a diagnosis of cancer.	Listen attentively.
		Provide support, concern, care, and hope.
	Patient will contact the local unit of the American Cancer Society for information and support.	Refer patient to a local chapter of the American Cancer Society.

Discharge planning and patient/family education

Provide the patient with the following:

Suggested dietary guidelines following gastrectomy (Box 10-4)

Information on dumping syndrome (see Box 10-4)

Information on digestive do's and don'ts (see Box 10-3)

The telephone number of the local unit of the American Cancer Society

Evaluation

Patient consistently eats five or six small, nutritious meals every day.

No postoperative complications have occurred.

Patient has gained 5 pounds since discharge from the hospital.

Patient walks around one block every day.

A home health aide was not needed because patient and family manage care well.

Patient has joined a support group of the local unit of the American Cancer Society.

Patient has resumed normal social activities.

Box 10-4.

Patient Education

Suggested Guidelines Following Gastrectomy

Dietary Guidelines

Eat low-carbohydrate, high-fat, high-protein foods.

Eat five or six small meals a day.

Eat slowly.

Rest after meals.

Be relaxed.

Chew foods well.

Eat foods containing pectin (e.g., citrus fruits).

Take vitamin supplements.

Avoid the following:
  Extremely hot or cold foods
  Caffeine
  Milk products
  Alcohol
  Food that upsets stomach (e.g., spices)
  Acetylsalicylic acid
  Smoking
  Stressful situations

Symptoms and Prevention of Dumping Syndrome

Dumping syndrome occurs 15 minutes to 1 hour after eating and has the following symptoms:
  Weakness
  Perspiration
  Epigastric fullness
  Nausea/vomiting
  Abdominal cramping
  Faintness
  Flushing
  Diarrhea
  Palpitations

To prevent dumping syndrome, limit:
  High-fiber foods
  Complex carbohydrates (e.g. bread, rice, vegetables)
  Concentrated sweets, sugars, and salt
  Extremely hot or cold foods
  Fluids with meals or for 1 hour before or after
  Items containing milk at first

Adapted from Doenges ME, Moorhouse MF, and Geissler AC (1989). Nursing care plans, ed 2, Philadelphia, FA Davis, p. 409 and Burtis G, Davis J, and Martin S (1988). Applied nutrition and diet therapy, Philadelphia, WB Saunders, pp. 533-534.

Additional instructions for the individual patient and/or family:

CANCER OF COLON

Cancer of the colon is very common in older adults. It is the third most common type of cancer in both men and women.

▶ **PATHOPHYSIOLOGY, SIGNS, AND SYMPTOMS**

The cancer may start from a polyp (there are also benign polyps) or an ulcer on the wall of the colon. The exact cause is not known, although it has been suggested that a high-fat, low-residue, low-bulk diet may contribute to the development of cancer of the colon because it causes food residues to be retained in the bowel longer and thus exposes the tissue to carcinogens (certain chemicals in food) for a longer period of time. Other causes, in particular colon polyps, may be genetic or familial. Typical symptoms include the following:

Constipation
Blood in the feces
Flatulence
Cramping abdominal pain
Bowel obstruction
Nausea and vomiting

▶ **DIAGNOSTIC PROCEDURES**

The American Cancer Society recommends the following diagnostic procedures, primarily to rule out malignancies of the colon or to detect them early:

Digital rectal examination by a physician annually after age 40
Guaiac test on feces annually after age 50
Proctoscopy every 3 to 5 years for those over age 50, after there have been two annual examinations that were normal

Flexible sigmoidoscopy, colonoscopy, and/or barium enema as determined by the physician, if there is a family history of cancer of the colon. (Biopsy may be done to determine whether polyps are cancerous)

▶ **MEDICAL MANAGEMENT**

Surgery is the primary treatment, with excision of the portion of the colon involved. If the tumor is in the cecum, ascending colon, or transverse colon, the remaining sections of colon can be sutured together with little change in function. If the tumor is in the descending, or sigmoid, colon, a permanent colostomy will be required because that tissue and the rectum will be removed.

▶ **PROGNOSIS**

If the cancerous tumor has not infiltrated the intestinal muscle wall and if nearby lymph nodes are not involved, the prognosis is very good. Many people live a long normal life with a permanent colostomy. If adjacent tissues are involved, radiation and chemotherapy may be used but are not very effective.

▶ **NURSING MANAGEMENT—NURSING CARE PLAN**
Cancer of the Colon

Assessment

SUBJECTIVE DATA
Increasing constipation
Pain in lower abdomen

OBJECTIVE DATA
Bright red blood in the feces
No bowel movements

Nursing Care Plan		
Nursing diagnosis	**Expected outcomes**	**Nursing interventions (rationale)**
See the nursing care plan for patients with cancer of the stomach or colon in the preceding section on cancer of the stomach.		

Discharge planning and patient/family education
Provide the patient with the following:
Suggested guidelines following colon resection (Box 10-5)
Information on digestive do's and don'ts (see Box 10-3)
The telephone number of the local unit of the American Cancer Society

Evaluation
Patient has learned to care for colostomy (if sigmoid colon/rectum resection).
Normal bowel elimination has returned.
See evaluation for cancer of the stomach for postoperative care.

Box 10-5.

Patient Education

Suggested Guidelines Following Colon Resection (Without Colostomy)

Eat a bland diet for several weeks (e.g., ground meats, soft cooked vegetables, puddings, gelatin desserts, milk).

Avoid fried foods (e.g., steak), raw vegetables or fruits, herbs and spices, alcohol, caffeine, black pepper, popcorn, nuts, celery.

Take a stool softener daily or use a rectal suppository if needed to have a soft bowel movement.

Do not have an enema, and do not strain while having a bowel movement.

Be as physically active as you feel able to be.

Additional instructions for the individual patient and/or family:

DIVERTICULOSIS

Diverticulosis is a condition in which small outpouchings or sacs protrude from the gastrointestinal tract. These outpouchings, called diverticula, may occur anywhere along the gastrointestinal tract but are most often found in the sigmoid colon. Diverticulosis is very common in older adults, especially those who are obese. It is more common in men than in women.

▶ PATHOPHYSIOLOGY, SIGNS, AND SYMPTOMS

Diverticula are generally due to a weak part of the muscle in the bowel. They are not malignant. Possible causes are thought to be poor muscle tone of the intestinal wall and straining due to chronic constipation caused by lack of bulk in the diet, both common problems in many older adults. A congenital weakness of the muscle wall may
also be involved. There are usually few symptoms, although symptoms and complications may occur if the diverticula become infected as a result of fecal substances being retained in the sacs. The symptoms may include the following:

Cramping pain or tenderness in the lower left abdomen
Nausea
Vomiting
Abdominal distension
Diarrhea
Intestinal spasm
Fever and chills
Intestinal obstruction or perforation (in severe cases)
(Williams, 1990, p. 443)
Flatulence
Heartburn
Constipation
Occult blood (small amounts) in feces (rare)

▶ DIAGNOSTIC PROCEDURES

The diverticula can be seen on x-ray with a barium enema. They can also be visualized by sigmoidoscopy and colonoscopy. Because there are normally few symptoms, the disease is usually discovered while the bowel is being examined for other possible problems. A yearly guaiac test for occult blood is recommended for all adults over the age of 40 as a simple, safe, and inexpensive screening tool for many gastrointestinal problems.

▶ MEDICAL MANAGEMENT

In the absence of infection (diverticulitis), bleeding, abscess, obstruction, or perforation, the primary treatment, if any is needed, is dietary. A high-fiber, high-bulk, low-residue diet is recommended to aid in the passage of stool and to prevent constipation. "Some studies have indicated that fibers of a coarse type have a more significant effect on stool weight, increased intestinal transit, and reduced intraluminal pressure in the colon than do the five types of brain" (Williams, 1990, p. 445).

If acute diverticulitis occurs, dietary fiber should be reduced, the patient should be on bed rest, and antibiotics may be given. Obstruction, abscesses, or perforation will require surgery (removal of the portion of the colon involved, with temporary colostomy).

▶ PROGNOSIS

The prognosis is excellent if dietary guidelines are followed, constipation is reduced, and complications (infection, perforation, or obstruction) do not occur.

▶ NURSING MANAGEMENT—NURSING CARE PLAN
Diverticulosis

Assessment

SUBJECTIVE DATA
Chronic constipation
Straining at stool

OBJECTIVE DATA
Positive guaiac stool test
Black, tarry stools

	Nursing diagnoses	Expected outcomes	Nursing interventions (rationale)
N U R S I N G C A R E P L A N	Potential for infection related to fecal residue in diverticula	No infection will occur.	Teach patient about nutritious, high-fiber diet (increases size of intestinal lumen so intestines contract more and contents go through more quickly) (see Box 10-6). Teach patient about signs and symptoms of infection (see Box 10-6).
	Pain related to presence of diverticula in sigmoid colon	Pain will be relieved.	Teach patient about complications of diverticulosis. Provide medications as ordered.
	Constipation related to inactivity and low-fiber diet	Patient will have a medium to large soft, brown bowel movement without straining at least every 2 days.	See interventions for constipation in the next section of this chapter.

Discharge planning and patient/family education
Provide the patient with copies of Boxes 10-3 and 10-6.
Evaluation
No symptoms or complications have occurred.
Patient eats a high-fiber, high-bulk, low-roughage diet.
Patient has lost 10 pounds in 1 month.
Patient limits alcohol intake to special occasions.
Patient has a large, soft, brown bowel movement each morning after breakfast.
Patient is careful not to strain, bend, lift, or wear tight clothes.

Box 10-6.

Patient Education

Suggested Guidelines for Patients with Diverticulosis

Dietary Suggestions

Eat high-residue, high-bulk foods:
  Whole wheat breads
  Fresh fruits (apples, bananas, prunes, pears, peaches, plums)
  Vegetables (beans, carrots, peas, cabbage)
  Bran cereals
  Whole rye breads
  Oatmeal

Increase fluid intake.

Avoid high-roughage foods (e.g., celery, nuts, popcorn).
Avoid spicy foods.
Avoid alcohol.
Avoid large meals.
Lose weight (if needed).

Other Suggestions

Avoid stress and tension.
Do not strain while having a bowel movement.
Do not bend or lift.
Do not wear tight clothes.
Avoid strong laxatives.
Take bulk laxatives (e.g., psyllium).

Call your physician if these symptoms appear:
  Pain in left lower abdomen
  Red, black, or tarry stools
  Fever and chills
  Nausea and vomiting
  Severe constipation (no stool for 3 to 4 days)

Additional instructions for the individual patient and/or family:

CONSTIPATION

Constipation is a decrease in the number of bowel movements, often accompanied by difficult or painful defecation. It is a symptom rather than a disease, but it is a major problem for many older adults, especially those who are frail, dependent, immobile, and/or cognitively impaired. Some older persons have had a problem with constipation all of their lives and it becomes much more severe in old age. Others have minimal problems, probably because they eat well and are active both physically and mentally.

▶ PATHOPHYSIOLOGY, SIGNS, AND SYMPTOMS

Bowel elimination patterns are very individualized. It is not abnormal if an individual does not have a bowel movement every day. Having a bowel movement less often than every 4 days is usually considered abnormal, but most people do not feel well if they do not have a bowel movement at least every 2 or 3 days. Constipation can be a symptom of several major physiologic problems, for example, intestinal obstruction due to a neoplasm of some type, a rectocele in the female, cecal volvulus, or a strangulated hernia in the male in which a portion of the intestinal tract extends through the wall of the abdomen. Or it can be the result of inadequate fluid or food, primarily bulk, in the diet or lack of exercise. Other common causes of constipation, especially in older people, are as follows:

Decreased peristalsis (possibly due to medications being taken, e.g., aspirin, tranquilizers, and hypnotics, or to lack of potassium in the diet)
Decreased abdominal muscle mass and tone
Obesity
Lack of teeth or dentures (for adequate chewing)
Depression (possibly related to decreased diet and activity)
Enlarged prostate
Rectal pathology (e.g., tumor or stricture)
Delaying defecation when the urge occurs because of inability physically to get to the bathroom
Anxiety and/or stress
Common symptoms of constipation are the following:
   No stool for 3 or 4 days
   Hard, dry stool
   Abdominal distension
   Hemorrhoids that often bleed
   Straining to have a bowel movement
   Headache
   Lethargy
   Mental confusion
   Nausea and vomiting
   Abdominal pain or tenderness

▶ DIAGNOSTIC PROCEDURES

The exact cause of constipation is sometimes difficult to diagnose in older people. Older adults, and possibly their family or physician, may believe that their constipation is due to lack of bulk in the diet, inactivity, or the aging process, whereas there is really a more serious cause. Therefore any change in bowel habits needs to be investigated.

▶ MEDICAL MANAGEMENT

After any specific pathologic or anatomic cause has been ruled out (e.g., neoplasm or volvulus), the treatment may be very individualized and is based on the age, physical condition, mobility, and dietary patterns of the individual.

The best treatment is probably the most simple one: a proper diet and adequate exercise. Specific recommendations include the following:
   High-residue, high-bulk diet (e.g., whole wheat and bran bread, vegetables, fruits, legumes)
   Low-fat diet
   Exercise (simple walking is probably the best and safest—around one or two blocks if physical condition permits and physician has recommended)
   Reduced stress, anxiety, depression
   Bulk laxatives, if needed, rather than strong laxatives
   Rectal suppositories, if needed
   Fleet's enema—saline or oil retention (rather than a large amount of water or soapsuds solution)—as a last resort

▶ PROGNOSIS

Chronic constipation continues to be a consistent and bothersome daily problem for many older adults. If an individualized routine of diet, exercise, and bulk laxatives is found to be effective, it should be continued wherever the patient is—at home, in the hospital, or in a nursing home.

▶ **NURSING MANAGEMENT—NURSING CARE PLAN**
  Constipation

Assessment

SUBJECTIVE DATA

"My bowels haven't moved in a few days."
"I can't eat anything until I have a bowel movement."
"It sure does hurt."
"Please give me an enema."

OBJECTIVE DATA

Distended abdomen
No bowel movement recorded in 3 days
Mass palpated in left lower quadrant of abdomen
*Has been going to the bathroom every few minutes
  without having a bowel movement*

	Nursing diagnoses	Expected outcomes	Nursing interventions (rationale)
N U R S I N G C A R E P L A N	Constipation related to inadequate bulk in diet and limited mobility	Patient will increase high-residue, high-bulk foods and water in the diet.	Assess quantity and quality of food intake at each meal. Assess types of high-residue foods preferred. Provide high-residue foods at all three meals each day. Provide at least 2000 ml of fluid every 24 hr.
		Patient will walk for a total of 20 min at least 3 days a week after having a medical checkup.	Encourage patient to gradually increase walking distance (e.g., around house, around yard, around one and then two blocks). Teach patient to mark on calendar the amount walked on what days.
		Patient will have a medium to large, soft, brown bowel movement at least every 2 to 3 days.	Assess bowel elimination daily (amount, consistency, shape, color, odor). Teach patient how to observe and record type of bowel movements.

Discharge planning and patient/family education
Provide the patient with copies of Boxes 10-3 and 10-7.
Evaluation
Patient eats three regular meals a day and includes high-residue and high-bulk foods in the diet every day.

Patient drinks eight 8-ounce glasses of fluid every day.
Patient has worked up to walking for 20 minutes 3 days a week.
Patient has started having a large, soft, brown bowel movement every morning.

Box 10-7.

Patient Education

Preventing Constipation

Eat three regular meals every day.

Include the following types of food in your diet:
  Whole wheat bread (instead of white bread)
  Bran bread
  Whole wheat or bran cereals
  Vegetables (especially carrots, spinach)
  Fruits (especially prunes, bananas)

Drink at least eight 8-ounce glasses of fluid every day (include fruit juices such as apple, prune, and cranberry).

Walk for 20 minutes at a steady pace at least 3 days a week.

Try to have a bowel movement at the same time every day.

Go to the bathroom when you feel the urge—do not delay.

Do not strain while having a bowel movement.

Do not take harsh laxatives or have enemas unless absolutely necessary.

Additional instructions for the individual patient and/or family:

FECAL INCONTINENCE

Fecal incontinence, the inability to retain a bowel movement or know when one occurs, is a problem for some older people, especially those who have had a neurologic problem such as a cardiovascular accident. Fecal incontinence can cause skin problems (e.g., irritation and ulcers), self-image problems (especially if the person is ambulatory and alert), and caregiver stress (both for professionals and for family members in the home, especially the latter). Fecal incontinence, along with urinary incontinence, is quite often a major factor in the decision to institutionalize an older family member. However, the condition can be managed quite well in the home with adequate professional support and supplies.

▶ PATHOPHYSIOLOGY, SIGNS, AND SYMPTOMS

There are many reasons for fecal incontinence. The most common causes in older adults are as follows:

> *Tumors and/or surgery involving the rectum and anal opening*
> *Diseases or conditions involving the neurologic system that affect nerve impulses in the rectum (e.g., stroke, Alzheimer's disease, tumors)*
> *Decreased mental status due to severe depression, delirium, or dementia*
> *Diarrhea due to diet, chemicals, medications, and/or constipation*

The most common symptoms are the inability to recognize when a bowel movement occurs and the expelling of feces in bed or clothes.

▶ DIAGNOSTIC PROCEDURES

The rectum and sigmoid colon need to be examined to rule out a pathologic cause. Neurologic causes need to be determined by a complete neurologic evaluation, including a computerized axial tomography (CAT) scan and an electroencephalogram.

▶ MEDICAL MANAGEMENT

If the cause is an anatomic problem of the rectum or anus, surgery may be needed. If the problem is neurologic, however, management most likely will be long-term. A diet that makes the feces more solid and firm may help to prevent fecal incontinence, but the most effective treatment is probably toilet training, which is outlined in Box 10-8.

▶ PROGNOSIS

Even though cure may not be possible, there are many nursing measures that can be instituted to help the patient and family manage the problem of fecal incontinence.

Box 10-8.

Bowel training program for fecal incontinence

Assess exact times, amounts, and frequency of fecal incontinence 24 hours a day for 7 days.

Record the above on a chart, noting the times fecal incontinence occurs the most often.

If patient is in bed, place on a bedpan in high Fowler's position 20 minutes before the usual time of fecal incontinence.

If patient is ambulatory, assist to the bathroom 20 minutes before the usual time of fecal incontinence. Place the patient's feet flat on the floor. Press slightly over the lower abdomen.

Provide the patient with consistent amounts of high-residue, high-bulk foods three times a day at the same times every day.

Administer a bulk laxative if the feces is too soft or a stool softener once or twice a day if the feces is hard.

► **NURSING MANAGEMENT—NURSING CARE PLAN**
Fecal Incontinence

Assessment

SUBJECTIVE DATA

Not aware of having had a bowel movement
"I hate for you to have to do that." (clean up)

OBJECTIVE DATA

Feces on bed, hands of patient, chair, floor
Does not eat all of food at most meals

	Nursing diagnoses	Expected outcomes	Nursing interventions (rationale)
N U R S I N G C A R E P L A N	Bowel incontinence related to major neurologic deficits	Fecal incontinence will cease.	Institute a bowel training program as shown in Box 10-8. Teach other caregivers (e.g., family) about the program.
	Potential impaired skin integrity	The skin will remain intact and free from redness and edema.	Observe for fecal incontinence every 30 min 24 hr a day. When fecal incontinence occurs, cleanse skin carefully with warm soapy water, pat dry, and apply a very small amount of powder or cornstarch to reddened areas where skin touches skin. Use waterproof pads on bed and waterproof pants if patient is ambulatory. Change as soon as they become moist. Observe skin around rectum and buttocks daily.
	Toileting self-care deficit related to lack of mobility	No fecal incontinence will occur.	Offer bedpan or assist to bathroom at designated intervals. Assist to cleanse self if needed.
	Situational low self-esteem related to fecal contents and odor on self	Patient will always be clean and free of fecal odor.	Check for fecal incontinence every 30 min and clean patient as soon as incontinence occurs. Open windows in room if possible.
		Patient will accept assistance of caregiver for cleansing.	Approach cleansing following fecal incontinence in an accepting manner. Show support and concern by smiling, if appropriate, and gentle cleansing. Continue to use waterproof pants.

Discharge planning and patient/family education

Teach patient and/or family the importance of keeping the skin clean and dry and how to use a bowel training program (see Box 10-8).

Evaluation

Episodes of fecal incontinence have decreased to once or twice a week.
Patient eats three regular meals every day.
Skin remains intact.
Waterproof pants make patient feel more secure.

REFERENCES

Burtis G, Davis J, and Martin S (1988). Applied nutrition and diet therapy, Philadelphia, WB Saunders Co.

Deters GE (1987). Problems of digestion. In Lewis SM and Collier IC, editors: Medical-surgical nursing, ed 2, New York, McGraw-Hill.

Doenges ME, Moorhouse MF, and Geissler AC (1989). Nursing care plans, ed 2, Philadelphia, FA Davis.

Elrod R (1987). Problems of ingestion. In Lewis SM and Collier IC, editors: Medical-surgical nursing, ed 2, New York, McGraw-Hill.

Williams SW (1990). Essentials of nutrition and diet therapy, St Louis, Mosby−Year Book, Inc.

CHAPTER 11

Genitourinary System

Laura Talbot

URINARY INCONTINENCE

Urinary incontinence, the unintentional leakage of urine, is classified as either acute or persistent. Acute incontinence is a temporary condition usually associated with an acute infection or illness and will resolve once health is restored. Persistent incontinence continues even after the resolution of an acute illness. The five types of persistent incontinence are stress incontinence, urge incontinence, reflex incontinence, total incontinence, and functional incontinence. An individual can have more than one type of persistent incontinence, which makes resolution difficult.

▶ PATHOPHYSIOLOGY, SIGNS, AND SYMPTOMS

The signs and symptoms of incontinence depend on the type of incontinence the individual has. Box 11-1 lists the types along with a description of each.

▶ DIAGNOSTIC PROCEDURES

Urodynamic studies are used to evaluate the patient for a detrusor reflex.
  Cystometrogram (CMG)—evaluates the neuromuscular mechanism of the bladder
  Rectal electromyography—records urine flow rate and electromyogram activity
  Urethra pressure profile—records pressures along the uretha
  Electromyography of sphincter activity reveals muscle or nerve disorders.
Urinalysis and culture are used to detect bacterial infection.

Box 11-1.

Types of incontinence

Stress incontinence—the inability to prevent the release of urine with increased intraabdominal pressure
Urge incontinence—loss of urine after only a brief sensation of urgency
Reflex incontinence—involuntary loss of urine without the sensation to void
Total incontinence—continuous leakage of urine without warning or abdominal distension
Functional incontinence—bladder and sphincter function is intact but loss of urine occurs before the individual reaches an appropriate receptacle (such as happens with the confused individual)

▶ MEDICAL MANAGEMENT

Pharmacologic management:
  Flavoxate, imipramine, oxybutynin, propantheline, and dicyclomine are used to decrease detrusor contractility.
  Phenylephrine, ephedrine, phenylpropanolamine, and bethanechol are used to increase bladder neck tone and detrusor activity by stimulating the alpha-sympathetic nervous system.
  Beta-blocking agents are used to improve control by inhibiting the beta receptors to the urethral sphincter.
  Antibiotics are used if the incontinence is due to a urinary tract infection.
  Estrogen therapy is used for the postmenopausal woman if the incontinence is due to an estrogen deficiency.

Surgical management:

    Marshall-Marchetti-Krantz procedure is a method of correcting female stress incontinence by suspending the bladder neck and urethra to the posterior surface of the pubis.

    Modified peyrera bladder neck suspension is another method of correcting female stress incontinence by suspension of the bladder and urethra without open pelvic surgery. A vaginal dissection and a small suprapubic incision are used.

Artificial urinary sphincter is the implantation of a hydraulically activated cuff to the bladder neck or bulbous urethra for bladder control.

Transurethral Teflon injections are used to increase the urethral resistance when damage to the sphincter muscles has occurred.

▶ PROGNOSIS

Management is directed toward treating the underlying cause. If the underlying cause can be resolved, many times the incontinence will subside. The problem is identifying the etiology of the incontinence or addressing the patient with more than one cause, which complicates the investigation.

▶ NURSING MANAGEMENT—NURSING CARE PLAN
Urinary Incontinence

Assessment

SUBJECTIVE DATA
Dysuria
Urgency associated with involuntary loss of urine

OBJECTIVE DATA
Polyuria
Nocturia
Abnormal urodynamic studies

	Nursing diagnoses	Expected outcomes	Nursing interventions (rationale)
N U R S I N G C A R E P L A N	Knowledge deficit related to incontinent garments, bladder training, Kegel exercises, and catheter devices	Patient will verbalize an understanding of ways to manage urinary incontinence that will include an interactive discussion on incontinent garments, bladder training, Kegel exercises, incontinent pads, and catheter devices.	Assess the patient's present knowledge base. Discuss incontinent garments on the market that make it easier for patients with arthritis or other dexterity problems to remove their clothing. Teach pelvic floor (Kegel) exercises (Box 11-2). Set up a bladder training schedule to assist the patient (especially the confused patient) and significant other in establishing elimination habits. Provide literature on incontinent pads. Many manufacturers provide free samples to use on a trial basis. Teach patient about catheter devices for both internal and external use. (Internal devices should be used as a last resort because of the potential for infection. External devices are available for both men and women and are another alternative in managing incontinence.)
	Impaired skin integrity related to skin breakdown from urine on the skin	Skin will remain intact. Patient will verbalize an understanding of methods of preventing skin problems.	Assess the skin for color, moisture, rashes, odor, or lesions to obtain a baseline. Encourage good personal hygiene. A sitz bath can provide temporary relief when skin breakdown has occurred.

Nursing Care Plan—Urinary Incontinence—cont'd

Nursing diagnoses	Expected outcomes	Nursing interventions (rationale)
Body image disturbance related to the fear of being incontinent in a public area	Patient will verbalize feelings and discuss ways to prevent incontinence in public.	Change incontinent pads frequently to decrease the soiled pad's contact with the skin. Apply protective skin ointment to act as a skin barrier. Teach signs and symptoms of a skin infection that would need professional intervention. Assess patient's present feelings and fears associated with incontinence. Be available so that the patient can express feelings. Explore the impact incontinence has on the patient's sexuality. Discuss solutions such as emptying the bladder before intercourse. Plan outings in which the bathroom can easily be located, or prior to the outing map out all bathroom locations for quick access.

Discharge planning and patient/family education

Arrange for a home health nurse to survey the home for environmental factors that could be contributing to the incontinence. For example, the distance to the toilet may be too far and a bedside toilet could prevent some incontinent episodes.

Refer patient to an incontinence support group so that feelings and solutions can be shared. The following list will assist in contacting a support group.

   HIP is an acronym for Help for Incontinent People. HIP provides information on incontinence through its newsletter and audiocassettes. In addition, HIP puts out a book titled Resource Guide of Continence Aids and Services *to assist patients in finding supplies in the privacy of their home. For more information contact HIP, PO Box 544, Union, SC 29379.*

   The Simon Foundation is an organization for continence. The membership fee is $15 and includes a quarterly newsletter called The Informer. *The organization promotes awareness, research, and education about continence. For more information write The Simon Foundation, Box 815, Wilmette, IL 60091.*

   Continence Restored, Inc., is a nationwide support group. To find a local support group, send a self-addressed envelope to Continence Restored, Inc, 785 Park Ave, New York, NY 10021.

Teach patient self-examination of the skin.

Tell patient to consult physician if skin infection occurs.

Patient should examine skin on a regular basis. If a rash occurs, it should be treated immediately by applying the protective ointment and changing soiled clothing more frequently. If the rash continues to spread or becomes red and inflamed with drainage, the physician should be called.

Evaluation

Patient verbalizes an understanding of ways to manage urinary incontinence that includes a working knowledge of incontinent garments, bladder training, Kegel exercises, incontinent pads, and catheter devices.

Skin remains intact.

Preventive methods are implemented.

Patient verbalizes feelings of fear of becoming incontinent in public. Ways to prevent accidents are discussed.

Box 11-2.

Kegel exercises

Identify the pelvic floor muscles. Instruct the patient to stop the urinary stream while voiding and then restart it. Do this each time the bladder is emptied. Gradually the patient will have full awareness of the muscles involved.

Have the patient do the maneuver while not voiding, squeezing for at least 5 seconds.

Recommendations are to do the exercise 100 times a day over the next 3 months to see whether improvement occurs.

CYSTITIS

Cystitis is inflammation or infection of the bladder. The most common cause is an ascending urinary tract infection predominantly caused by *Escherichia coli* (a gram-negative bacterium). Other gram-negative organisms that may be involved are *Klebsiella pneumoniae*, *Proteus mirabilis*, *Enterobacter aerogenes*, and *Pseudomonas aeruginosa*.

Older people are particularly at risk because they often have chronic diseases such as diabetes and gout. Other factors that increase risk are low estrogen levels in women, prostate enlargement in men, and a declining immune system.

▶ PATHOPHYSIOLOGY, SIGNS, AND SYMPTOMS

With the invasion of pathogens into the urinary tract the bladder becomes irritated. It loses its elasticity, which causes frequency of urination and a sensation of urgency.

If the bladder neck and urethra become involved, dysuria develops.

Urinary frequency, nocturia, urgency, and dysuria are commonly seen in older adults when no infection exists. This makes a urinary tract infection (UTI) difficult to diagnose on the basis of these complaints. Yet many times confusion and incontinence, which are not common symptoms, are caused by a UTI.

▶ DIAGNOSTIC PROCEDURES

Gram stain—preliminary screen to determine whether the bacteria involved are gram positive or gram negative

Urine culture and sensitivity—to determine number of bacteria (greater than 100,000/ml) and their drug sensitivity

Urinalysis:

Color—cloudy, dark yellow; may be blood in urine

pH—more than 7

Nitrate—positive

Glucose oxidase—positive

Microscopic observations—bacteria, struvite, many white blood cells, red blood cells

▶ MEDICAL MANAGEMENT

Antimicrobial therapy based on the results of the urine culture and sensitivity test is the treatment of choice for uncomplicated UTI. If the UTI is due to an obstruction, anatomic abnormalities, or renal calculi, therapy is directed toward correcting the underlying cause.

▶ PROGNOSIS

The prognosis is good with proper treatment, but UTI often reoccurs.

▶ **NURSING MANAGEMENT—NURSING CARE PLAN**
  Cystitis

Assessment

SUBJECTIVE DATA

Painful or burning urination
Suprapubic pain
Low back pain

OBJECTIVE DATA

Urgency, frequency, nocturia
Urine culture positive for bacteria

	Nursing diagnoses	Expected outcomes	Nursing interventions (rationale)
N U R S I N G C A R E P L A N	Knowledge deficit (methods of preventing a urinary tract infection) related to a possible recurrence of a UTI	Patient will verbalize an understanding of ways to prevent a UTI that will include an interactive discussion on fluid intake, diet, and products to avoid.	Discuss products and procedures that contribute to UTIs (Box 11-3). Encourage the patient to drink at least 2000 to 3000 ml of fluid per day unless contraindicated by a preexisting condition. Discuss the use of an acid-ash diet to acidify the urine. Teach the signs and symptoms of UTI such as frequency, burning on urination, urgency, and nocturia. Be sure to include topics specific to older people such as confusion and incontinence.
	Infection related to bacteria in the urinary tract	Urine culture will be negative for bacterial growth.	Assess character of the urine. Note color, odor, amount, and clarity. Monitor vital signs, especially temperature. Be alert to oral temperatures greater than 99° F. (Older people have subnormal temperatures.) Check culture and sensitivity to be sure pathogen is sensitive to the antibiotic prescribed. (Note: more than three different organisms in a clean catch specimen suggest a contaminated specimen.) Instruct patients to take antibiotics as prescribed and to continue to take the medication until it is gone even though they start to feel better. Encourage patient to drink juices such as cranberry and apple that acidify the urine (discourages bacterial growth).

Discharge planning and patient/family education

Teach patient how to use a dipstick (Microstix-Nitrite) to screen urine at home for infection.

One means of preventing urinary tract infections is to keep the pH of the urine on the acid side, which discourages the growth of bacteria. Patients can acidify their urine in the following ways:

Take ascorbic acid.

Drink cranberry juice.

Include meats, eggs, nuts, cheese, and whole grains in your diet.

Arrange for follow-up urine cultures on an outpatient basis.

Teach patient how to obtain a clean catch urine specimen (Box 11-4).

Evaluation

Urine culture is negative for bacterial growth.

Patient verbalizes methods to prevent the recurrence of a urinary tract infection.

Box 11-3.

Ways to prevent urinary tract infections

Avoid bubble baths, feminine hygiene sprays, and perfumed products.

Avoid tub baths. Take showers instead.

Wipe from front to back, especially after a bowel movement.

Void at the first urge so as not to overdistend the bladder.

Empty bladder frequently during the day and at night.

Empty bladder immediately after sexual intercourse.

Box 11-4.

Obtaining a clean catch urine specimen

Wash hands with soap and water.

Remove sterile container from the wrapper. Remove the sterile cap, being careful not to touch the inside of the lid or cup. Lay the cap down with the inner surface up.

Clean around the urinary meatus with an antimicrobial solution.

Women: Separate the labia with one hand. Use the other hand to hold the cup. Start urinating into the toilet. Insert the cup into the stream of urine, collecting the remainder of the urine excreted.

Men: Retract the foreskin to expose the glans penis. Clean the urinary meatus. Start urinating into the toilet. Insert the cup into the stream of urine. Collect the remainder of the urine except for the last few drops.

Recap the container without touching the rim or inside of the cup. Take the specimen to the laboratory immediately.

PYELONEPHRITIS

Pyelonephritis is a pyogenic, frequently bilateral, infection of the kidney. A bacterial infection is often the cause, but other contributors are metabolic diseases, renal disease, urinary obstruction, and trauma.

▶ PATHOPHYSIOLOGY, SIGNS, AND SYMPTOMS

Acute pylonephritis is usually the result of an ascending infection. Escherichia coli *is a frequent offender among women, but other pathogens are* Klebsiella, Proteus, *and* Enterobacter. *Patients with indwelling catheters are likely to colonize uncommon organisms such as Serratia. The presenting symptoms are fever, chills, flank or abdominal pain, nausea, frequency of urination, dysuria, and costovertebral tenderness.*

Chronic pyelonephritis produces atrophy and calcyceal deformity of the kidneys. It has an insiduous onset and is often associated with some type of renal obstruction.

▶ DIAGNOSTIC PROCEDURES

Gram stain—to determine whether bacteria are gram negative or gram positive

Urine culture and sensitivity—to determine number of bacteria (greater than 100,000/ml) and their drug sensitivity

Urinalysis:

pH—alkaline

Microscopic observations—bacteria, white blood cell cast, red blood cells, granular casts

Intravenous urogram—to evaluate kidneys for structural defects

▶ MEDICAL MANAGEMENT

Antimicrobial medication based on culture and sensitivity of urine sample is the treatment of choice. Long-term therapy may be necessary to eradicate the infection. Follow-up urine cultures are necessary to evaluate the effectiveness of treatment.

▶ PROGNOSIS

Acute pyelonephritis can progress to chronic pyelonephritis with repeated infections. Yet chronic pyelonephritis can occur without a history of acute pyelonephritis. End-stage renal failure may follow. The prognosis will then depend on the severity of the renal failure.

▶ NURSING MANAGEMENT—NURSING CARE PLAN
Pyelonephritis

Assessment

SUBJECTIVE DATA
Chills
Flank or abdominal pain
Nausea
Frequency of urination
Dysuria

OBJECTIVE DATA
High fever
Costovertebral tenderness
Urine culture positive for bacteria

	Nursing diagnoses	Expected outcomes	Nursing interventions (rationale)
N U R S I N G C A R E P L A N	Knowledge deficit related to preventive measures associated with pyelonephritis	Patient will verbalize an understanding of ways to prevent the reoccurrence of pyelonephritis that will include an interactive discussion on fluid intake, medications, and follow-up screening.	Assess patient's knowledge of pyelonephritis to obtain a baseline from which to begin teaching. Teach patient to take the full course of antibiotics even though symptoms subside. Discuss the need to drink at least 2000 to 3000 ml of fluid every day to dilute urine. Emphasize the need for follow-up screening of urine to prevent a reoccurrence of the infection. Teach methods to prevent reinfection (see Box 11-6).
	Alteration in comfort: Pain related to physical symptoms of pyelonephritis	Patient will verbalize a decrease in flank pain and dysuria.	Assess the nature of the pain to obtain a baseline. Administer a urinary analgesic such as phenazopyridine hydrochloride (Pyridium) as needed for dysuria. Administer a systemic analgesic for flank pain. Administer antimicrobial therapy to eradicate the bacterial infection. Explain signs and symptoms of reinfection, which is a common occurrence. Teach patient preventive measures: increased fluid intake, good personal hygiene, emptying the bladder regularly to avoid overdistension. Provide comfort measures such as positioning, heating pad, and diversional techniques. Be alert to pain that does not subside and consult with the physician.

Continued.

Nursing Care Plan—Pyelonephritis—cont'd

Nursing diagnoses	Expected outcomes	Nursing interventions (rationale)
Infection related to bacterial infection of the kidney	Urine culture will be negative for bacterial growth.	Administer antimicrobial medication on the basis of urine culture and sensitivity to ensure proper medication for the offending organism. Ensure a well-lighted path to the bathroom for patients with nocturia. Provide juices and water to encourage an increase in fluid intake (unless contraindicated by a preexisting condition). Teach patient how to obtain a clean catch urine specimen, and provide written instructions (see Box 11-4).
	Intravenous urogram will show no structural changes in the kidney.	Assist in preparing for diagnostic studies such as an intravenous urogram.

Discharge planning and patient/family education
Teach patient that serial urine cultures may need to be done on a regular basis to screen for reoccurrence.
Teach patient how to obtain a clean catch urine specimen (see Box 11-4).
Teach patient the signs and symptoms of a reoccurrence of infection.
Instruct on medications (see Box 11-5).
Teach patient how to prevent reinfection (Box 11-6).
Arrange for outpatient follow-up by physician.

Evaluation
Patient verbalizes an understanding of ways to prevent a recurrence of pyelonephritis.
Patient verbalizes a decrease in flank pain and dysuria.
Urine culture is negative for bacterial growth.
Intravenous urogram shows no structural changes in the kidney.

Box 11-5.

Instructions for taking the urinary analgesic phenazopyridine hydrochloride

The purpose of this medication is to decrease the burning when you urinate.
For best results take this medicine 30 minutes before meals or 2 hours after meals.
This medication can upset your stomach. If this occurs, take with food or milk.
Do not be alarmed when this medicine turns your urine a red-orange color.

Box 11-6.

Patient Education
Methods to Prevent Reinfection

Wear cotton underwear because nylon holds in moisture.

Urinate immediately after sexual intercourse.

Shower instead of taking a tub bath.

Avoid bubble baths, feminine hygiene sprays, and perfumed products.

Always wipe from front to back, especially after a bowel movement.

Do not wait to urinate. Void at the first urge so as not to overdistend your bladder.

Additional instructions for the individual patient and/ or family:

CALCULI (KIDNEY AND BLADDER)

Urolithiasis is the formation along the urinary tract of calculi composed of urinary crystalline salts. Calcium phosphate is the most frequent component, but other salts that form stones are oxalate, uric acid, and cystine or a combination of calcium, magnesium, and ammonium phosphate.

▶ PATHOPHYSIOLOGY, SIGNS, AND SYMPTOMS

Symptoms occur when the urine flow is partially obstructed or blocked by the stone. A stone in the kidneys or ureters causes sudden, severe, sharp pain. With the pain the patient will have nausea, vomiting, diaphoresis, and pallor. Intermittent pain indicates that the stone is causing intermittent obstruction, many times while moving down the ureter. Vesical calculi (bladder stones) cause urinary frequency, pain, intermittent urine stream, hematuria that increases with exercise, and decreased bladder capacity.

▶ DIAGNOSTIC PROCEDURES

Urinalysis—microscopic observation of bacteria, white blood cell cast, red blood cells

KUB (kidney, ureter, and bladder)—visualization of the stone on x-ray
Intravenous pyelogram—locates radiolucent stones; denotes the extent of the obstruction

▶ MEDICAL MANAGEMENT

Renal calculi—analgesic, forced fluids, smooth muscle relaxants, cystoscopic basket extraction, percutaneous fragmentation and extraction through nephroscope, lithotripsy, surgery for urine blockage, i.e., pyelolithotomy, nephrolithotomy, ureterolithotomy, nephrectomy
Vesical calculi—analgesic, antispasmodic, appropriate fluid intake, lithotripsy, litholapaxy, cystoscopic basket extraction, surgical removal of stone if too large to pass by suprapubic approach (cystolithotomy)

▶ PROGNOSIS

If calculi are allowed to go untreated, serious complications can occur as a result of the back flow of urine. The patient may develop a chronic infection and suffer severe impairment of renal function with possible loss of the kidney.

▶ **NURSING MANAGEMENT—NURSING CARE PLAN**
  Calculi

Assessment

SUBJECTIVE DATA

Pain located in the flank, abdomen, inner thigh, and/
  or genitalia
Nausea/vomiting

OBJECTIVE DATA

Hematuria, fever, chills
Frequency and hesitancy of urination
Visualization on x-ray

	Nursing diagnoses	Expected outcomes	Nursing interventions (rationale)
N U R S I N G C A R E P L A N	Alteration in comfort: Pain related to renal or bladder stone	Patient will verbalize a decrease in pain.	Assess the nature of the pain to obtain a baseline. Administer analgesic as needed for pain. Provide heat to flank by applying moist heat or giving a hot bath. Provide various fluids to encourage a high intake. Encourage ambulation to promote stone passage. Prepare patient for surgery if stone does not pass.
	Knowledge deficit related to medication, fluids, and the prevention of stone recurrence	Patient will verbalize an understanding of fluid intake, medication, and ways to prevent stone recurrence.	Assess patient's knowledge level and willingness to learn to obtain a baseline for teaching. Teach patient ways to increase fluid intake to 3 to 4 liters/day, which will dilute urine. Instruct patient on medication. Include purpose, dosage, side effects, and special instructions. Explain to patient ways to prevent stone recurrence (see Box 11-7). Teach patient the signs and symptoms of a kidney stone.
	Alteration in pattern of elimination related to stone blocking urine flow	Patient will resume previous pattern of elimination.	Assess patient's usual elimination pattern to have a baseline pattern. Monitor intake and output to ensure that intake is high and that output approximates intake. Provide a variety of fluids so patient is taking in at least 3000 ml/day unless contraindicated by a preexisting condition. (This is necessary to assist in washing out the stone.)
		Stone will pass.	Encourage ambulation to assist in passage of stone. Strain all urine and send for crystallographic analysis so appropriate therapy can be instituted. Monitor intermittent bladder irrigation and strain for stones in the bladder.

Discharge planning and patient/family education

Arrange for outpatient follow-up by physician.

Instruct patient on the use of analgesic.

Teach patient to strain all urine and save the stone *for analysis.*

Tell patient to drink 3 to 4 liters of fluids a day (unless contraindicated).

Teach patient preventive measures based on the composition of the stone (Box 11-7).

Teach patient the signs and symptoms of a recurrence of kidney and/or bladder stone.

Evaluation

Pain is decreased.

Patient verbalizes an understanding of fluid intake, medications, and ways to prevent stone recurrences.

Previous elimination pattern is resumed. Stone is passed.

Box 11-7.

Preventing recurrence of stones of various compositions

Uric acid calculi

Alkalinization of the urine:

Potassium acetate, potassium citrate, or sodium bicarbonate may be prescribed to change the pH of your urine.

Dipsticks may be purchased to test the pH of your urine.

Encourage fluids. Drink at least 3 to 4 liters a day. If you have a fever or perspire in excess, you must increase your fluid intake even more.

Take allopurinol as prescribed by your physician.

Modify your diet by drinking more milk and eating more fruits (except for cranberries, plums, and prunes) and vegetables (e.g., green vegetables and legumes), which alkalinize the urine.

Magnesium ammonium phosphate stone

Caused primarily by urinary tract infections.

See Box 11-3.

Idiopathic hypercalciuria

Drink at least 1 cup of fluid an hour around the clock. If you have a fever or perspire in excess, you must increase your fluid intake even more.

Take hydrochlorothiazide as prescribed by your physician.

Limit your intake of calcium to moderate amounts.

BENIGN PROSTATIC HYPERPLASIA

Benign prostatic hyperplasia (BPH) is the enlargement of the prostate gland commonly seen in men between the ages of 40 and 50. This enlargement of the gland causes varying degrees of bladder outlet obstruction. It is believed to be related to the hormonal changes associated with aging.

▶ PATHOPHYSIOLOGY, SIGNS, AND SYMPTOMS

As the prostate enlarges, patients experience changes in their pattern of urinary elimination. Symptoms of obstruction are hesitancy, decreased force of urinary stream, postvoid dribble, frequency of urination both at night and during the day, and the sensation of a full bladder even after voiding. At first the bladder will compensate and there will be a spontaneous improvement in the frequency and force without improvement in the BPH, but eventually the compensatory mechanism will no longer be effective. The bladder will become noncompliant and hypotonic. The result will be residual urine in the bladder after urination and an increased susceptibility to infection. Overflow incontinence will occur with this overdistended bladder, resulting in involuntary leakage of urine.

▶ DIAGNOSTIC PROCEDURES

Rectal examination—shows enlarged prostate gland with a rubbery consistency
Cystoscopy—provides evaluation of prostate size
Postvoiding cystogram—evaluates residual urine

▶ MEDICAL MANAGEMENT

Surgery is the preferred method of alleviating the symptoms. One of the following procedures is used:

Transurethral resection of the prostate (TURP)—A resectoscope is used to remove all or part of the gland within the prostatic capsule.

Suprapubic prostatectomy—This procedure is used for removal of a large benign hypertrophied gland. A midline vertical incision above the symphysis pubis is made. The prostate is approached through the bladder. This is an open removal of the prostate gland.

Retropubic prostatectomy—Through an abdominal incision, the prostate gland is reached below the bladder neck. This is an open removal of the prostate gland.

▶ PROGNOSIS

The prognosis is excellent with the TURP. This procedure requires no incision, and sexual potency is usually maintained.

▶ NURSING MANAGEMENT—NURSING CARE PLAN
Benign Prostatic Hyperplasia

Assessment

SUBJECTIVE DATA
Difficulty initiating voiding
Hesitancy and decreased force of urine stream
Overflow incontinence
Postvoid dribbling

OBJECTIVE DATA
Decreasing kidney function
Renal calculi
Recurrent kidney and/or bladder infections
Urinary frequency, urgency, nocturia

	Nursing diagnoses	Expected outcomes	Nursing interventions (rationale)
N U R S I N G C A R E P L A N	Knowledge deficit related to BPH	Patient will verbalize an understanding of BPH that will include discussion on the major concepts of BPH and prevention and early detection of complications.	Assess patient's knowledge level and ability to learn, to have a baseline for teaching. Teach major concepts of BPH so patient will understand what is causing it. Teach patient about the signs and symptoms of the early complications of BPH (Box 11-8) such as decreasing force of urine stream and frequency of urination both during the day and at night. Encourage patient to increase fluids unless contraindicated by a preexisting condition. Discuss the signs and symptoms of a urinary tract infection such as burning on urination and frequency, hesitancy, and urgency of urination.

Nursing Care Plan—Benign Prostatic Hyperplasia—cont'd

Nursing diagnoses	Expected outcomes	Nursing interventions (rationale)
Altered patterns of urinary elimination related to enlarged prostate gland	The patient's bladder will not become overdistended, and the urine culture will be negative for bacteria.	Assess current elimination pattern. Note frequency of urination (for both day and night), force of stream, and signs and symptoms of a urinary tract infection. Palpate bladder for overdistension. Perform intermittent catheterization as needed for an overdistended bladder. Monitor intake and output to ensure that intake is approximately equaling output. Collect urine specimen for culture and sensitivity testing if an infection is suspected. Monitor serum creatinine and blood urea nitrogen to evaluate kidney function.
Urinary retention related to bladder obstruction from enlarged prostate	Patient will have a nonpalpable bladder.	Assess the patient's ability to perform self-catheterization. (A preexisting condition such as arthritis may prevent the patient from performing the procedure.) Teach patient and/or significant other self-catheterization in case of inability to void. Limit caffeine-containing drinks, which cause bladder irritation. Perform a postvoid catheterization to evaluate the amount of urine left in the bladder after urinating. Teach patient to void every 2 to 4 hr to prevent the bladder from becoming overdistended.

Discharge planning and patient/family education

Arrange for outpatient follow-up by physician and/or visiting nurse.

For further information about prostate problems read The Prostate Book *by Stephen N. Rous, MD (W.W. Norton & Co, Inc, 500 Fifth Ave, New York, NY 10110).*

Teach patient self-catheterization if needed (see Box 11-9).

Provide a referral to a home health nurse for assistance in urinary catheterization if needed.

Evaluation

Patient verbalizes an understanding of benign prostatic hyperplasia. An interactive discussion on the major concepts of BPH, early detection of complications, and therapy options took place between the nurse and patient.

Bladder is nonpalpable.

Bladder is nondistended upon palpation.

Urine culture is negative for bacteria.

Box 11-8.

Patient Education

Benign Prostatic Hyperplasia

Benign prostatic hyperplasia can alter your pattern of urinary elimination. If you notice any of the following changes, report them to your doctor:

Difficult to begin voiding

Urine stream is weak

Going to the bathroom more frequently

Urine leakage

The sensation of a full bladder after you have just gone to the bathroom

Frequent voiding at night

Additional instructions for the individual patient and/or family:

Box 11-9.

Patient Education

Self-Catheterization

Assemble all equipment: soap, water, catheter, lubricant.

Wash hands.

Sit on a stool or toilet.

Clean the penis with soap and water.

Grasp the end of the catheter and lubricate the tip.

Insert the catheter into the urethra until urine flows. Do not force the catheter in. If unable to insert into bladder, notify your physician.

Let the urine flow into the toilet or jar until the flow stops. The urine should be clear yellow with a mild odor.

Remove the catheter from the urethra.

Additional instructions for the individual patient and/or family:

UTERINE PROLAPSE

Uterine prolapse is the displacement of the uterus from its normal position. The usual cause is trauma from childbirth. In those who are nulliparous, it is believed to be of congenital etiology.

▶ PATHOPHYSIOLOGY, SIGNS, AND SYMPTOMS

The prolapse occurs insidiously. If the cervix projects outside the vagina, it becomes exposed and unprotected.

The exposed tissue becomes dry and irritated, leading to bleeding ulcerations.

▶ DIAGNOSTIC PROCEDURES

The method for diagnosing a prolapsed uterus is bimanual pelvic examination. The uterus will feel lower than normal in the vagina upon palpation. With complete prolapse the uterus and cervix extend outside the introitus with inversion of the vaginal canal.

► **MEDICAL MANAGEMENT**

The usual procedure is vaginal hysterectomy or colpo-cleisis. A vaginal pessary is used to hold the uterus in place when surgery is not desired.

► **PROGNOSIS**

The prognosis is excellent with surgery. The older person who is a poor surgical risk has the option of the vaginal pessary or colpocleisis, which involves obliteration of the vagina.

► **NURSING MANAGEMENT—NURSING CARE PLAN**
   Uterine Prolapse

Assessment

SUBJECTIVE DATA

The patient stating that she "feels something falling down up there."

OBJECTIVE DATA

Protrusion of the uterus from the vagina
Palpating the uterus low in the vagina

	Nursing diagnoses	Expected outcomes	Nursing interventions (rationale)
N U R S I N G C A R E P L A N	Knowledge deficit related to prolapsed uterus, surgical intervention, and follow-up care	Patient will verbalize an understanding of the disease process, surgical intervention, and follow-up care.	Assess the patient's knowledge of uterine prolapse to get a baseline from which to begin teaching. Teach patient about the care of a uterus that has complete prolapse. If the uterus is protruding, it may need to be reinserted into the vagina to prevent trauma. Support the patient in her decision on medical therapy. Instruct the patient on home care following a hysterectomy (Box 11-10).
	Alteration in comfort: Pain related to surgery for prolapsed uterus	Patient will verbalize a decrease in pain. There will be no facial grimacing.	Assess the level of pain to get a baseline of the intensity of the pain. Administer the analgesic before the pain gets out of control and analgesia is less effective. Use diversional tactics to get the patient's mind off pain. Position patient so she is as comfortable as possible. With an abdominal incision, instruct patient to use pillows over incision when coughing.
	Body image disturbance related to removal of reproductive organ	Patient will verbalize a positive self-concept.	Be available for patient to express her feelings regarding the loss of her reproductive organ. Encourage discussion between patient and sexual partner regarding the surgery. Discuss questions and concerns that patient may have, especially myths and misconceptions regarding changes in sexuality or loss of femininity.

Box 11-10.

Patient Education

Home Care Following a Hysterectomy

Avoid sexual intercourse, douching, or inserting anything in the vagina for 6 weeks.

Avoid heavy lifting for 6 weeks.

Do not strain when having a bowel movement.

Eat foods high in fiber to avoid constipation.

Walk daily. Try to increase your distance slowly.

Call your physician if you notice an increase in pain, a fever, or an increased or foul smelling vaginal discharge. If you have an abdominal incision, look for redness, swelling, or discharge.

Additional instructions for the individual patient and/or family:

Box 11-11.

Patient Education

Taking a Narcotic Analgesic

Do not drive or operate any heavy machinery. This medication causes drowsiness.

This medication may cause constipation. To prevent this from occurring, eat a diet high in fiber, drink plenty of

water, and exercise as tolerated.

Do not drink alcoholic beverages while taking this medication.

Get up slowly. Dizziness may occur and cause you to fall.

Additional instructions for the individual patient and/or family:

Discharge planning and patient/family education
Arrange for outpatient follow-up by physician and/or visiting nurse.
Refer patient to a support group.
Teach patient correct information regarding the surgery, outcome, and home care (see Boxes 11-10 and 11-11).

Evaluation
Patient verbalizes an understanding of the disease process, surgical intervention, and follow-up care.
Patient verbalizes a decrease in pain. There is no facial grimacing.
Patient verbalizes a positive self-concept.

CANCER (KIDNEY, BLADDER, PROSTATE, UTERUS, CERVIX, VAGINA)

Cancer is a malignant growth characterized by its tendency to spread to surrounding tissue and metastasize to other areas of the body. The etiology of cancer is unknown, but there are high correlations between cancer and cigarette smoking, radiation, genetic predisposition, viruses, carcinogenic chemicals, and certain drugs. In addition, age, gender, ethnic group, and residence in certain geographic areas are factors in the development of some types of cancer.

▶ PATHOPHYSIOLOGY, SIGNS, AND SYMPTOMS

The signs and symptoms of the cancer depend on the location of the neoplasm (Table 11-1) plus the extent of the tumor and its metastasis.

▶ DIAGNOSTIC PROCEDURES

Kidney cancer—excretory urography, nephrotomography, ultrasonography, renal arteriography, cyst puncture, abdominal computerized tomography (CT) scan, microscopic cell study, cytologic cell study

Bladder cancer—cystogram, intravenous pyelogram, urinary cytology, cystoscopy and biopsy, pelvic CT scan, ultrasound, bimanual examination

Prostate cancer—rectal examination to palpate firm prostatic nodules, needle biopsy of nodule, test for elevated serum acid phosphatase, radioactive immunoassay, bone marrow aspiration

Uterine cancer—Papanicolaou test, uterine curettage, pelvic examination

Cervical cancer—Papanicolaou test, cervical punch biopsy, colposcopy, endocervical curettage

Vaginal cancer—Papanicolaou test, biopsy by Schiller's test

▶ MEDICAL MANAGEMENT

Treatment is based on the location of the cancer (Table 11-2).

▶ PROGNOSIS

The prognosis depends on the stage of the cancer when detected. Many patients with neoplasms discovered in the early stage have a long survival time. Early detection and prompt intervention are the key.

Table 11-1. Symptoms of cancers of the genitourinary system

Location	Symptoms
Kidney	Painless hematuria, flank pain, fever, palpable mass
Bladder	Painless hematuria, frequency, burning, dysuria, pyuria, palpable mass
Prostate	Urinary frequency, dysuria, hesitancy, pyuria, hematuria
Uterus and cervix	Inappropriate bleeding and/or discharge from the uterus
Vagina	Inappropriate bleeding, vaginal discharge, dyspareunia

Table 11-2. Treatment of cancers of the genitourinary system

Location	Therapy
Kidney	Radical nephrectomy with lymph node dissection, nephroureterectomy, radiotherapy, chemotherapy
Bladder	Topical and systemic chemotherapy, radiation therapy, cystectomy (bladder removal) with possible urinary diversion
Prostate	Radical perineal or retropubic prostatectomy, radiotherapy, hormonal therapy
Uterus and cervix	Total abdominal hysterectomy, radiotherapy, chemotherapy
Vagina	Radical surgery (radical hysterectomy, vaginectomy and pelvic lymph node dissection), radiotherapy

► **NURSING MANAGEMENT—NURSING CARE PLAN**
Cancer

Assessment

SUBJECTIVE DATA
Denial
Pain

OBJECTIVE DATA
Unusual bleeding or discharge
Change in bowel or bladder habits
Unexplained weight loss
A lesion that does not resolve

	Nursing diagnoses	Expected outcomes	Nursing interventions (rationale)
N U R S I N G C A R E P L A N	Anxiety related to the threat of death	Patient will express a decreased level of anxiety.	Assess the patient's present level of anxiety so that the intensity of the anxiety can be addressed. Provide a calm, stress-free environment to decrease sensory stimulation. Encourage the patient to verbalize feelings about the recent diagnosis to help decrease anxiety. Provide comfort and reassurance by staying with the patient and letting the patient talk, cry.
	Alteration in comfort: chronic pain related to the advanced stages of cancer	Patient will state that the pain is at a manageable level. Methods that help to reduce pain will be implemented.	Assess the degree of pain patient is experiencing to get a baseline of the pain experience. Administer an analgesic before pain becomes unmanageable. Teach patient noninvasive methods of pain relief such as relaxation, cutaneous stimulation, and distraction. Evaluate how the pain experience is affecting the patient's lifestyle and discuss ways to assist.
	Knowledge deficit related to early detection of cancer	Patient will verbalize methods to detect cancer in its early stages.	Assess patient's knowledge of methods to detect cancer early. Instruct patient on the guidelines for the screening of cervical cancer and prostate cancer (Box 11-12). Teach patient the early signs and symptoms of cervical cancer, uterine cancer, and prostate cancer. Teach patient the risk factors associated with each type of cancer.

Discharge planning and patient/family education

Refer patient to a support group and/or counselor for help in dealing with diagnosis of cancer.

Refer patient to a hospice for assistance with pain management at home.

Teach patient methods of relaxation, cutaneous stimulation, and guided imagery for use in pain management.

Arrange for follow-up screening by health care professional (see Box 11-12).

For information about cancer call or write the American *Cancer Society, 777 Third Avenue, New York, NY 10017—(800) 4-CANCER.*

For printed material write the Office of Cancer Communication, National Cancer Institute, Bldg 31, Rm 10A18, Bethesda, MD 20205.

Evaluation

Patient expresses a decreased level of anxiety.

Patient states that the pain is at a manageable level.

Methods that help to reduce pain have been implemented.

Patient verbalizes methods to detect cancer in its early stages.

Box 11-12.
Early detection of cancer

Cervical cancer

An annual Pap smear and pelvic examination are recommended.

Prostate cancer

A rectal examination to evaluate the prostate should be done annually starting at age 40.

RENAL FAILURE

Renal failure is the impairment of renal function, resulting in the kidney's inability to concentrate urine, eliminate waste, or regulate electrolyte concentrations. There are two classifications of renal failure, acute and chronic. Acute renal failure is usually caused by inadequate renal perfusion, obstruction along the urinary tract, or renal diseases (e.g., glomerulonephritis). Chronic renal failure is caused by renal disease or other chronic systemic diseases such as diabetes, gout, or lupus erythematosus.

▶ PATHOPHYSIOLOGY, SIGNS, AND SYMPTOMS

Acute renal failure has three phases: oliguric phase, diuretic phase, and then recovery phase. In the oliguric phase urine output drops to less than 400 ml/day (or the patient will have high output failure in which nitrogen is retained but fluid is excreted). Elements that are usually excreted by the kidney are retained. This produces an increase in urea, creatinine, uric acid, potassium, and magnesium in the blood. Physical symptoms will be urine that is scant and bloody, nausea, vomiting, lethargy, and drowsiness. In the next phase, the diuretic phase, the patient's urine output starts to increase and glomerular filtration begins to occur. In the recovery phase renal function improves over a period of 3 to 12 months.

Chronic renal failure also has three phases: diminished renal reserve, renal failure, and uremia. In diminished renal reserve the patient may be asymptomatic or have a few symptoms such as urinary frequency caused by the inability to concentrate the urine. In renal failure nitrogenous compounds are retained, resulting in elevated serum creatinine and blood urea nitrogen (BUN). In the uremia phase, there is further renal decline. Azotemia increases with fluid and electrolyte imbalance. This results in the symptoms of uremia, which include mental status changes, anemia, renal osteodystrophy, neurologic abnormalities, anorexia, nausea, vomiting, gastrointestinal ulcerations with bleeding, pruritus, and crystallized perspiration on the skin known as uremic frost.

▶ DIAGNOSTIC PROCEDURES

Acute renal failure is indicated by the following:
  Urinalysis—tubular cells, tubular cell casts, granular casts
  Serum creatinine—progressive rise
  BUN—elevated
  Serum potassium, chloride, phosphate, and magnesium—elevated
  Serum sodium, calcium, bicarbonate—decreased
  Arterial blood gases (ABG)—acidosis
Chronic renal failure shows the following:
BUN—elevated
ABG—metabolic acidosis
Serum calcium—decreased
Alkaline phosphatase, serum potassium—elevated
Urinalysis—proteinuria, hematuria, white blood cells, red blood cells, and leukocyte, fatty, granular, hyaline and/or waxy casts
Hematocrit and erythrocyte indices—normochromic, normocytic anemia
Creatinine clearance—10 to 50 ml/min

▶ MEDICAL MANAGEMENT

Acute renal failure: treatment of the underlying cause, limiting all substances that require excretion by the kidney, fluid restriction, limiting sodium and potassium intake, daily weight, renal dialysis
Chronic renal failure: dietary and fluid management based on patient's condition, regulation of electrolytes, renal dialysis, kidney transplantation

▶ PROGNOSIS

The prognosis depends on the underlying disease process and its complications. In acute renal failure the patient usually does not die of renal failure but of associated complications related to the primary cause of the renal failure. The outcome of chronic renal failure has been improved by the use of dialysis and renal transplant.

► **NURSING MANAGEMENT—NURSING CARE PLAN**
Renal Failure

Assessment

SUBJECTIVE DATA
Mental status changes: confusion, lethargy

OBJECTIVE DATA
Oliguria, anuria
Pruritus
Hypertension

	Nursing diagnoses	Expected outcomes	Nursing interventions (rationale)
N U R S I N G C A R E P L A N	Alteration in pattern of urinary elimination related to renal decline	Patient will maintain or improve renal status as evidenced by increased urine output and decreasing serum creatinine and BUN.	Measure intake and output to ensure that there is a balance. Monitor urine specific gravity to evaluate urine concentration. Obtain a daily weight to evaluate the patient's fluid status. Monitor serum creatinine and BUN to evaluate renal filtration. Prepare patient for renal dialysis, which assists patient in filtering the blood.
	Potential fluid volume excess related to the kidneys not excreting fluid	Patient will have no signs and symptoms of fluid volume excess.	Assess the patient for signs and symptoms of fluid volume excess such as increased weight, altered mental status, increased blood pressure, edema, distended neck veins, and adventitious breath sounds. Monitor vital signs, especially blood pressure, which indicates fluid retention. Monitor weight for an increase due to fluid retention. Evaluate hemodynamic monitoring equipment. Note central venous pressure and pulmonary capillary wedge pressure for indications of fluid excess. Monitor intake and output to be sure there is a balance in fluid intake and output.
	Knowledge deficit related to renal failure and its management	Patient will verbalize an understanding of renal failure that will include a demonstration and interactive discussion on diet, fluid restrictions, and self-monitoring skills.	Teach patient, at the appropriate level, the major concepts of renal failure so patient has a basic knowledge of the disease process. Reinforce dietitian's teaching on diet therapy. Instruct patient on use of fluid restriction to decrease possibility of hypervolemia. Teach patient self-monitoring skills such as how to weigh self (Box 11-13), measure and record intake and output, and monitor blood pressure (Box 11-13) so complications can be quickly reported.

Discharge planning and patient/family education

Arrange for follow-up by physician and/or visiting nurse.

Provide referral to a dialysis unit.

Demonstrate to the patient how to measure and record intake and output.

Be sure to discuss with patient what is included in output (e.g., vomitus and diarrhea as well as urine).

Teach the patient the early signs of a fluid imbalance.

Refer to dietitian for dietary counseling.

Arrange for follow-up by home health nurse on self-monitoring skills.

Evaluation

Patient maintains or improves renal status as evidenced by increased urine output and decreasing serum creatinine and BUN.

The signs and symptoms of fluid volume excess did not occur.

The patient verbalizes an understanding of renal failure that includes a demonstration and interactive discussion on diet, fluid restrictions, and self-monitoring skills.

Box 11-13.

Patient Education

Renal Failure

When taking blood pressure, remember:
Take your blood pressure at same time each day.
Use the same arm.
Exercise increases blood pressure, so do not exercise prior to taking your blood pressure.
Relax before you take your blood pressure; stress can also cause an increase.

When weighing yourself, be sure to:
Weigh at the same time every day
Wear approximately the same clothing; for example, always weigh yourself either with or without shoes.
Calibrate the scale to zero to obtain an accurate reading each time.

Additional instructions for the individual patient and/or family:

BIBLIOGRAPHY

Benign prostate hyperplasia and incontinence (1989). *The Informer,* summer ed, Wilmette, Ill, The Simon Foundation.

Burtis G, Davis J, and Martin S (1988). Applied nutrition and diet therapy, Philadelphia, WB Saunders Co.

Talbot L (1990). Nursing management of adults with renal disorders. In Beare PG and Myers JL, editors: Principles and practice of adult health nursing, ed 4, St Louis, The CV Mosby Co, pp 1013-1027.

Talbot L and Marquardt M (1989). Critical care assessment, St Louis, The CV Mosby Co.

Thompson J, McFarland G, Hirsch J, et al (1989). Mosby's manual of clinical nursing, ed 2, St Louis, The CV Mosby Co.

CHAPTER 12

Nervous System

Danna Strength

ALZHEIMER'S DISEASE

Alzheimer's disease is the most common of the neurodegenerative diseases. It is progressive and causes pathologic changes in the brain that lead to dementia, a "slowly progressive and irreversible organic brain syndrome" (Burgess, 1990, p. 700). Alzheimer's disease affects approximately 1 million older adults in the United States (Donohoe, 1990, p. 1097). Men and women are affected equally. It is estimated that the prevalence is as high as 20% by age 80 (Brunner, Suddarth, Bare, et al, 1988, p. 1482).

▶ PATHOPHYSIOLOGY, SIGNS, AND SYMPTOMS

Although the etiology is unknown, possible causes include environmental, hereditary, and immunologic factors. The degeneration occurs in the cerebral cortex, with cortical atrophy and loss of neurons. Microscopic examination reveals neurofibrillary tangles and senile plaques in brains of patients diagnosed with Alzheimer's disease. As nerve cells from the cerebral cortex are lost, there is a corresponding reduction in cerebral blood flow (Brunner, Suddarth, Bare, et al, 1988).

Clinical manifestations occur in three stages with some areas of overlapping (Box 12-1). Stage one symptoms, which may last for a period of 2 to 4 years, include some memory loss, forgetfulness, and absentmindedness. The patient may also experience time and spatial disorientation, decreased ability to concentrate, mistakes in judgment, changes in affect, and lack of spontaneity. In addition, there may be disturbances of perception, carelessness, delusions of persecution, muscle twitching, and seizure activity. The changes are subtle and may go unrecognized or be downplayed. Patients often become depressed during this stage when they realize that something is wrong with them.

The disorder is more frequently diagnosed in stage two as symptoms grow progressively worse and are more difficult to conceal. In this stage, which may extend over a longer period of time than stage one, clinical manifestations include increasing forgetfulness of both recent and remote events and intellectual changes such as inability to calculate (acalculia), to read (alexia), and to write (agraphia). Personality and behavioral changes also occur, as evidenced by increasing withdrawal and loss of socially acceptable behaviors. These changes are complicated by agnosia (inability of the patient to attach meaning to sensory impressions), astereognosis (inability to recognize objects by touch), and auditory agnosia (inability to recognize familiar sounds or words), which affects comprehension. Restlessness, wandering, and sleep disorders also occur during this stage. Important papers and personal possessions are misplaced, bills go unpaid, and personal hygiene is neglected. There is an element of paranoia in that families are accused of taking papers or possessions and neighbors are accused of meddling if they offer assistance. Stage two is probably most difficult for families because of the progressive inability of the patient to function and the increasing demands on family members' time and energy.

The third stage usually lasts no longer than a year and results in death, frequently as a result of aspiration pneumonia. In this stage the severity of both the mental and physical symptoms has increased. The patient loses the ability to perform self-care activities, no longer recognizes family members, and has lost the ability to communicate in a meaningful way with others. A decrease in appetite leads to emaciation and increased muscular weakness, and the patient becomes helpless and bedridden.

Box 12-1.

Stages of Alzheimer's disease

Symptoms of stage one

Memory loss
Time disorientation
Spatial disorientation
Affect changes
Mistakes in judgment
Absentmindedness
Decreased concentration abilities
Lack of spontaneity
Perceptual disturbances
Carelessness in actions
Transitory delusions of persecution
Epileptiform seizures
Muscular twitchings

Symptoms of stage two

Forgetfulness of recent and remote events
Increased inability to comprehend
Complete disorientation
Restlessness at night
Increased aphasia
Agnosia
Astereognosis
Apraxia

Perseveration phenomena
Hyperorality
Insatiable appetite without weight gain
Alexia
Auditory agnosia
Socially acceptable behaviors are forgotten
Hypertonia
Unsteady gait
Agraphia

Symptoms of stage three

Marked irritability
Paraphasia
Seizures
Hyperorality
Loss or diminution of emotions
Bulimia
Visual agnosia
Hypermetamorphosis
Apraxia
Decreased appetite
Bedridden
Emaciated
Helpless
Unresponsive or coma

From Williams L (1986). Alzheimer's: The need for caring, J Gerontol Nurs 12(2):23. Reprinted with permission.

▶ DIAGNOSTIC PROCEDURES

Diagnosis is made on the basis of a detailed history, a physical, and a mental status assessment (Table 12-1). A variety of diagnostic tests are then performed. These include an electroencephalogram (EEG), an electrocardiogram (ECG), computed tomography (CT), and magnetic resonance imaging (MRI). Other medical conditions such as depression, head injury, and brain tumors that mimic the symptoms of Alzheimer's disease must be ruled out before a definitive diagnosis can be made.

▶ MEDICAL MANAGEMENT

There are no medical interventions to cure or arrest the progression of Alzheimer's disease. Treatment is directed toward providing safety, meeting self-care needs, and meeting nutritional requirements. Pharmacologic agents such as haloperidol (Haldol), thiothixene (Navane), loxapine (Loxitane), and thioridazine (Mellaril) are pre-scribed to control the behavioral aspects of the disorder (Bauvette-Risey, 1989). Family therapy is supportive. Caregivers need factual information regarding the progression of Alzheimer's disease, as well as assistance in locating community support groups. Families may also need information and counsel in determining the appropriateness of institutional care.

Research presently being conducted offers hope for the future. These endeavors are directed toward determining the exact etiology, developing specific diagnostic procedures, and developing additional medications that will prove effective in the management of Alzheimer's disease.

▶ PROGNOSIS

The prognosis is poor. The disease often lasts from 5 to 20 years, and the physical, psychological, and financial problems encountered by the caregivers are immeasurable.

Table 12-1. Mental status assessment

I. GENERAL APPEARANCE: Underweight _____ Overweight _____ Emaciated _____ Clean _____ Unkempt _____ Needs bath _____ Clothing appropriate to season/occasion _____ Peculiarity of dress/ cosmetics _____ Explain and describe _____

_____

II. MOTOR STATUS: Posture erect _____ Stooped _____ Slouched _____ Muscular twitching _____ Grimacing _____ Posturing _____ Gait coordinated _____ Gait unsteady _____ Gait stiff _____ Shuffling _____ Other/describe _____

_____

III. ACTIVITY: WNL _____ Seizures _____ Lethargic _____ Purposeful _____ Disorganized activity _____ Restless at night _____ Bedridden _____ Other/describe _____

IV. FACIAL EXPRESSION: Alert _____ Tense _____ Sad _____ Crying _____ Happy _____ Angry _____ Flat _____ Other/describe _____

V. MOOD: Angry _____ Depressed _____ Sad _____ Calm _____ Happy _____ Agitated _____ Labile _____ Other/describe _____

VI. ENVIRONMENT: Interest in family _____ Friends _____ Social activities _____ Environment _____

VII. ORIENTATION: Oriented to time _____ Place _____ Person _____ Preoccupied _____ Distractable _____ Immediate memory _____ Recent memory _____ Distant memory _____ Complete disorientation _____

VIII. THOUGHT PROCESSES: Able to complete sentences _____ Jumps from topic to topic _____ Spontaneous _____ Mute _____ Logical _____ Illogical _____ Loose associations _____ Meaningless repetition of words _____ Decreased concentration ability _____ Mistakes in judgment _____

IX. THOUGHT CONTENT: DESCRIBE

Obsessions _____ _____

Compulsions _____ _____

Delusions _____ _____

X. DANGER ASSESSMENT:

Suicidal thoughts _____ _____

Suicidal plans _____ _____

Recent suicidal gesture

and/or attempt _____ _____

XI. INSIGHT: Aware of present impairment _____ What makes you think so? _____

_____

Aware of treatment need _____ What makes you think so? _____

_____

Adapted with permission from Frances Richardson, Harris College of Nursing, Texas Christian University, Fort Worth, and Harris Methodist HEB, Bedford, Tex.

▶ **NURSING MANAGEMENT—NURSING CARE PLAN**
Dementia of the Alzheimer's Type (DAT)

Assessment

The assessment may be performed over a period of several days. The nurse may need additional time to collect and evaluate subjective and objective data because the patient may be unable to cooperate in providing information for the nursing history. In the early stages, memory deficits and impairments in judgment may be difficult to recognize and evaluate on the basis of limited contact with the patient.

SUBJECTIVE DATA
History
Physical
Mental status evaluation (see Table 12-1)
OBJECTIVE DATA
Memory loss
Impaired judgment

Wandering, especially at night
Sleep disorders, e.g., insomnia
Inability to perform activities of daily living (ADL)
Decreased recognition of family/friends
Decreasing communication
Urinary and fecal incontinence

	Nursing diagnoses	Expected outcomes	Nursing interventions (rationale)
N U R S I N G C A R E P L A N	Altered thought processes related to degeneration of nerve cells	Patient will be oriented to person, place, and time; thought processes will be supported.	Use clock with large numbers and daily calendar marked with events. Speak in a slow manner and low tone, using simple short sentences. (Low tone is more easily heard and simple sentences are more easily comprehended.) Correct faulty perceptions (e.g., clarify who you are, provide reality orientation to day and location). Use patient's full name when speaking to the patient. Place patient's name in large print on door to room and place mementos in shadow boxes outside door (orients to sense of person and place). Paint bathroom door in bright (even neon) colors (attracts attention to bathroom when location is forgotten). Allow additional time for response. (Older people need more time to process thought.) Clarify responses, if needed, in a gentle manner. Provide assistance with decision making (selection of clothes to wear, participation in activities).
	Potential for injury related to decreased awareness/failure to recognize hazards	Safe environment will be provided.	Secure car keys if patient is prone to wandering and a hazard to self and others. Provide safe environment. Remove small throw rugs. Install grab bars in bathroom facilities. Assign room away from outside doors or stairs. Lock outside doors so patient cannot open them.

Nursing Care Plan—Dementia of the Alzheimer's Type (DAT)—cont'd

Nursing diagnoses	Expected outcomes	Nursing interventions (rationale)
		Keep rooms well lighted—baths, halls, dining areas.
		Use night-light in bathroom and hallways.
		Keep bed in low locked position.
		Secure identification bracelet on arm.
		Ensure that shoes and socks are worn and patient is appropriately dressed for weather (in case of wandering).
		Assess ability to swallow.
		Cut food in small pieces if needed (decreases likelihood of choking).
		Allow maximum independence in protected environment.
Bathing, dressing, feeding, toileting self-care deficit related to memory loss/decreasing functional level	Patient will continue self-care activities until third stage.	Develop and write down routine for performing self-care. (Activities can be checked off when performed.)
		Place personal hygiene items in view of patient or in a labeled drawer.
		Check to see whether items are returned to proper place after use. (Maintaining consistency in environment is important.)
		Allow rest periods between self-care activities.
		Compliment patient when tasks are completed (increases self-esteem and feeling of accomplishment).
		Assist in performance of ADL when needed.
		Send soiled clothing to laundry/family for care.
Impaired verbal and written communication related to memory loss/personality changes	Patient will communicate needs, wishes, desires.	Assess ability to comprehend, speak, and write.
		Reduce distracting environmental stimuli (TV, radio) when talking (assists in focusing on conversation).
		Use patient's name at beginning and end of sentences (keeps patient oriented).
		Use short simple sentences (easier to comprehend).
		Give one-step commands/directives/explanations.
		Maintain eye contact.
		Allow additional response time. (Older adults need additional time to process information and to respond.)
		Avoid causing agitation/frustration (leads to increased confusion, decreased functioning).
		Maintain a calm, reassuring attitude.

Continued.

Nursing Care Plan—Dementia of the Alzheimer's Type (DAT)—cont'd

Nursing diagnoses	Expected outcomes	Nursing interventions (rationale)
Altered family processes related to progressive deterioration of mental and physical abilities	Family processes will be supported.	Assess family's roles, relationships, strengths. (Alzheimer's disease is demanding on family, and personal strengths need to be developed.) Involve family in developing plan of care (leads to increased compliance of family members). Allow family to express concerns/personal pain. Assist family in understanding disease process (helps family to know their feelings are normal). Encourage family to talk and touch loved one. (Expressions of acceptance and love are needed by patient.) Refer family to a local therapeutic support group (Alzheimer's Disease and Related Disorder Association).

Discharge planning and patient/family education

Assess home environment.

Keep patient active and involved with family/friends.

Assist family to develop coping mechanisms.

Encourage family to join a support group. For the address and phone number of a local group, write to Alzheimer's Disease and Related Disorder Association, 360 North Michigan Ave, Chicago, IL 60601.

Encourage family to schedule respite care on a regular basis.

Encourage family to obtain legal guardianship.

Provide patient/family education on patient safety (Box 12-2) and ways to improve communications. See Box 12-6 (p. 242) for communication tips (some information designed for patients with cerebrovascular ac-

cident also applies to patients with Alzheimer's disease).

Evaluation

Patient is oriented to day, time, place, and person.

Thought processes/memory are maintained with cues and clarification.

No injuries occur; safety devices are used.

Patient performs self-care at expected level in relation to stage of disease.

Patient understands simple communications.

Patient complies with verbal directives.

Patient verbalizes contentment when interacting with family.

Family discusses feelings with nurse.

Family joins therapeutic support group.

Box 12-2.   # Patient/Family Education

Patient Safety

Have patient wear an identification band with name, address, phone number.

Install an alarm system or special locks on doors.

Secure car keys.

Ensure that patient is always appropriately dressed for weather (in case of wandering).

Place all medications in a locked medicine cabinet.

Place all cleaning compounds/poisons in a locked cabinet.

Keep a bathroom or hallway light on at night.

Keep environment free of unnecessary furniture, and do not rearrange living area.

Bedroom should be on ground floor if at all possible. If bedroom is upstairs, install stair guard.

Additional instructions for the individual patient and/or family:

HUNTINGTON'S DISEASE

Huntington's disease, formerly called chorea, is a genetic disorder that is characterized by involuntary choreiform movements and dementia. It is a progressive, autosomal dominant disease with no effective treatment. Most patients do not develop symptoms until the fourth decade of life, and men are affected slightly more often than women. It is estimated that 25,000 people in the United States have clinical symptoms of the disorder (Donohoe, 1990, p. 1108). Offspring of an affected parent have a 50% chance of developing the disorder.

▶ PATHOPHYSIOLOGY, SIGNS, AND SYMPTOMS

The causative gene is located on chromosome number 4. Neuronal deterioration and abnormalities in neurotrans-mission in the caudate nucleus and putamen are thought to be the cause of the movement disorder. Cognitive impairment is related to loss of cells in the cortex, the area of the brain associated with perception, reasoning, and thinking. Signs and symptoms are choreiform movements, intellectual dysfunction, and emotional changes. The symptoms are progressive in nature. Speech changes from slurred to unintelligible, and choreiform movements lead to eventual loss of ambulation. Bizarre facial grimaces are associated with Huntington's disease. Intellectual dysfunction includes progressive impairment in thought processes, reasoning, and judgment, and memory loss, leading to eventual dementia. Patients exhibit paranoid thinking, irritability, anger, and depression. Suicide is not an uncommon end to the disease.

▶ **DIAGNOSTIC PROCEDURES**

Diagnosis is based on data from the history and physical examination. Differential diagnosis is directed toward ruling out Sydenham's chorea and Wilson's disease. In Huntington's disease the lack of association with rheumatic fever and the absence of hepatolenticular degeneration and Kayser-Fleischer rings, both of which are present in Wilson's disease, are important in the differential diagnosis.

▶ **MEDICAL MANAGEMENT**

Medical management is directed toward control of involuntary movements and behavioral traits. Haloperidol (Haldol), one of the butyrophenones, is a dopamine blocker and aids in the control of both movement and behavior. Another classification of drugs that exhibits some effect on the disorder is the phenothiazines, which are antipsychotic/neuroleptic drugs that block dopamine receptors. Examples are chlorpromazine (Thorazine) and thioridazine (Mellaril). These drugs are started in lower doses in older patients. Genetic counseling is indicated, and a multidisciplinary approach is needed to provide support to patients and their families.

▶ **PROGNOSIS**

The prognosis is poor, and death usually results within 1 to 6 years.

▶ **NURSING MANAGEMENT**

An essential of management is genetic counseling for children of patients with Huntington's disease. Refer to the nursing care plan for dementia of the Alzheimer's type (pp. 226-228) for additional specifics on nursing management.

PICK'S DISEASE

Pick's disease is a progressive disorder characterized by cerebral atrophy that results in degeneration of cognitive abilities, personality, and emotions. It primarily affects the frontal, temporal, and parietal lobes of the brain, and it is transmitted as an autosomal dominant trait. Clinically, Pick's disease is similar to Alzheimer's disease, and distinction between the two disorders is most frequently made on autopsy.

Pick's disease is an extremely rare disorder. The peak frequency of onset is at about age 54, although it may occur earlier in life, as early as the 20s. Onset decreases markedly after age 54, and by age 75 new cases are extremely rare (Heston and White, 1983, pp. 59-60). Pick's disease is more common in women than in men, and there is a familial tendency.

▶ **PATHOPHYSIOLOGY, SIGNS, AND SYMPTOMS**

Cerebral atrophy of the frontal and temporal lobes is marked. There is a line of demarcation between the affected and normal portion of the brain. Histologically, the nerve cells are pale and swollen and contain round cytoplasmic globules called Pick bodies (Davies, 1988, p. 13). Clinical manifestations include incomprehensible and repetitive speech, progressive loss of intellectual abilities, changes in personality such as flattened affect and decreased initiative, and loss of memory. Early intellectual impairment is characterized by distractability and inability to deal with new problems. The physical state deteriorates in conjunction with central nervous system changes.

▶ **DIAGNOSTIC PROCEDURES**

Diagnosis is made on the basis of symptoms, age of onset, and family history of the disorder. Computed tomography (CT) scans and magnetic resonance imaging (MRI) are of diagnostic value, but definitive diagnosis is made at autopsy on the basis of the microscopic appearance of the brain.

▶ **MEDICAL MANAGEMENT**

Treatment is supportive because there is no known cure. Families benefit from individual psychotherapy or group therapy, but therapy is of limited value to patients since their flattened affect and mental deterioration interfere with therapist/patient interactions.

▶ **PROGNOSIS**

The prognosis is poor. Death occurs after an average duration of 4 years.

▶ **NURSING MANAGEMENT**

Refer to the nursing care plan for dementia of the Alzheimer's type (pp. 226-228) for specifics on nursing management.

CREUTZFELDT-JAKOB DISEASE

Creutzfeldt-Jakob disease is a progressive encephalopathy characterized by degeneration of the pyramidal and extrapyramidal tracts. It is generally thought to be caused by an unidentified slow virus, but genetic factors may also be involved because there is a familial tendency. Creutzfeldt-Jakob disease is an extremely rare disorder that affects about 1 million persons (Davies, 1988, p. 13). The onset occurs in the middle years, earlier than the onset of Pick's disease, and the disease progresses rapidly.

▶ **PATHOPHYSIOLOGY, SIGNS, AND SYMPTOMS**

The cerebral cortex, basal ganglia, and spinal cord are typically involved in the degenerative process. Widespread microscopic vacuoles are present in the involved structures of the brain and give them their spongy appearance. The disease is characterized by progressive dementia, muscle wasting that results in weakness of the legs, dysarthria, involuntary movements, neurasthenia, and somnolence (Porth, 1982, p. 638).

▶ **DIAGNOSTIC PROCEDURES**

In the initial stage the electroencephalogram (EEG) is normal, but as the disease progresses the EEG is characterized by paroxysmal spikes with delta and theta slow-wave activity.

▶ **MEDICAL MANAGEMENT**

Treatment is supportive and symptomatic. There is no known cure for the disease. The usual course of the disease rarely exceeds 1 year.

▶ **NURSING MANAGEMENT**

Refer to the nursing care plan on dementia of the Alzheimer's type (pp. 226-228) for specifics on nursing management.

PARKINSON'S DISEASE

Parkinson's disease is a chronic, progressive disorder of the central nervous system. It is the second most common neurologic condition in older adults (Bauvette-Risey, 1989). The onset is usually between ages 60 and 80, and men are affected more frequently than women.

▶ **PATHOPHYSIOLOGY, SIGNS, AND SYMPTOMS**

The etiology is unknown; however, Parkinson's disease may be caused by arteriosclerosis, it may be a sequela of encephalitis, or it may be drug induced. Parkinson's disease is a disorder of the extrapyramidal tract. It is characterized by loss of cell pigment of the substantia nigra of the basal ganglia, which includes the corpus striatum, globus pallidus, subthalmic nucleus, and red nucleus. Two neurotransmitters, dopamine and acetylcholine, are also involved in this disorder of movement. Dopamine acts as an inhibitor on the extrapyramidal tract and is deficient in the striatum. This deficiency leads to the

symptoms of Parkinson's disease. Acetylcholine levels are normal in these patients, but the balance between dopamine and acetylcholine is disturbed, producing aggravation of the symptoms (Bauvette-Risey, 1989).

The cardinal symptoms are tremor, rigidity, akinesia, and postural difficulties (Figure 12-1), which are characteristic symptoms of extrapyramidal tract disorders. Tremor usually occurs at rest and is referred to as pill-rolling tremor. Rigidity, due to hypertonicity of muscles, is referred to as cogwheel rigidity. Akinesia (absence of spontaneous movement) is coupled with bradykinesia (slowing of voluntary movement). Postural difficulties are apparent in the gait of the individual. Steps are small and shuffling, with the body leaning forward and the head down. Steps become faster (propulsive gait) and the individual does not swing the arms. Rigidity of the facial muscles leads to a blank, fixed expression referred to as masked facies. Facial rigidity and rigidity of the throat muscles lead to difficulties in mastication and swallowing. Speech is slow and measured and spoken in a monotonous voice. The individual also experiences perspiration and drooling, which add to constipation. There is a high prevalence of dementia in individuals with Parkinson's disease.

▶ **DIAGNOSTIC PROCEDURES**

There is no known test to confirm the diagnosis of Parkinson's disease. The diagnosis is made on the basis of a complete history and physical and by ruling out other neurologic conditions.

▶ **MEDICAL MANAGEMENT**

Major pharmacologic agents used to control the symptoms of Parkinson's disease are dopaminergics, anticholinergic agents, and dopamine agonists (Table 12-2). Sinemet, a combination of carbidopa and levodopa, has largely replaced L-dopa as the drug of choice because the combination has fewer side effects and carbidopa permits an increased concentration of levodopa to cross the blood-brain barrier. Physical therapy and occupational therapy are ordered in conjunction with the pharmacologic program. In patients with severe disabling tremor or levodopa-induced dyskinesia, stereotaxic surgical procedures may be considered to destroy parts of the thalamus, thereby reducing tremor and rigidity (Brunner, Suddarth, Bare, et al, 1988).

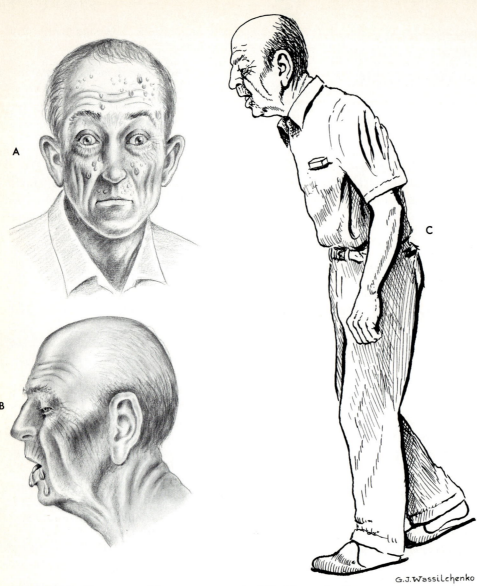

Figure 12-1. Characteristic features of patient with Parkinson's disease. **A,** Excess sweating. **B,** Sialorrhea. **C,** Shuffling gait. (From Rudy EB [1984]. Advanced neurological and neurosurgical nursing, St Louis, Mosby–Year Book, Inc, p. 269. Reprinted with permission.)

G.J.Wassilchenko

Table 12-2. Drugs used in management of Parkinson's disease

Drug	Action	Side effects	Drug	Action	Side effects
Dopaminergics			**Anticholinergic agents**		
Levodopa (L-dopa)	Replaces dopamine in central nervous system (CNS)	Nausea and vomiting Decreased blood pressure Dry mouth Decreased appetite Delusions	Trihexyphenidyl (Artane) Benztropine mesylate (Cogentin) Procyclidine (Kemadrin) Biperiden (Akineton)	All anticholinergic agents listed have similar action: Block action of acetylcholine Relieve tremor and rigidity	All anticholinergic agents have similar side effects: Dry mouth Blurred vision Urinary retention Confusion Tachycardia Rash Constipation
Carbidopa/levodopa (Sinemet)	Replaces dopamine in CNS and decreases side effects of levodopa	Same as with levodopa though lessened			
			Dopamine agonists		
			Bromocriptine (Parlodel)	Stimulates dopamine receptors	Confusion Decreased blood pressure Nausea and vomiting Hallucinations

▶ **NURSING MANAGEMENT—NURSING CARE PLAN**
Parkinson's Disease (PD)

Assessment

SUBJECTIVE DATA

History of the following:
  Weakness, tiredness, and fatigue
  Tremor of hands at rest
  Change in speech
  Change in handwriting
  Difficulty in movement (starting to walk, turning in bed)

OBJECTIVE DATA

Tremor of hands at rest
Tremor of feet (sometimes) at rest
Pill-rolling movements of hands—aggravated when nervous or stressed

Rigidity—"lead pipe" muscle rigidity; two-joint flexor muscles are most affected
Akinesia—frozen in place and unable to move
Bradykinesia—most disabling of major symptoms
Postural instability—stooped posture, head bent forward
Gait—shuffling, propulsive, little swinging of arms, combined with stooped posture
Masked facies—little or no expression of emotions, few wrinkles in face
Slow/monotonous speech
Dysphagia
Excessive perspiration
Excessive salivation

NURSING CARE PLAN

Nursing diagnoses	Expected outcomes	Nursing interventions (rationale)
Ineffective airway clearance related to muscle weakness	Patient will remain free of respiratory complications/aspiration pneumonia.	Assess patient's ability to cough and keep own airway clear every day. (With the decrease in structure and function of respiratory muscles in older persons there is decreased strength for breathing and coughing.)
		Auscultate breath sounds every 4 hr (increased likelihood for respiratory complication due to age-related changes and intercostal muscle rigidity in patients with PD).
		Monitor vital signs every hour.
		Maintain hydration at 3000 ml/24 hr (po if able to swallow) unless this amount is contraindicated. (Inadequate fluid intake and increased salivation add to constipation.)
		Encourage deep breathing and coughing every hour. (Restricted expansion of chest wall due to intercostal muscle rigidity predisposes to respiratory complications.)
		Keep patient in upright sitting position as much as possible.
		Keep suction at bedside. (Muscle weakness leads to dysphagia and frequent choking.)
		Instruct family/patient in signs and symptoms of respiratory complications. (Muscle weakness and difficulty in swallowing and coughing lead to increased danger of aspiration pneumonia.)

Continued.

Nursing Care Plan—Parkinson's Disease (PD)—cont'd

Nursing diagnoses	Expected outcomes	Nursing interventions (rationale)
Potential for injury related to postural difficulties/gait disturbances/progressive neuromuscular degeneration	Patient will continue in physical therapy to maintain mobility.	Assess patient's ability to ambulate in own environment. (Postural instabilities lead to an increase in frequency of falls in older adults.) Assess environment for hazards every shift. Remove environmental hazards every shift. Supervise gait retraining program daily. Stand with broad base. Look up. Swing arms.
	Patient will use assistive devices in ambulation.	Instruct patient in use of assistive devices. (Cane or walker may be used to increase stability.) Collaborate with physical therapy on exercise program every week. Instruct patient to avoid hurrying (counteracts propulsive gait).
Altered nutrition: less than body requirements, related to dysphagia	Patient will express decreased anxiety regarding swallowing/choking.	Assess ability to swallow. Assess ability to feed self. Arrange small, frequent meals (avoids fatigue of eating in frail older patients). Weigh weekly. Perform weekly calorie counts. (Calorie intake may decrease because of chewing and swallowing difficulties.) Provide high-protein, high-bulk, high-roughage diet. (Soft solids and thick liquids are easier to swallow than thin liquids.) Use large absorbent napkins/towels at mealtime rather than bibs (maintains dignity and self-esteem in older adults). Assist with oral hygiene before meals. (Cleanse dentures thoroughly.) Provide rest periods before meals. Talk with patient before meals (promotes relaxation and enhances pleasure of meal). Prepare all foods for eating—cutting, opening packages. (Avoid small pieces or foods that crumble or break apart—can be "lost" because of decreased sensation in mouths of older persons.) Remain with patient during meals (increased fear of choking associated with dysphagia). Keep patient sitting up or in low Fowler's position for 30 min after meals. (Older people fre-

Nursing Care Plan—Parkinson's Disease (PD)—cont'd

Nursing diagnoses	Expected outcomes	Nursing interventions (rationale)
		quently have a dilated esophagus, which allows easy regurgitation.)
Self-care deficit related to loss of spontaneity and slowness of movement	Patient will perform activities of daily living (ADL) with assistance.	Place call light within easy reach. Assess ability to perform ADL. Allow for rest periods during care. Encourage patient to bathe and dress daily. Avoid laces, buttons on clothing. (Use Velcro when possible because rigidity increases difficulty in dressing self.) Provide elevated toilet seats and grab bars (allows for easier "push off" and increases safety). Provide elevated seats for straight-backed *arm* chairs. (Elevated chairs with arms allow for "push off.") Perform eye care every 2 hr (decreased blinking in PD). Acknowledge patient's accomplishments in self-care (increases self-esteem).
Knowledge deficit related to treatment regimen/home care	Patient will comply with pharmacologic management.	Assess readiness to learn. Provide information about the disorder. (Increased understanding of treatment program leads to increased compliance.) Encourage patient to keep appointments with physicians, physical therapists, and speech therapists. Instruct patient in medication schedule and side effects of drugs. (Many drugs have psychiatric side effects in older persons.) Refer family to a support group.

Discharge planning and patient/family education

Ensure that both patient and family have an understanding of the drug therapy program, including side effects of medications.

Provide information about purchasing of and reimbursement for assistive devices (e.g., walkers, canes, and other helpful appliances).

Assess home environment for safety and needed alterations (e.g., grab bars, raised commode seats, straight-back chairs with arms).

Stress the importance of eating a well-balanced diet even though this may be difficult because of problems with chewing and swallowing.

Ensure follow through on laboratory (blood) tests and physician appointments.

Provide the information in Box 12-3.

Evaluation

No respiratory complications occur.

Patient maintains physical therapy schedule.

Number of falls is decreasing with assistive devices.

Patient swallows without choking.

Admission weight is maintained.

Patient spaces self-care activities/rest periods.

Patient seeks assistance with ADL when needed.

Patient takes medication on schedule.

Patient performs self-assessment for side effects.

Family receives information and support from attending meetings. Local chapter can be contacted through Parkinson's Support Group of America, 11376 Cherry Hill Rd, No. 204, Beltsville, MD 20705.

Box 12-3.

Patient/Family Education

General Guidelines for Parkinson's Disease

Sleep on a firm mattress and use a bed board.

Exercise 20 minutes daily to maintain joint mobility (walk, swim, or ride a stationary bicycle).
When walking try to do the following:
  Maintain erect posture—hold head up.
  Lengthen stride.
  Pick feet up with each step.
  Swing arms loosely.

Sit in straight-back chair with high seat and arm rests to push up and out as you lean forward with heels back under chair.

Avoid fatigue. Frequent rest periods are helpful.

Maintain outpatient physical therapy program.

Make a constant effort to swallow saliva frequently.

If eating becomes a problem, use a stabilized plate and cup and built-up eating utensils. (Physical therapist can assist in obtaining these assistive devices.)

Eat a well-balanced diet high in fiber. Include foods such as the following:

Apples	Cereal—raisin bran
Applesauce	Oatmeal
Beans, black	Squash
and lima	Tomatoes
Brussels	
sprouts	

Speak in short sentences and exaggerate enunciation (helps prevent slurring of speech).

Avoid any drugs not prescribed by your physician.

For additional information contact the American Parkinson's Disease Association, 116 John St, New York, NY 10038.

Additional instructions for the individual patient and/or family:

TRANSIENT ISCHEMIC ATTACK

A transient ischemic attack (TIA) is a focal cerebral dysfunction of vascular origin. It is temporary, with a rapid onset of symptoms that last no longer than 24 hours (Bauvette-Risey, 1989, p. 320). TIAs should be thoroughly investigated and treated promptly because they are usually a precursor to a major stroke within 6 months.

CEREBROVASCULAR ACCIDENT

A cerebrovascular accident (CVA), commonly referred to as a stroke, is an alteration in the cerebral circulation that produces a decrease in the blood supply of the brain. The diminished oxygen supply may lead to necrosis of brain tissue with neurologic deficits unless normal circulation is restored immediately. The most common causes are thrombus, embolus, and hemorrhage. CVA is the second leading cause of death in adults over age 72 (Graves, 1988, p. 67) and the third leading cause of death in this country (Kinney and Schenk, 1990; Schenk, 1990). A CVA occurs 10 times more frequently in adults over age 75 than in those 55 to 59 (Bauvette-Risey, 1989, p. 319).

▶ **PATHOPHYSIOLOGY, SIGNS, AND SYMPTOMS**

The pathophysiology of a cerebrovascular accident must be examined in relation to the causative factors.

Thrombus—The lumen of one of the cerebral arteries becomes occluded, usually because of atherosclerosis. Thrombosis is the most common cause of a CVA.

Embolus—The embolus/emboli may come from any part of the body and lodge in an artery, usually in a narrowed part of an artery. Cerebral emboli frequently occur secondary to prosthetic heart valves, myocardial infarctions, or atrial fibrillation and during cardioversion for atrial fibrillation.

Hemorrhage—Hypertension, atherosclerotic changes, and congenital arteriovenous malformations are major factors that may cause a cerebral artery to rupture. When the rupture occurs, blood supply to the brain is decreased and surrounding tissue is compressed, leading to neurologic deficits.

Box 12-4.

Risk factors for cerebrovascular accidents

Age—occur at any age, but primarily in older adults
Hypertension—greater than 160/90 mm Hg.
Atherosclerosis/arteriosclerosis
High serum cholesterol and/or triglycerides
Obesity
Sedentary lifestyle
Smoking
Diabetes mellitus
Cardiac disorders—myocardial infarction, atrial fibrillation
Family history

Box 12-5.

Clinical manifestations of middle cerebral artery syndrome

Aphasia
Decreasing level of consciousness
Headache
Hemiplegia
Homonymous hemianopsia
Unilateral neglect of paralyzed side
Paresis
Possible Cheyne-Stokes respirations

Many of the risk factors (Box 12-4) associated with CVAs are to some extent controllable and are similar to the risk factors associated with cardiovascular disease.

Signs and symptoms are dependent on which cerebral artery was involved and the portion of the brain supplied by that artery. The middle cerebral artery is the most frequently occluded artery. Clinical manifestations are presented in Box 12-5. General clinical manifestations of a CVA are headache and nucchal rigidity (particularly from cerebral hemorrhage), slurred speech, aphasia, visual disturbance, numbness, tingling, sensory loss, impairment of motor function ranging from weakness to paralysis, confusion, memory deficits, loss of consciousness, and possible seizure activity.

▶ **DIAGNOSTIC PROCEDURES**

Diagnosis is made on the basis of a history (if possible) and a thorough physical examination. Additional diagnostic tools include radiographic examinations, EEGs, lumbar puncture, Doppler ultrasonography, and routine laboratory studies (Table 12-3).

▶ **MEDICAL MANAGEMENT**

Pharmacologic management of a cerebrovascular accident includes anticoagulant therapy unless the etiology is hemorrhagic, antihypertensive agents and diuretics, steroids for cerebral edema, and anticonvulsants if seizure activity is likely. Additional medical management is aimed toward prevention of complications and rehabilitation.

Table 12-3. Diagnostic tools—cerebrovascular accident

Test	Purpose
History and physical	Provides symptomatic basis for diagnosis
Cerebral angiography	Locates specific lesion
Brain scan	Demonstrates ischemia
CT scan	Identifies hematomas, infarcts, lesions
Doppler ultrasonography	Detects areas of impaired blood flow
EEG	Locates area of abnormal electrical discharges
Lumbar puncture	Reveals bloody cerebrospinal fluid if hemorrhagic
Laboratory tests—complete blood count, electrolytes, cholesterol, triglycerides, urinalysis	Provide benchmark for additional data

► **NURSING MANAGEMENT—NURSING CARE PLAN**
Cerebrovascular Accident (CVA)

Assessment

SUBJECTIVE DATA	*Unequal pupils*
HISTORY OF THE FOLLOWING:	*Aphasia*
Hypertension	*Visual loss*
Headache	*Bladder/bowel incontinence*
Nucchal rigidity	*Neurologic deficits*
Vertigo	*Alteration in level of consciousness*
OBJECTIVE DATA	*Convulsions*
Increased blood pressure	*Decerebrate posturing*

	Nursing diagnoses	Expected outcomes	Nursing interventions (rationale)
N U R S I N G C A R E P L A N	Impaired physical mobility related to weakness/hemiplegia	Patient will report an increase in strength and endurance.	Teach patient to perform range of motion (ROM) activities on unaffected side. Teach patient to self-assist in performance of ROM activities on affected side (may be more difficult in older adult with muscle atrophy and decreased muscle strength). Support stronger leg in performance of transfer activities.
		Patient will develop no complications of immobility.	Turn every 2 hr using turning sheet (avoids shearing forces that lead to skin breakdown; skin of older adult is very thin and fragile). Assess skin integrity every 2 hr. (Thinning of the epidermis in older adults leads to increased likelihood of injury and breakdown.) Use elbow and heel protectors. Place patient on egg crate/alternating pressure mattress. Use foot boards/padded splints/ tennis shoes to prevent foot drop (can occur within first 24 hr of CVA). Avoid prolonged periods of hip flexion (keep head of bed low) and knee flexion (prevents contractures of hip and knee). Use trochanter rolls to prevent external rotation. *Caution:* Use of trapeze bar may increase intracranial pressure (ICP), which is to be avoided.
	Altered nutrition: less than body requirements, related to dysphagia	Patient will ingest adequate dietary intake to maintain weight.	Assess difficulty in swallowing. Assess and document bowel sounds every 4 hr. Weigh patient daily before breakfast. Assist in selection of high-protein, high-calorie diet. (Dietary consultation may be necessary.)

Nursing Care Plan—Cerebrovascular Accident (CVA)—cont'd

Nursing diagnoses	Expected outcomes	Nursing interventions (rationale)
		Perform oral hygiene before meals. (Cleanse dentures well.)
		Provide foods with texture, and place them in unaffected side of mouth (easier to stimulate swallowing reflex).
		Place patient in semi-Fowler's or high Fowler's position for feeding. (Older persons have a dilated esophagus, and fluids could easily be regurgitated and aspirated.)
		Place food on back of tongue in unaffected side of mouth. (Older adults have decreased oral sensation, and CVA further decreases sensation on affected side.)
		Keep patient in position for 30 min postfeeding. (Suction machine should be available.) If nasogastric tube is in place, follow specific directions in procedure manuals.
Impaired verbal communication related to expressive or receptive aphasia	Patient will demonstrate increasing ability to express self and understand others.	Assess type of aphasia—expressive or receptive.
		Consult with physician regarding speech therapy when condition has stabilized.
		Speak clearly in simple words or sentences using low voice if receptive aphasia. (Low tones are perceived better by older adults than higher frequencies.)
		Use flash cards, drawings, gestures, pantomime for/with communication. (Visual aids reinforce verbal communication and increase association of words and image.)
		Address frustration over difficulties in communication, but ignore abusive and profane language.
		Provide alternative means of communication if expressive aphasia (pen and pencil, word computer).
		Allow additional time for processing of thought and sending message. (Longer response time is needed for older adults, and time is increased in expressive aphasia.)
		Select a few common words for daily practice if expressive aphasia.
		Praise patient for continued efforts in speaking.

Continued.

Nursing Care Plan—Cerebrovascular Accident (CVA)—cont'd

Nursing diagnoses	Expected outcomes	Nursing interventions (rationale)
Unilateral neglect related to homonymous hemianopsia/hemiplegia	Patient will demonstrate increasing awareness/use of affected side.	Assess effect of unilateral neglect on ability to perform self-care and function safely in environment. (Older adults have impaired motor coordination, and problem may be increased by CVA.) Compensate (initially) for deficit by speaking to patient from and arranging needed items on unaffected side. Force (gradually) recognition of affected side by approaching, speaking, arranging needed items on affected side (draws attention to affected side and forces recognition). Stimulate affected side by touching, rubbing with different textured materials. (Touching should be firm because older adults have decreased sensation.) Instruct patient to bathe and dress affected side first. Teach patient to inspect affected side of mouth during meals for "pocketing" of food. (Food may become "lost" as a result of decreased sensation caused by aging and effects of CVA.) Teach patient to inspect position of affected extremities. Teach patient to inspect environment for hazards prior to ambulation. Place affected arm in sling during ambulation (prevents shoulder subluxation).
Altered patterns of urinary elimination related to incontinence/retention catheter	Patient will report decrease in frequency of incontinence.	Offer bedpan/urinal every 2 hr for voiding. (Bladder size decreases in old age.) Encourage fluid intake of 3000 ml/24 hr unless on fluid restriction (difficult because older people have a decreased sense of thirst). Monitor for signs and symptoms of urinary tract infection every 4 hr (especially if patient has indwelling catheter). Maintain strict intake and output (if retention catheter). Keep perianal area clean and dry. Place sheet/towel over absorbent pads. (Absorbent pads should never come in contact with patient's skin.) Offer bedpan *promptly* when requested by patient.

Nursing Care Plan—Cerebrovascular Accident (CVA)—cont'd		
Nursing diagnoses	Expected outcomes	Nursing interventions (rationale)
		Encourage use of bathroom rather than bedpan/urinal, allowing time for ambulation. Ensure privacy. Reduce drinks with caffeine (may already be taking a diuretic). Treat as an adult. (Use last name and words such as protective pad rather than diaper.)
Self-care deficit: ability to perform ADL, related to neuromuscular impairment	Patient will demonstrate increasing ability to perform self-care activities (ADL) with less assistance. Patient will develop no complications.	Note: Interventions are presented in the nursing care plan for intracranial tumors (pp. 245-248).
Altered thought processes related to neurologic degeneration	Patient will respond appropriately to directions and will be oriented to event, person, and time.	Note: Interventions are presented in the nursing care plan for dementia of the Alzheimer's type (pp. 226-228).

Discharge planning and patient/family education
Teach patient and family the following:
  ROM exercises
  Proper positioning—lying, sitting, standing
  Transfer techniques
Promote self-care to the optimal level.
Promote continence of bladder and bowel.
Assess home environment for safety.
Assist to arrange for special equipment in the home (e.g., wheelchairs, ramps, walkers).
Assist to eliminate controllable factors, such as:
  Cigarette smoking
  Elevated blood pressure
  Elevated levels of cholesterol
  Excessive stress
  Lack of exercise

Patient/family education should include the communication tips in Box 12-6 and the information on the management of hypertension in Box 12-7, as well as the general guidelines for CVA and intracranial surgery in Box 12-11 (p. 249).

Evaluation
Patient performs own ROM four times daily.
No complications due to immobility develop.
Admission weight is maintained.
Patient makes wishes known to staff.
Patient communicates in a satisfactory manner with family.
Patient bathes and dresses affected side first.
Patient is beginning to use affected side in performance of ADL.
Patient is continent of bladder/bowel during daytime.

Box 12-6.

Patient/Family Education

Communication Tips

Measures designed to improve communication include the following:

Speak in low tones and use short, simple sentences.

Face the patient (CVA) on the uninvolved side.

Decrease distractions while communicating, for example, large number of people, radio, and TV.

Reinforce spoken word with visual clues, for example, flash cards, hand gestures, and pantomime.

Use same words repeatedly on a daily basis.

Encourage patient to draw, point, or write if unable to express self verbally.

Allow plenty of time for patient to formulate response.

Recognize that fatigue decreases ability to speak and express oneself.

Continue outpatient speech therapy sessions.

For additional information contact:
American Speech-Language-Hearing Association
10801 Rockville Pike
Rockville, MD 20852

Additional instructions for the individual patient and/or family:

Box 12-7.

Patient/Family Education
Management of Hypertension

Continue to take blood pressure medication as prescribed even though you may be feeling better.

Report to your physician for monthly checks of blood pressure. You may need to report more frequently when first diagnosed.

Avoid foods high in sodium content, such as the following:
  Bacon (regular or Canadian)
  Canned soup
  Cheddar cheese
  Corn flakes
  Crackers (graham or soda)
  Cured ham/pork sausage
  Pretzels
  Regular breads
  Regular margarine
  Salad dressings (French, Italian)
  Salted butter
  Saltine crackers
  Sardines (in oil)
  Soy sauce

Check salt/sodium content on label before buying.

Avoid sudden changes in position. Example: lying or sitting to standing.

Exercise regularly. Walk daily. If not possible, walk 20 to 30 minutes three times a week.

Lose weight if obese.

Stop smoking.

Avoid exposure to high temperatures. If taking a diuretic, perspiring heavily may lead to dehydration.

Notify physician if impotency develops. Medication for blood pressure may cause impotency and can be changed to correct it.

Additional instructions for the individual patient and/or family:

INTRACRANIAL TUMORS

Intracranial tumors may be benign or malignant. These space-occupying lesions may arise in the brain, meninges, or skull (primary tumors), or they may have metastasized from other organs of the body (secondary tumors). In metastatic lesions the primary site is frequently the lungs or breasts. Intracranial tumors occur most frequently in the fifth, sixth, and seventh decades of life. The most common brain tumor in the older adult is glioblastoma multiforme.

▶ PATHOPHYSIOLOGY, SIGNS, AND SYMPTOMS

Intracranial tumors may develop as a well-defined mass, or cellular proliferation can infiltrate tissue spaces without forming a well-defined mass (Hickey, 1986, p. 461). It is important to remember that some benign brain tumors may prove fatal because of their location and inaccessibility to surgery. Neurologic deficits occur as the neoplastic proliferation either compresses brain tissue or invades it (see Box 12-8 for classification of brain tumors). Signs and symptoms are dependent on the location of the tumor but generally include complaints of headache, visual disturbances, nausea and vomiting, personality changes, memory loss, drowsiness, disorders of movement, papilledema, unsteady gait, hemiparesis, olfactory disturbances, and seizure activity.

▶ DIAGNOSTIC PROCEDURES

Diagnosis is made on the basis of a thorough history, a physical examination, and a neurologic assessment. Commonly ordered diagnostic tests include chest and skull x-rays, electroencephalogram (EEG), computed tomography (CT) scan, cerebral angiography, visual-field and funduscopic examination, and visual-evoked responses (VER) (Table 12-4). Lumbar punctures are seldom performed because of the danger of brainstem herniation from increased intracranial pressure.

▶ MEDICAL MANAGEMENT

Medical management is symptomatic prior to surgery and includes mild analgesics for headache, corticosteroids for cerebral edema, anticonvulsants for grand mal seizure activity, and stool softeners to avoid straining with resultant increase in intracranial pressure. The majority of patients with brain tumors undergo surgery, conventional or laser, and this may be followed by chemotherapy and/or radiation, if needed.

Box 12-8.

Classification of brain tumors

Tumors originating in the brain tissue

Gliomas—infiltrating tumors that may invade any portion of the brain; most common type of brain tumor

  Astrocytomas (grades 1 and 2)
  Glioblastomas (grades 3 and 4 astrocytomas)
  Ependymomas
  Medulloblastomas
  Oligodendrogliomas
  Colloid cysts

  } Subclassified according to cell type

Tumors arising from covering of brain

Meningioma—encapsulated, well-defined, growing outside the brain tissue; compresses rather than invades brain

Tumors developing in or on the cranial nerves

Acoustic neuroma—derived from sheath of acoustic nerve
Optic nerve spongioblastoma polare

Metastatic lesions

Most commonly from lung and breast

Tumors of the ductless glands

Pituitary
Pineal

Blood vessel tumors

Hemangioblastoma
Angioma

Congenital tumors

From Brunner LS, Suddarth DS, Bare BC, et al (1988). Textbook of medical-surgical nursing, Philadelphia, JB Lippincott Co, p. 1466. Reprinted with permission.

Table 12-4. Diagnostic methods to confirm intracranial tumors

Test	Findings
Chest x-ray	May reveal primary tumor
Skull x-ray	Deviation of structures
EEG	Dysrhythmia
CT scan	Location and size of mass
Cerebral angiography	Vascular pattern of mass
Visual-field exam	Defects in visual field
Funduscopic exam	Evidence of papilledema
VER	Abnormalities of waveform
Lumbar puncture (performed with caution)	Malignant cells
	Increased spinal fluid protein
	Increased cerebrospinal fluid pressure

▶ NURSING MANAGEMENT—NURSING CARE PLAN
Intracranial Tumor/Cranial Surgery

Since most patients have a neurosurgical procedure performed, this section on nursing management will focus on the patient experiencing a craniotomy, with less emphasis on chemotherapy and radiation (see Box 12-12 for patient/family education on chemotherapy and radia- *tion). It is imperative that nurses be alert to neurologic crises and avert them if at all possible. These crises include cerebral edema, which leads to increased intracranial pressure (Box 12-9), alterations in level of consciousness (LOC), and seizure activity (Box 12-10).*

Assessment

SUBJECTIVE DATA
History of the following:
  Headache
  Visual disturbance/diplopia
  Nausea and/or vomiting
  Drowsiness
  Decreased hearing
  Dizziness
  Unsteady gait
  Weakness/hemiparesis

OBJECTIVE DATA
Aphasia
Difficulty in hearing
Dysphagia
Unequal pupils
Nystagmus
Differences in grip
Paralysis
Personality changes
Loss of equilibrium
Changes in affect
Grooming

	Nursing diagnoses	Expected outcomes	Nursing interventions (rationale)

N U R S I N G C A R E P L A N	Potential for injury related to infection, alteration in level of consciousness/increased intracranial pressure/seizure activity	No injury/infection will result from neurologic crises.	Maintain a patent airway. (Adequate gas exchange maintains intracranial homeostasis.)
			Keep head and neck in neutral position (prevents an increase in intracranial pressure [ICP]; see Box 12-9).
			Perform oral suctioning as needed. (Unconscious patients have an increase in secretions; coughing reflex may be decreased or lost.) Never suction nasally.
			Suction tracheostomy as needed, using sterile technique.
			Maintain head of bed as ordered.
			  Supratentorial craniotomy—30 degrees
			  Infratentorial craniotomy—flat
			Keep bed in low position with side rails up when not performing care.
			Avoid use of restraints if possible. (Fighting restraints will increase ICP.)
			Perform baseline assessment upon admission to postanesthesia room or intensive care unit.
			Observe for leaks and/or infection at insertion site of any line every 4 hr.
			Determine patency and proper connection of drainage tubes.
			Maintain *accurate* intake and output every hour, extending to every 8 hr. (Fluids may be restricted to prevent cerebral edema.)

Continued.

Nursing Care Plan—Intracranial Tumor/Cranial Surgery—cont'd

Nursing diagnoses	Expected outcomes	Nursing interventions (rationale)
Potential for injury related to infection, alteration in level of consciousness/increased intracranial pressure/seizure activity—cont'd		Monitor urine specific gravity. Record amount, color, and consistency of any drainage (may have ventriculostomy) every hour, extending to every 8 hr. Maintain strict aseptic technique in handling central venous catheter/changing tubing or dressing. Observe for alterations in level of consciousness (LOC) every 15 min. Observe for signs and symptoms of increased ICP every 15 min (see Box 12-9). (Monitoring devices provide continuous measurement. Sustained increase above 15 mm Hg [200 mm H_2O] is abnormal.) Observe for seizure activity (may be due to irritation from surgery or cerebral edema). (See Box 12-10.) Record observations of neurologic crisis. Monitor neurologic assessment/vital signs every 15, 30, or 60 min, or as indicated. Monitor temperature, pulse, respiration, and blood pressure. (Increased systolic blood pressure and decreased pulse rate are late signs of increased ICP; respiratory arrest may occur as a result of cerebral edema.) Assess pupil size reactions. (Older adults have a decrease in pupil size—unequal pupils indicate increased ICP.) Test motor function. (Weakness in extremities may be due to age or residual from surgery. Increased weakness on one side indicates increased ICP.) Test hand grip bilaterally. Test leg movement bilaterally. Observe for paralysis/unusual movement. Test for response to painful stimuli. (Decreased response to painful stimuli indicates increased ICP.) Test reflexes. Observe for abnormal posturing. (Decorticate and decerebrate posturing indicate increased ICP.) Observe for leakage of spinal fluid—rhinorrhea and/or otorrhea. (Use aseptic technique to avoid infection/meningitis.)

Nursing Care Plan—Intracranial Tumor/Cranial Surgery—cont'd		
Nursing diagnoses	**Expected outcomes**	**Nursing interventions (rationale)**
Potential for injury related to infection, alteration in level of consciousness/increased intracranial pressure/seizure activity—cont'd		Apply sterile, loose, dry dressing to upper lip and external ear if rhinorrhea/otorrhea occur. (Do not pack nose or ear canal.) Maintain precautions with hypothermia blanket.
Bathing/hygiene, dressing/grooming, feeding/toileting self-care deficit related to neuromuscular dysfunction/immobility	No complications will occur from self-care deficits.	Turn, position every 2 hr. (Avoid "packing" with pillows—may result in increased temperature.) Avoid supine position. (An unconscious patient should never be left alone on back.) Utilize arm bolsters, bed cradle, sand bags, splints, and turn sheets. Perform ROM exercises every 4 hr (prevents deformities, stimulates circulation). Inspect skin/pressure areas for skin breakdown every 2 hr. Apply TED (thromboembolic disease) hose—reapply every 8 hr after bathing legs. Perform leg exercises every 2 hr (prevents contractures, stimulates circulation). Test Homan's sign every 4 hr. (Fluid restrictions lead to increased coagulation of blood and thrombus formation.) Keep linens clean, dry, and wrinkle free. Remove any crust formation around eyes as necessary. Instill liquid tears every 2 hr. (Blinking reflex may be lost, leading to drying of cornea with resultant blindness.) Perform oral hygiene every 2-4 hr. Lubricate lips every 2 hr. Perform nasal care every 2-4 hr. (Do not suction nasally or insert anything into nasal passages.) Provide for general hygiene (bathe, comb and shampoo hair, shower). Maintain patent closed urinary drainage system. (Full bladder produces increased restlessness.) Perform catheter care every 4 hr. Begin bladder/bowel program, if indicated. Avoid straining with bowel elimination (leads to increased ICP). Administer nasogastric feedings if ordered. Monitor patient/total parenteral nutrition for incompatibilities. Obtain accurate daily bed weight before breakfast (if unable to stand).

Continued.

Nursing Care Plan—Intracranial Tumor/Cranial Surgery—cont'd

Nursing diagnoses	Expected outcomes	Nursing interventions (rationale)
Bathing/hygiene, dressing/grooming, feeding/toileting self-care deficit related to neuromuscular dysfunction/immobility—cont'd Knowledge deficit related to patient/family ability to provide home care	Patient/family will comply with rehabilitation program.	Monitor laboratory reports for electrolyte imbalance. Assist with transfer—bed to chair. Instruct in use of assistive devices. Alert family to possible personality changes. Instruct patient/family on medication schedule and side effects. Instruct in importance of continued therapy programs–physical, occupational, speech. Teach seizure precautions/care to family.

Discharge planning and patient/family education

Prevent complications—rehabilitation begins on admission.

Multidisciplinary approach is necessary. Includes nursing and medical staff and music, occupational, physical, and speech therapy personnel.

Assess ability to perform ADL.

Assist in obtaining needed assistive devices.

Assess home environment for safety and needed adaptations.

Patient/family support group is needed as well as provisions for respite care.

Provide patient/family education on communication tips (see Box 12-6), guidelines for cerebrovascular accident and intracranial surgery (Box 12-11), chemotherapy and radiation (Box 12-12), and seizure precautions (Box 12-13).

Evaluation

No signs and symptoms of infection occur.

Early signs and symptoms of neurologic crises are recognized: altered LOC, increased ICP, seizure activity.

No injuries occur during seizure activity.

Patient accepts care from care giver.

No complications occur as a result of self-care deficit.

Patient complies with home care management.

Box 12-9.

Signs and symptoms of increased intracranial pressure

Lethargy
Decreased level of consciousness
Decreased response to stimuli
Pupil inequality (size)
Decreased pupillary reactions (speed)
Papilledema
Progressive weakness and/or paralysis of extremities
Restlessness, anxiety, and irritability
Decreased respirations, progressing to apnea
Increased blood pressure and widening pulse pressure
Decreased pulse rate
Increased temperature
Emesis
Seizure activity
Onset of abnormal posturing

Box 12-10.

Pertinent data to be recorded for seizure activity

Frequency, number, and duration
Presence or absence of aura
Starting point and progression
Parts of body involved
Eye movement
Length of tonic and clonic phase
Position of head, body, and extremities
Changes in position after onset
Clenching of teeth
Biting of tongue
Frothing of mouth
Pupil activity and eye deviation
Skin color
Diaphoresis
Character of respirations
Incontinence
Changes in motor power after seizure
Duration of sleep postseizure

Box 12-11.

Patient/Family Education

Guidelines for Cerebrovascular Accident and Intracranial Surgery

Set short-term achievable goals.

Break tasks down into single components.

Keep tasks relevant to needs and interests of patient.

Keep environment highly structured and repetitive.

Avoid fatigue—as agitation and frustration increase, performance decreases.

Avoid behaviors/events that increase agitation. These may include too many visitors and loud noise (arguing, music, voices).

Avoid alcohol use. Even small amounts may increase agitation and confusion and interfere with action of seizure medication.

Take all medications as prescribed. Follow directions for taking medications for high blood pressure and seizure activity daily in regularly spaced doses. Mark when taken on medication calendar.

Continue any prescribed therapy—occupational, physical, and speech—until discontinued by physician.

Seek support group for patient and family.

Keep scheduled appointments with physician.

Call physician with any questions or on regression of behavior.

Physician's telephone number _____

Additional instructions for the individual patient and/or family:

Box 12-12.

Patient/Family Education
Chemotherapy and Radiation

Keep all scheduled appointments with physician.

Do not take any drugs (even aspirin) without approval of your physician.

Keep all outpatient appointments for chemotherapy or radiation.

Protect yourself from infection by avoiding crowds and children.

Do not wash off skin markings used for radiation therapy.

Do not use cosmetics, lotions, or powders on site receiving radiation treatments.

Avoid rubbing, scratching, or shaving the area receiving treatment.

Avoid exposure to sunlight.

Remain alert for any signs of bleeding in stool, urine, or vomitus.

Observe your skin for bruising.

Avoid foods that are irritating to the mouth, such as citrus fruit or juices, and heavily spiced foods.

Eat small, frequent meals. Chilled foods and drinks are more easily tolerated.

Avoid alcohol and smoking because these are irritants to the mouth and throat.

Mouth may be rinsed with Viscous Xylocaine. Glycerine swabs are soothing but increase drying of mouth.

Notify your physician of any difficulties or unusual symptoms you may be experiencing.

Physician's telephone number _____

Additional instructions for the individual patient and/or family:

Box 12-13.

Patient/Family Education

Seizure Precautions

Stay with the patient having a seizure.

Call for assistance.

Place the patient flat on the bed or floor.

Protect from injury by performing the following actions:
Loosen belt, collar, and tie.
Move furniture and other objects to protect head and extremities.
Do not attempt to force open clenched teeth.
Do not attempt to restrain.

Do not place fingers in the patient's mouth during seizure activity.

Do not use a glass thermometer to take temperature of a patient who is prone to seizure activity.

Seizure medication must be taken as prescribed by physician. Do not cease to administer/take because patient is feeling better and experiencing no seizures.

Difficulty in walking or keeping balance should be reported to physician immediately.

Helmets (football-type) can be worn during waking hours to protect from injury.

After seizure, turn patient to side to permit drainage from mouth.

Remember that the patient may be very tired and sleepy after a seizure.

Physician's telephone number _____

Additional instructions for the individual patient and/or family:

REFERENCES

Bauvette-Risey J (1989). Nervous system. In Burggraf V and Stanley M, editors: Nursing the elderly: A care plan approach, Philadelphia, JB Lippincott Co, pp 313-355.

Brunner LS, Suddarth DS, Bare BC, et al (1988). Textbook of medical-surgical nursing, Philadelphia, JB Lippincott Co. pp 1463-1528.

Burgess AW (1990). Psychiatric nursing: In the hospital and the community, Norwalk, Conn, Appleton & Lange, pp 699-722.

Davies P (1988). Alzheimer's disease and related disorders: An overview. In Aronson MK, editor: Understanding Alzheimer's disease: What it is, how to cope with it, future directions, New York, Scribner's, pp 3-14.

Donohoe K (1990). Nursing management of adults with degenerative disorders. In Beare PG and Myers JL, editors: Principles and practice of adult health nursing, St Louis, Mosby−Year Book, Inc, pp 1097-1117.

Graves M (1988). Physiologic changes. In Hogstel MO, editor: Nursing care of the older adult, New York, John Wiley & Sons, Inc, pp 63-89.

Heston LL and White JA (1983). Dementia: A practical guide to Alzheimer's disease and related illnesses, New York, WH Freeman & Co. pp 52-67.

Hickey JV (1986). The clinical practice of neurological and neurosurgical nursing, Philadelphia, JB Lippincott Co. pp 461-482.

Kinney M and Schenk E (1990). Problems of the nervous system. In Phipps WJ, Long BC, and Woods NF, editors: Medical-surgical nursing: Concepts and clinical practice, ed 4, St Louis, Mosby−Year Book, Inc.

Porth C (1982). Pathophysiology: Concepts of altered health states, Philadelphia, JB Lippincott Co. pp 363-642.

Rudy EB (1984). Advanced neurological and neurosurgical nursing, St Louis, Mosby−Year Book, Inc, p 269.

Schenk E (1990). Problems of the nervous system. In Phipps WJ, Long BC, and Woods NF, editors: Medical-surgical nursing: Concepts and clinical practice, ed 4, St Louis, Mosby−Year Book, Inc.

Williams L (1986). Alzheimer's: The need for caring. J Gerontol Nurs 12(2):23.

BIBLIOGRAPHY

Anderson GP (1989). A fresh look at assessing the elderly, RN 89(6):28-40.

Brunner LS and Suddarth DS (1986). The Lippincott manual of nursing practice, Philadelphia, JB Lippincott Co.

Burnside IM (1988). Nursing and the aged: A self-care approach, New York, McGraw-Hill.

Campbell VG (1989). Neurologic system. In Thompson JM, McFarland GR, Hirsch JE, et al, editors: Mosby's manual of clinical nursing, ed 2, St Louis, Mosby−Year Book, Inc, pp 239-375.

Carpenito LJ (1989). Nursing diagnosis: Application to clinical practice, Philadelphia, JB Lippincott Co.

Christ MA and Hohloch FJ (1988). Gerontologic nursing, Springhouse, Pa, Springhouse.

Dudas S (1990). Nursing management of adults with cerebrovascular disorders. In Beare PG and Myers JL, editors: Principles and practice of adult health nursing, St Louis, Mosby−Year Book, Inc, pp 1117-1143.

Gee ZL and Passarella PM (1985). Nursing care of the stroke patient: A therapeutic approach, Pittsburgh, AREN-Publications.

Hamilton GP (1988). Health care of the older adult. In Brunner LS, Suddarth DS, Bare BG, et al, editors: Textbook of medical-surgical nursing, Philadelphia, JB Lippincott Co, pp 141-168.

Hartshorn J (1990). Nursing management of adults with intracranial disorders. In Beare PG and Myers JL, editors: Principles and practice of adult health nursing, St Louis, Mosby−Year Book, Inc, pp 1184-1196.

Hogstel MO and Taylor-Martof M (1988). Perioperative care. In Hogstel MO, editor: Nursing care of the older adult, ed 2, New York, John Wiley & Sons, Inc, pp 335-353.

Kim MJ, McFarland GK, and McLane A (1991). Pocket guide to nursing diagnoses, ed 4, St Louis, Mosby−Year Book, Inc.

Lederer JR, Marculescu GL, Mocnik B, and Seaby N (1991). Care planning pocket guide: A nursing diagnosis approach, ed 4, Redwood City, Calif, Addison-Wesley Nursing.

Lubkin IM (1986). Chronic illness: Impact and interventions, Boston, Jones & Bartlett.

Luckmann J and Sorensen KC (1987). Medical-surgical nursing: A psychophysiologic approach, Philadelphia, WB Saunders Co.

Mastrian KG (1984). The patient with a degenerative disease of the nervous system. In Rudy EB, editor: Advanced neurological and neurosurgical nursing, St Louis, Mosby−Year Book, Inc, pp 265-287.

Nelson MK (1990). Organic mental disorders. In Hogstel MO, editor: Geropsychiatric nursing, St Louis, Mosby−Year Book, Inc, pp 177-212.

Pajk M (1984). Alzheimer's disease: Inpatient care, Am J Nurs 84(2):216-232.

Phipps WJ, Long BC, Woods NF, and Cassmeyer VL (1991). Clinical manual of medical-surgical nursing, ed 2, St Louis, Mosby−Year Book, Inc.

Spencer RT (1986). Drugs affecting the nervous system: Central nervous system drugs. In Spencer RT, Nichols LW, Lipkin GB, et al, editors: Clinical pharmacology and nursing management, Philadelphia, JB Lippincott Co, pp 493-523.

Steffl B (1989). Discharge planning and the elderly. In Burggraf V and Stanley M, editors: Nursing the elderly: A care approach, Philadelphia, JB Lippincott Co, pp 17-35.

Strength DE (1986). Independent, interdependent, dependent, and non-nursing actions and judgments concerning the care of adult comatose patients with craniocerebral trauma in a shock-trauma unit, unpublished dissertation, The Catholic University of America, Washington, DC.

Tucker SM, Canobbio MM, Paquette EV, and Wells MF (1988). Patient care standards: Nursing process, diagnosis, and outcome, St Louis, Mosby−Year Book, Inc.

Waterhouse HP (1986). Drugs affecting the nervous system: The psychoactive drugs. In Spencer AT, Nichols LW, Lipkin GB, et al, editors: Clinical pharmacology and nursing management, Philadelphia, JB Lippincott Co, pp 493-523.

CHAPTER 13

Discharge Planning

Marta A. Browning

By the year 2030 almost 22% of the U.S. population will be older adults (American Association of Retired Persons and Administration on Aging, 1990). Currently, this growing population cohort accounts for 31% of total health care expenditures and for 42% of all days of care in hospitals (Weinrich, Boyd, and Nussbaum, 1989). Older adults compose over half the census of medical-surgical units, and their length of stay averages 8.9 days, 3.5 days longer than that of persons under 65 years of age (American Association of Retired Persons and Administration on Aging, 1990). Twenty-five percent of hospitalized older adults are readmitted to the hospital at least two times within 12 months of their discharge date (Johnson, 1990). Ninety-five percent of older adults aged 65 to 84 and 78% of older adults aged 85 and over live in the community in their own homes or with relatives or friends who serve as companions and, at times, caregivers (American Association of Retired Persons and Administration on Aging, 1990). Fifteen percent of older adults suffer severe cognitive impairment that affects their ability to carry out activities of daily living, but even within this group 75% live at home (Gillies, 1986). Most older adults have one or, more often, several chronic illnesses, and 8% of aging Americans experience sequelae of these illnesses severe enough to render them homebound (Folden, 1990). Just a brief review of statistics such as these commands active involvement of nurses in the development and coordination of health care services that will ensure continuity of care for vulnerable older adults as they progress through cycles of health-illness-rehabilitation.

Provision of continuity of care is accomplished through a process called discharge planning. The primary goals of such planning are to maintain the majority of older adults in their own homes or residences of choice and to prevent rehospitalization. The prevention of avoidable or premature hospitalization and of readmission should be a major focus of care for older adults. Researchers rate the current quality of discharge planning as poor and recognize that its low priority ranking among health professionals results in delayed and inadequate assessment, poor documentation, and fragmented implementation of posthospital services (Naylor, 1990). Johnson's study (1989) of 50 pairs of aged patients and their nurses on two medical units revealed that nurses viewed discharge planning as a separate activity, secondary in importance to meeting the physical needs of patients. Nurses cited a lack of educational preparation in gerontology, high patient loads, and a shortage of nursing staff as factors contributing to their inability to perform adequate discharge planning tasks. Patients in this study ranked all discharge planning activities as "very important" or "extremely important" to them and stressed the need to include families in planning for postdischarge care. Patients cited the frustration of having instructions read to them as they were wheeled out the hospital door or being given no opportunity to ask questions, request clarification of instructions, or demonstrate mastery of self-care procedures before discharge (Johnson, 1989). In Naylor's study (1990) of hospitalized older adults 85% of the patients were considered high risk and in need of discharge planning, but only 20% received such planning from the social services department.

Nurses play a very important role in smoothing the transition of patients from acute care hospitals to their community-based residences. Nurses also participate in the coordination of services between hospitals and nursing facilities, which is an essential component of continuity of care for older persons.

DISCHARGE PLANNING: A CONCEPT CLARIFIED

Discharge planning is the process of ensuring continuity of care (Corkery, 1989). The objective of discharge planning is to create progressive levels of health services designed to meet the individualized needs of patients as these needs change with health status. The discharge plan is interdisciplinary and collaborative in nature. Table 13-1 identifies the health care professionals involved in discharge planning and describes their roles. Discharge plans are implemented in two major ways. The first

method of implementing discharge plans is through teaching the patient and his or her family or caregivers to manage their own health care needs. The second method of implementing discharge plans is through patient referral to a variety of agencies and/or institutions that can meet their needs at a given point in time.

Though the process of discharge planning is commonly associated with a patient's release from an acute care hospital, it is an appropriate and essential part of other transitions as well. Table 13-1 illustrates a number of situations in which discharge planning should be implemented.

Functions of Discharge Planning

Programs. Zarle (1989) described the overall goal of a discharge planning or continuing care program as ensuring that patients who enter acute care institutions have a planned program to meet their continuing care needs and a defined follow-up plan when they leave the hospital. She described a number of functions performed by the discharge planning program (Box 13-1).

Legal Basis for Discharge Planning

Prior to 1982 acute care institutions were reimbursed by the federal government for services provided to Medicare and Medicaid patients by a system of retrospective payment. Because all services were reimbursed, there was little incentive to limit the length of hospital stays or to examine closely the types of services being provided. It was assumed that services were best provided in a hospital after the patient had been formally admitted.

In 1982 a prospective method of reimbursement was introduced to constrain the escalating cost of health care under federally insured programs. This system of pay-

Table 13-1. Shifts in levels of health care services requiring provision of continuity of care through discharge planning referrals

Health care provider #1	Direction of referral	Health care provider #2
Intensive care unit (ICU), acute care hospital	⟷	Medical-surgical unit, same hospital
Emergency room, acute care hospital	⟷	Home health agency
Acute care hospital	⟷	Rehabilitation hospital or center
Acute care hospital	⟷	Home health agency
Acute care hospital	⟷	Nursing facility
Nursing facility	⟷	Home health agency
Acute care hospital	⟷	Skilled nursing facility
Home health agency	⟷	Nursing facility
Acute care hospital	⟷	Board and care or group home facility
Acute care hospital and home health agency	⟷	Community care options/programs for frail older adults
Acute care hospital and home health agency	⟷	Adult day care hospital or center
Acute care hospital and home health agency	⟷	Outpatient services Private physicians Therapy services (physical therapy, speech therapy, occupational therapy) Health maintenance organizations, preferred provider arrangements
Acute care hospital and home health agency	⟷	Patient and/or caregivers functioning independently
Acute care hospital and home health agency	⟷	Hospice
Hospice	⟷	Bereavement services

Box 13-1.

Functions of a discharge planning program

Identification of patients with posthospital needs

Identification of patients who may require extended stays in acute care or alternative institutions

Identification of patients and/or families with unique social circumstances that would affect plans for timely discharge

Education of professional staff about continuing care assessment and referral

Coordination of discharge planning services

Provision of data and information for administrative policy making

Monitoring and evaluation of discharge planning activities

Maintenance of records and documentation of discharge planning activities

ment was based on the use of Diagnostic Related Groups (DRGs) that linked reimbursement to days of stay and mix of services. This shift in reimbursement method dramatically altered the reward system for institutions and shifted the fiscal incentive from lengthy hospital stays and overutilization of services to promotion of early discharge and the provision of many traditional inpatient services in outpatient or community-based settings. Home care services became critical for the care of patients who were being discharged "sicker and quicker," and high-technology services, once seen only in hospitals, moved into homes to be managed by patients and caregivers under the guidance of visiting nurses and members of the allied health professions. Private insurers rapidly followed the federal government's lead in cost containment. Today, effective discharge planning that moves patients out of the hospital quickly is critical to the institution's fiscal health and its survival in the marketplace.

Thus discharge planning activities are mandated by

professional health care organizations and are required by federal law for hospitals participating in the Medicare programs. Table 13-2 illustrates some of these requirements and guidelines.

Organization of Discharge Planning Services

Discharge planning or continuing care services may be provided through a variety of organizational constellations. Rorden and Taft (1990) describe four basic categories.

The separate discharge planning unit. Separate discharge planning units occupy their own office space and are assigned specific staff members. Usually the discharge planning team is headed by a nurse or a social worker. Referrals are made to this unit by physicians and other health professionals on the basis of formal criteria established by the institution.

Table 13-2. Regulatory basis for discharge planning

Regulatory or professional organization	Guidelines	Regulatory or professional organization	Guidelines
Heinz-Stark Bill, 1986 Medicare Quality Protection Act	Requires hospitals to: Provide discharge planning Develop a uniform needs assessment instrument Provide patients with written notification of their Discharge Planning Rights, including right of appeal if they believe they are discharged too soon or posthospital services are not available Give patient written notice of the utilization review committee's denial for continued stay and notify patient that Medicare will no longer pay for continued stay Provide appeals process for patient to contact the local Peer Review Organization (PRO) by noon of the day following receipt of the notice of discharge to avoid fiscal liability for continued days of stay	American Hospital Association	Identification of patients who require discharge planning Continuity of medical care and/or other care Initiation of discharge planning on a timely basis Assessment of availability of posthospital services to meet posthospital needs Individualized discharge counseling and instruction from the nurse Identifies essential elements for planning, which include: Early identification of patients likely to need posthospital care Assessment, counseling, and education of the patient and family Development and implementation of a discharge plan Postdischarge follow-up Monitoring of discharge planning by the hospital's Quality Assurance Program
Joint Commission on Accreditation of Healthcare Organizations (JCAHO)	Standards state that hospitals must provide: Policies and procedures on discharge planning	American Nurses' Association	Standards of Practice call for a staff nurse to be discharge planner for every patient

Data compiled from Corkery (1989), Rorden and Taft (1990), and Zarle (1987).

Decentralized discharge planning unit. Decentralized discharge planning units also have separate offices, but the discharge planners are deployed to specific patient care units where they initiate patient referrals back to the centralized discharge planning unit.

Coordinated discharge planning alliance. A coordinator or liaison officer, often a nurse, is designated to receive referrals and to contact other professionals involved in care of the patient for information and/or consultation on development of the discharge plan. Professionals such as nurses, physical therapists, occupational therapists, speech therapists, and nutritionists participate on the discharge planning team on an as needed basis.

Informal professional alliance. In large institutions only 10% of patients may be served by the formal discharge planning group, leaving as many as 90% of patients without clear access to discharge planning services. In such cases the nurse must function as a discharge planning coordinator who works with the physician to obtain medical orders that involve social workers, nutritionists, and allied health professionals in the patient's care.

Members of Discharge Planning Teams

A number of individuals may participate in the discharge planning process as members of discharge planning teams or as representatives of administrative interests through groups such as Utilization Review and Quality Assurance Committees. A list of discharge planning participants and their role in the process is contained in Table 13-3.

Table 13-3. Participants in discharge planning

Category of personnel	Role played in discharge planning	Category of personnel	Role played in discharge planning
Patient, patient's family, patient's caregivers, or significant others	Responsible for collaborating with the physician and other members of the discharge planning team to identify the services that will be needed and the most acceptable method for obtaining them. Also responsible for providing accurate and complete information regarding finances, living situations, and willingness and availability of support systems to provide posthospital care for the patient. Responsible for contacting community resources and for keeping follow-up appointments with physicians, outpatient therapies, and/or other programs providing rehabilitative support.		home care. May serve as a clinical nurse specialist who provides specialized patient education. Coordinates discharge planning for patients not referred to discharge planning department.
Physician	Responsible for setting discharge planning goals for patients and for authorizing posthospital care through verbal and written orders.	Social workers	Responsible for psychosocial assessment of the posthospital needs of patient, family, and/or caregiver. Helps patients to secure funding through entitlements to meet their health care needs and make referrals to appropriate welfare programs if the patient's income level is at or below the poverty line. Collaborate with patients and family members to identify and access appropriate community resources.
Nurses	Responsible for identifying posthospital needs of patients and for referring those requiring posthospital health care services to the discharge planning unit. Responsible for preparing patient and family for discharge. May serve as discharge planner or discharge liaison nurse for		Responsible for securing placement for older adults in nursing homes or other community-based residential care facilities such as board and care homes, group homes, personal care homes, congregate housing, or life care communities. Also instrumental in securing enrollment of patients in programs such as adult day care, community care options sponsored by area agencies on aging, congregate meal or home-delivered meal programs, and if necessary, adult protective services.

Table 13-3. Participants in discharge planning—cont'd

Category of personnel	Role played in discharge planning	Category of personnel	Role played in discharge planning
Physical therapists, occupational therapists, speech therapists, respiratory therapists	Responsible for management of illness and disability to limit long-term effects of disease processes. Responsible for education of patient and caregivers in the independent management of assistive devices and activities of daily living. Refer patients for continuing care by community-based therapists.	Clergy or psychologists	Clergy are often involved with hospice patients and are available to patient, family, and other caregivers to provide support in the management of grief and loss. Psychologists provide counseling to patient and/or family as needed.
Nutritionists	Responsible for the evaluation of need for special diets. May serve on nutrition support team and order supplies for enteral feedings if needed by patient at home. Instruct patient and caregivers in implementation of special diets. Refer patients for continuing dietary supervision posthospitalization.	Utilization review coordinators	Serve administrative interests of hospital to see that rules for maximum reimbursement through state and federal programs are met. Alert discharge planning staff that patients have been placed on alternate level of care status and are ready to leave the acute care setting.
Pharmacists	Advise physicians, nurses, and patients about drug management. Alert professionals to potential for drug interactions and probability of deleterious side effects for specific patients. Are especially helpful in collaborating with patient's visiting nurse and physician to select combinations of medications that increase ease of self-administration and reduce the numbers of pills/injections or the frequency of administration for drugs taken by older adults. May manage or coordinate home enteral nutrition, chemotherapy, or intravenous therapy programs.	Case managers of insurance companies	Oversee patient benefits and reimbursement for services provided by hospitals and home care agencies. Often responsible for authorizing the delivery of specific services. In determining follow-up home care services, may increase the level and intensity of service if persuaded that these activities will prevent or delay rehospitalization.
		Quality assurance personnel	Responsible for evaluating the quality of care received by patients during their hospital stay and for determining the appropriateness of discharge plans. Summaries of their evaluations can be used by discharge planning personnel to increase the effectiveness and scope of services provided by their department.

Data compiled from Corkery (1989), Rorden and Taft (1990), and Zarle (1987).

SPECIFIC RESPONSIBILITIES OF THE NURSE IN DISCHARGE PLANNING

Nurses are involved in the discharge planning process on many levels. They may serve as the patient's primary nurse (staff nurse) responsible for direct discharge planning activities with the patient (Box 13-2), they may serve in a specialized role as a discharge planner (Box 13-3), or they may serve as a home care liaison nurse (Box 13-4). A nurse serving in any of these capacities may be a member of a Discharge Planning, Quality Assurance, or Utilization Review Committee.

Identification of Older Adults Who Will Need Continuing Care Services after Discharge

All hospitalized patients should be carefully evaluated for continuing care needs, and most older adults will qualify at some level for continuing care services. Although the reality of staffing in modern hospitals makes referral of every patient a practical impossibility, certain factors should alert nurses to the need for in-depth evaluation of the patient for posthospital care (Box 13-5).

Box 13-2.
Discharge planning responsibilities of primary or staff nurse

Identifying patients needing continuing posthospital care

Teaching self-care activities to patients, families, caregivers

Obtaining physician orders for referral to other disciplines (therapists, nutritionist, social worker) for discharge preparation and teaching

Obtaining physician orders for referral of patient for home care services

Referring patients and families to other nurse specialists for predischarge teaching based on specialized needs. These may include enterostomal therapists for ostomy patients, nutrition support nurses for patients needing enteral nutrition, and clinical nurse specialists in the following:

Gerontology

Cardiovascular management

Oncology

Diabetes management

Respiratory/pulmonary care

Participating in discharge planning rounds or meetings

Referring patients needing discharge planning to the discharge planning department

Ensuring that patients take home sufficient medical supplies to last until their first home delivery by an outside vendor

Ensuring that patients are discharged with sufficient medication to last until caregivers can fill prescriptions at an outpatient pharmacy

Providing information for discharge planners to use in preparation of written referrals to posthospital health care facilities

Box 13-3.
Responsibilities of discharge planner

Directing and coordinating discharge planning activities

Conducting discharge planning meetings or rounds

Educating professional staff and employees regarding their roles, functions, and responsibilities in the discharge planning process

Interviewing and assessing clients and families referred for discharge planning

Collaborating with patients, families, and/or other caregivers in the selection of appropriate discharge planning services and securing permission from them for referral to appropriate posthospital agencies or institutions

Preparing written referrals or faxes for transmission to posthospital agencies

Placing telephone referrals

Examining inpatient admission, discharge, and transfer lists to identify potential continuing care patients who may not have been identified by staff in discharge planning meetings

Collaborating with physicians to secure services ordered for their patients

Collaborating with the social work department if extended care placement of patient is necessary

Identifying and evaluating community resources for posthospital care

Participating as a member of hospital utilization review or length of stay committee

Ordering durable medical equipment and/or medical supplies from appropriate vendors

Coordinating and obtaining authorization for services for third party payers

Developing policies, procedures, and protocols for the discharge planning program

Maintaining records and documentation of discharge planning services

Evaluating discharge planning services and coordinating results of that evaluation with the evaluations of the Quality Assurance Committee

---

Box 13-4.

Responsibilities of home care liaison nurses

Home care liaison nurses are employed by home care agencies. They are invited by the hospital to participate in the discharge planning program to augment the services of the discharge planning department. Their role is to manage the hospital-to-home transition for patients who are identified as candidates for home care services. Responsibilities include the following:

Identifying patients who meet Medicaid, Medicare, or third party criteria for home care services

Educating patients and families regarding specific home care services that will be provided on discharge and securing consent for commencement of services

All other responsibilities that are performed by the hospital discharge planner may be performed by the home care liaison depending on the nature of the hospital-home care agency contract.

Box 13-5.

Patient situations needing posthospital care

Patient is of advanced age accompanied by frailty (e.g., 80 years old and above).

Patient lives alone.

Address is in low-income or high-crime area or distant from any type of health care.

Family support system is uncertain, uninterested, or physically distant.

Conflict exists among caregivers regarding management of patient's care.

Patient suffers from confusion or altered mental status.

Patient needs assistive or adaptive devices, including respiratory equipment.

Patient requires assistance with activities of daily living (e.g., feeding, toileting, dressing, bathing, shopping, cleaning, laundry, cooking).

Caregiver is advanced in age and/or suffers from chronic illness.

Person identified as responsible caregiver is very young (e.g., English-speaking 12-year-old in a non–English speaking family system).

Patient's endurance is limited.

Medical condition is unstable.

Multiple medications are needed.

Self-care regimen will include performance of technical medical procedures (e.g., catheter care, wound care, tube feedings, ostomy care).

Patient has questionable hydration status, poor appetite, and/or needs specialized diet.

Patient has history of bowel and/or bladder problems (especially constipation).

Patient has no telephone.

Communication is impaired (e.g., aphasia, tracheostomy).

Patient is non–English speaking or uses and understands only limited English.

Sensory perception is altered.

Condition will require pain control and management of pain control medications.

Condition requires adaptation of home environment or requires support systems beyond the normal range of family caregiver means.

Elder neglect or abuse (physical, psychosocial or financial) is suspected.

Coping ability is questionable (e.g., external locus of control displayed by passive involvement in care).

Depression or other mental health problems exist in patient and/or caregiver.

Availability of transportation is limited.

Condition precipitates a change in social roles of patient and/or caregivers.

Response of patient or family caregivers to teaching is poor or uncertain. Nurses should be especially concerned about patients who do not ask questions or seek clarification of information presented. Passive acceptance of health education efforts is often caused by lack of understanding or low literacy.

Present hospitalization is a rehospitalization after recent discharge or patient has history of frequent emergency room visits or hospitalizations.

Multiple physicians are providing care and will continue to be involved in the patient's care.

Primary community physician used by patient is not associated with the hospital or is himself or herself an older adult who has not remained current by engaging in continuing education activities.

Patient has expressed dislike of acute care physician and preference for family doctor. This leads to noncompliance after discharge.

Patient has history of recent losses or life stresses.

Patient, family, and/or other caregivers express uncertainty about their ability to perform self-care activities and express fear of making an error that will prove deleterious to patient.

Prognosis is terminal and patient chooses to die at home.

Teaching as Part of the Discharge Planning Process

Education of the patient, family, and other caregivers in self-care management is the primary responsibility of the nurse in the discharge planning process. A full discussion of principles and theories of teaching-learning, strategies for enhancing the teaching-learning process, and preparation of teaching materials is beyond the scope of this manual. It is suggested that nurses avail themselves of continuing education opportunities to enhance their skills in health education. Often the nurse must provide health teaching under adverse conditions in an abbreviated period of time. If nurses develop skills in health education to the degree that they have developed skills in health assessment and performance of technical procedures, patient noncompliance and hospital readmissions can be greatly reduced. This manual provides suggested content and handouts for conveying basic information to patients preparing for discharge. Box 13-6 presents the essential factors to consider when teaching older adults. As nurses prepare older adults and their caregivers to assume the responsibility for self-care, the following considerations should be kept in mind.

Identification of caregiver and/or support person. It is extremely important to identify the support person who will be helping the older adult when he or she arrives at home. For example, sometimes an older adult's children make hospital visits, but they are nowhere to be found when the patient arrives at home and the care giving is left to a neighbor. Some older adults exaggerate the availability and willingness of support persons to serve as caregivers in order to be discharged to their homes instead of a nursing home. It is not unusual for the visiting nurse to arrive for follow-up visits and find older adults alone, isolated, and unable to manage self-care. Calls placed to inpatient colleagues reveal that a caregiver was present for teaching in the hospital but has now abandoned the patient because the complexities and demands of patient support were overwhelming.

Age of caregiver. Today people are living longer. It is not unusual for the old-old (age 80 and above) to be taken care of by caregivers above 60 years of age who are themselves debilitated. The opposite can also occur. Many older adults are left partially in the care of the very young (age 11 or 12) who fill in after school for parents who are at work. In non-English speaking families, a young person who speaks English is often the family's intermediary with the health care system. Nurses must plan patient teaching appropriate for the capacities of these specialized caregivers.

Fear. Older adults and caregivers view technical medical procedures such as catheter management, self-injection, tube feedings, ostomy care, management of Hickman lines, and intravenous manipulation with great trepidation. Many are afraid that a mistake will occur and they will be responsible for injury or death of the patient. These learners may also have negative feelings about handling body fluids, role changes, and loss of independence. Effective teaching requires that nurses identify these overt and covert concerns of patients, families, and caregivers.

Time. Effective teaching cannot be done the morning of discharge. Nurses must demand and get systems in their institutions that alert them to pending discharge early enough so that several days are available for patient and caregiver education. Patient education must be broken into easily digested modules that are taught and reinforced over a period of time. Patients and their caregivers must have time to think about material taught and to ask questions and return demonstrations of procedures. Older adults take fewer risks than young people. Aging generally brings about an increase in cautiousness and a desire to "get things right." Older adults learn best when allowed to absorb and integrate material at their own pace. A fear of being wrong or making mistakes may block learning and lead to noncompliance.

Conflicting learning demands. In large medical centers, especially teaching hospitals, the older adult and his or her caregivers will have been given follow-up instruction by a broad array of people. These include (but are

---

> **Box 13-6.**
>
> ### Essential factors to consider when teaching older adults
>
> Speak slightly slower and louder. Enunciate distinctly, and keep voice pitch low.
>
> Assess what is already known, individual motivation, and need to know.
>
> Teach in a quiet environment (e.g., turn off TV).
>
> Assess ability to see, hear, read, write, and manipulate equipment that will be needed in later care.
>
> Present information in small segments. Do not give instructions in a hurry.
>
> Limit each teaching session to 15 or 20 minutes.
>
> Teach when the patient is free of physical discomfort (e.g., pain, nausea).
>
> Provide clearly typed (or written) materials that are concise and in large black print (or writing).
>
> Do not ask or expect the patient to write instructions as you talk or demonstrate. Have patients write instructions in their own words.
>
> Provide time for practice and return demonstration of skills requiring manual dexterity.
>
> Give positive verbal and nonverbal rewards when appropriate.

Data compiled from Kim (1989).

not limited to) the medical student, the nursing student, the intern, the resident, the specialty fellow, the attending physician, the nutritionist, and ancillary and housekeeping personnel who offer unsolicited advice. Much information, particularly that given by physicians representing different specialty disciplines, is directly contradictory. Before nurses can commence effective teaching, they must ask what information has already been given and ask to see all written materials already in the patient's possession. Nurses must also ask for and listen to the patient's and caregiver's description of what they believe they are to do when they go home.

Literacy level. The United States is experiencing a crisis in literacy. Many citizens are illiterate and innumerate. In some cities illiteracy affects over 25% of the population. Many older adults, particularly minority patients, had limited educational opportunities when young and they have spent a lifetime compensating for and hiding an inability to read or to understand what is read even if they can identify the words. Therefore, it is extremely important for nurses to ask "How do you learn best?" and to present materials in a manner most compatible with patients' expressed desires. Patients with low-level literacy are often very bright and readily memorize procedures through demonstration and return demonstration. Both literate and low-literacy patients benefit from written materials that have large print and contain only what is essential.

Barriers to learning. Nurses must remember that many medications, particularly those provided for pain, affect a patient's state of consciousness and block learning. All barriers to learning must be carefully assessed. Some common examples of barriers to learning in older adults are presented in Box 13-7.

Box 13-7.
Barriers to learning in older adults

Sensory changes such as decreased vision and hearing
Pain
Bladder frequency and urgency
Limited endurance, resulting in fatigue that shortens the attention span
Physical inability to perform motor tasks
Environmental noise, which older adults find more distracting and disruptive than younger persons
Environmental temperature, particularly the distraction caused by drafts and chilling
Depression, which is probably present in half of ill older adults and leads to low energy levels that impede compliance even when the patient or caregiver understands instructions

---

Because older adults often have undergone changes in sensory perception, learning will be enhanced if nurses take a multisensory approach to the presentation of materials. Care should be taken to slow the rate of speech to 100 to 106 words per minute and to keep voice pitch low (Kim, 1989). Spoken instructions should be reinforced with written instructions if the patient is literate. Often it is helpful to older patients to have them write the instructions in their own words under the direction of the nurse.

Referral to others. The primary nurse will, at times, need to involve specialists in the education of his or her patient. Clinical nurse specialists, enterostomal thera-

---

Box 13-8.
Elements of a discharge summary

Discharge site
Where is the patient going?

Identification of caregiver or significant other
Who will be assisting the patient with management of self-care activities?

Summary of condition at discharge
A brief statement should be given regarding the patient's physical condition and specific self-care tasks. Included in this summary should be notations about functional status and ability to perform activities of daily living. Nurses should also describe the patient's mental status and level of coping skills at discharge.

Medications
Include names, doses, frequency of medications, and instructions given to patient and/or caregiver regarding their use.

Equipment or supplies
List equipment or supplies sent home with patient and instruction regarding their use.

Special teaching
Summarize teaching done prior to discharge, and indicate the patient's and/or caregiver's response to teaching.

Referrals and/or plans for follow-up
Indicate plans for follow-up care including names of physicians who will be supervising care and dates and location of follow-up appointments. If the patient has been referred to other institutions or health care agencies, the details of transfer or referral should be summarized. Contact people in referral institutions should be identified.

pists, allied health therapists, nutritionists, and respiratory therapists may need to be involved if the patient and family are to attain mastery of self-care skills. Primary nurses should maintain control over this kaleidoscope of professionals and ensure that they are not presenting contradictory material. Referrals should be made to visiting nurses for home care follow-up. These professionals specialize in patient-caregiver education and can ensure that the patient, family, and other caregivers have correctly adapted information presented in the hospital to their home environment.

Discharge from the hospital. When the patient is discharged from the hospital, the nurse will be responsible for preparing a discharge summary for the patient's chart. These discharge summaries play an important role in providing data for quality assurance evaluations conducted by acute care hospitals. Each institution will have its own format, but in general the elements found in Box 13-8 should be included.

DISCHARGE TO HOME CARE SERVICES

Eligibility for Home Care

Older adults are eligible for home care services under the Medicare program provided that they meet the criteria listed in Box 13-9. It is important to note that home care services are intermittent and part-time in nature. Patients requiring continuous full-time skilled services or custodial care would not be eligible for home care services.

Types of Services Provided by Home Health Agencies

Patients who meet the eligibility criteria for home care receive an extended array of services. Skilled services are provided by nurses, physical therapists, occupational therapists, and speech-language pathologists. In addition, the patient may receive supportive and counseling services from a medical social worker and personal care services from a home health aide. Table 13-4 describes specific services provided by the members of various disciplines.

Referral to a Home Care Agency

All older adults who have been hospitalized for an illness or injury that will cause an alteration in lifestyle should be considered for referral to a home care agency. If the nurse is not certain whether the patient will meet the eligibility criteria for home care (e.g., homebound or requiring skilled services intermittently), a referral can be made for a home care evaluation visit and the home health agency can make the determination regarding the patient's eligibility for service. At times, the nurse or discharge planner making the patient referral will request

---

> **Box 13-9.**
>
> **Eligibility for home care services under Medicare**
>
> The patient is confined to his or her home. The patient must be essentially homebound so that leaving home would require a considerable and taxing effort. Acceptable absences from home include those that are infrequent, are of short duration, or are for the purpose of receiving medical treatment.
>
> Services are provided under a plan of care established and approved by a physician, and the patient is under the care of a physician who is qualified to sign the physician certification and plan of care.
>
> The patient needs skilled nursing care on an intermittent basis, needs physical therapy or speech therapy, or has continued need for occupational therapy.

From Department of Health and Human Services (1989).

---

services of specific disciplines such as nursing or physical therapy. More often, the inpatient nurse or discharge planner will be uncertain about the specific services needed by the patient and family. In that case, a referral is made for a nursing evaluation. When such a referral is made, the visiting nurse makes an initial visit to the home to evaluate the specific needs of the patient and family in the home situation. At the conclusion of this visit, the nurse consults with the patient's physician, suggesting specific orders to be included on the plan of treatment and securing verbal orders for the involvement of other members of the interdisciplinary team such as the therapists, a social worker, or an aide. The visiting nurse will also order supplies and durable medical equipment needed by the patient and order any laboratory studies considered necessary by the physician.

Although nurses working in acute care settings do not need to be concerned with the intricacies of operationalizing home care services, they should bear in mind the needs of the visiting nurse who will continue in the community setting the care that his or her colleagues initiated in the hospital. The visiting nurse's initial contacts with the patient and family will be influenced by the type of information received from the referring institution. If the referral has come from an inpatient nurse through a discharge planner acting as intermediary, much clinical data may be lost in the transfer. Therefore, it is essential that visiting nurses, acute care nurses, and discharge planners work closely to develop referral forms that convey a clear picture of the patient's clinical status at time of transfer from one health care setting to another. Table 13-5 depicts the types of information to be included on a referral form.

Table 13-4. Specific services provided by home care agencies by discipline

Discipline providing service	Services provided	Discipline providing service	Services provided

Nurses
  Registered nurse
  Licensed practical nurse under supervision of a registered nurse
  Nursing student under supervision of a registered nurse
	Skilled observation and assessment of patient's condition
	Management and evaluation of patient care plan being implemented by nonskilled person (e.g., caregiver)
	Teaching and training of patient and/or caregivers to manage self-care
	Administration of medications (oral, parenteral)
	Tube feedings and replacement, adjustment, stabilization, and suctioning of tubes
	Nasopharyngeal and tracheostomy aspiration
	Catheter insertion, sterile irrigation, and replacement (suprapubic and urethral)
	Wound care (e.g., ulcers, burns, pressure sores, surgical sites, fistulas)
	Ostomy care
	Heat treatments
	Management and administration of medical gases (e.g., oxygen)
	Venipuncture
	Rehabilitation nursing procedures (e.g., bowel and bladder training program)
	Psychiatric nurse evaluation and therapy
		Speech-language pathologists
		
		Occupational therapists
		
		Medical social workers
			Ultrasound, shortwave, and microwave diathermy treatments
			Application of hot packs, infrared treatments, paraffin baths, and whirlpool baths
			Speech/voice production services
			Training of patient or caregivers to augment speech-language communication
			Rehabilitative speech and language skills for patients with aphasia
			Selection and teaching of task-oriented therapeutic activities designed to restore:
			Physical function
			Sensory-integrative function
			Training patient and caregiver to perform compensatory techniques to improve independence in activities of daily living
			Designing, fabricating, and fitting orthotic and self-help devices
			Vocational and prevocational assessment and training directed toward restoration of function in the activities of daily living lost due to illness/injury
			Developing and implementing individualized therapeutic activity programs for patients with diagnosed psychiatric illnesses
			Assessment of impact of social and emotional factors on patient's illness and response to treatment
			Assessment of ability of home care agency to implement the plan of treatment, given the patient's and family's financial resources, home situation, and available community support systems

Physical therapists	Skilled rehabilitative services Assessment of range of motion, strength, balance, coordination, endurance, functional ability of patient Therapeutic exercise program Gait evaluation and training Range of motion tests Range of motion exercises for patients manifesting medical complications		

Based on Medicare Home Health Agency Manual (Department of Health and Human Services, 1989).   *Continued.*

Table 13-4. Specific services provided by home care agencies by discipline—cont'd

Discipline providing service	Services provided	Discipline providing service	Services provided
Home health aides (under supervision of the registered nurse provider)	Identification of appropriate community resources for patient and caregiver Provision of counseling services required by patient Personal care services Bathing Dressing Hair care Nail care Oral hygiene Shaving Application of deodorant Skin care Foot care Ear care Feeding Assistance with elimination (including enemas) Routine catheter and colostomy care Assistance will ambulation Bed positioning Assistance with transfers Changing simple dressings	Medical suppliers	Assistance with medication ordinarily self-administered Routine care of prosthetic and orthotic devices Changing of bed linens Assistance with activities directly supportive of skilled therapy services (e.g., range of motion exercises, repetitive speed routines) Services incidental to and provided in conjunction with personal care services: Light cleaning Limited meal preparation Trash removal Limited shopping Catheters, needles, syringes, dressings, irrigating fluids Durable medical equipment (hospital beds, walkers, canes, commode chairs, wheel chairs)

Table 13-5. Components of effective referral forms for home care

Information component	Rationale for requesting information	Information component	Rationale for requesting information
Full name of patient	Give full name of patient for identification purposes.		with the patient. For example, is the physician a surgeon, an internist, a cardiologist?
Birth date of patient	Give date of birth for identification and age of patient.		If possible, one physician should be designated who assumes responsibility for the patient. Often visiting nurses must call four or five physicians who saw the patient during hospitalization before obtaining orders for care.
Patient's address, including zip code	Give complete address, including zip code and/or census tracts. Large urban areas often have several streets with the same name, and the zip code and/or census tracts help visiting nurses locate the sector of the city in which the patient resides.	Follow-up physicians	If the patient is being discharged from the hospital back to the care of a community-based physician, it is essential that the visiting nurse receive that information.
Patient's phone and/or number through which patient can be reached	Obtain patient's phone number and a backup phone number through which the patient can be reached. Often the patient's phone is disconnected or the patient has some disability that prevents him or her from answering the phone. Many older adults intend to be discharged to their own homes but in a few days find that they must move in with a relative and are thus lost to visiting nurses if a secondary phone number is not available.		Indicate whether a discharge summary has been transferred from inpatient physicians to the community-based physician. Often the visiting nurse is buffeted between physicians as he or she attempts to clarify discharge orders and secure home care authorizations.
		Acute care nursing contact	In many settings discharge planners are social workers. Often home health nurses need to clarify clinical data, and this is best done nurse-to-nurse. It is helpful to have the name of a nursing contact person who is familiar with the patient's course of treatment during hospitalization
Name, address, and phone number of caregiver	Caregivers may live with the patient or may reside outside the patient's home. Visiting nurses will want to schedule visits with the patient when the caregiver is available so that patient and caregiver can be taught self-management of care together.		
Health insurance, Medicare, Medicaid numbers	This information establishes the payment source for home care billing.	Brief history of course of hospitalization	It is not unusual for older adults to be confused and disoriented following hospitalization as a result of stress, medications, or medical condition.
Referring physician	The names of all physicians caring for the patient in the hospital should be given, along with a brief description regarding their role		Even well-oriented patients have difficulty accurately describing tests and procedures

Continued.

Table 13-5. Components of effective referral forms for home care—cont'd

Information component	Rationale for requesting information	Information component	Rationale for requesting information
	performed during the course of their hospital stay. Planning nursing care is difficult without accurate, objective information.	Treatments	All treatments should be clearly ordered and wounds or tube sites clearly described.
Diagnoses	Give all relevant diagnoses and information regarding the ones that continue to present problems for the patient. The patient may have been admitted to the hospital for congestive heart failure but at time of discharge may be more troubled by an exacerbation of arthritis. The hospital's primary diagnosis may not be the one that must assume priority for the visiting nurse.	Recent laboratory values	The visiting nurse does not have the patient's inpatient chart to refer to, and several days or weeks may pass before laboratory work is done again. Laboratory values at discharge are very important in establishing baseline information for nursing assessment.
		Diet	Diet orders are frequently overlooked on referrals. Visiting nurses need to know about special diets, appetite, and any chewing or swallowing difficulties.
Copy of nursing physical assessment	It is helpful for visiting nurses to have a copy of the patient's most recent physical assessment or systems review performed by nurses or physicians in the hospital. It is not unusual for an older person's condition to change dramatically in the time between referral and the first home visit 24-36 hr later. Historical physical assessment data allow the visiting nurse to identify emerging problems as he or she conducts an admission physical for home health services.	Equipment and supplies	Information should be given about durable medical equipment. Has the equipment been ordered through hospital vendors or is it to be the responsibility of the home health agency? Patients should be sent home with 24-48 hr of medical supplies (e.g., dressings) in case there is a delay in obtaining home delivery of needed materials.
Medications	List all medications and their dosage and frequency. Let the home health agency know whether the patient left the hospital with medications, prescriptions, or neither. Older patients are often sent home with prescriptions only. Many have limited finances or transportation difficulty, and several days may pass before medications can be obtained.	Summary of inpatient teaching instituted in hospital	It is helpful for the visiting nurse to know what the patient and family or other caregivers have been taught and how they responded to health education efforts. Armed with this information, the visiting nurse can plan his or her own teaching efforts to reinforce or expand information given in the hospital. It is helpful to know the type of handouts or instruction sheets that have been given to the patient so that these can be reviewed during the first home visit.

Table 13-5. Components of effective referral forms for home care—cont'd

Information component	Rationale for requesting information	Information component	Rationale for requesting information
Functional limitations	Identify any functional limitations that affect the patient's ability for self-care. Is the patient dependent on assistive devices such as wheelchairs, walkers, canes?	Social and support systems	Does the patient have an apparent support network? Has he or she had regular, interested visitors while in the hospital? Are there any special problems the visiting nurse should know about? The visiting nurse must enter all types of neighborhoods to deliver services. Especially in large cities, some neighborhoods or social situations are dangerous. Some family situations are rife with tension. Hospital personnel have an obligation to alert their community-based colleagues to potential dangers they may encounter on home visits.
Activity level	Is the patient up as tolerated or on complete bed rest?		
Mental status	Describe that patient's mental status clearly. It is important for visiting nurses to know whether the patient can comprehend instructions and remember to carry out self-care activities. Visit patterns and frequency of home visits will be closely correlated with changes in the patient's mental status or level of depression.	Summary of major nursing diagnoses	Identification of nursing diagnoses still active at time of discharge will help visiting nurses to plan nursing assessment for the first home visit.

DISCHARGE TO OTHER INSTITUTIONAL SETTINGS

Patients can be discharged home with self-management, home with assistance of family members, or home with the assistance of community support systems. Occasionally, however, patients cannot immediately return home. Some will require temporary placement in a facility for rehabilitation and short-term recuperation, and a few will require long-term care that can be provided only in a nursing home. Members of the discharge planning team will work closely with the patient and family members to ensure that transfers to other alternative care facilities are acceptable and compatible with the patient's and family's long-term goals. Referral to these facilities is primarily managed by the discharge planning department

in cooperation with the social work staff. Primary nurses working with the patient should ensure that basic patient information is transferred to the new facility to enable their nursing and allied health colleagues in those institutions to continue care commenced in the hospital. Sometimes a copy of the patient's chart and/or physician's discharge summary is transferred with the patient. It is suggested that discharge planning departments work closely with institutions to which they commonly refer patients to develop referral data forms that meet the needs of the receiving institution's staff. Certainly, at a minimum, information normally contained in a nursing discharge summary, nursing assessment and diagnosis data, and the medical orders should be immediately transferred. Table 13-6 identifies some of the common alternate care facilities.

Table 13-6. Types of alternate care facilities

Type of alternate care facility	Purpose	Type of alternate care facility	Purpose
Chronic care hospital	Assists patients who have slowly progessing diseases and terminal or irreversible chronic care conditions.	Congregate housing	Provides community-based residence that has a full range of support and social services available. Older adults live in their own apartments but share bathing and dining facilities.
Rehabilitation hospital	Provides an intensive program of restorative therapy after injury, illness, or disease. The patient is expected to return home after discharge.	Life care communities	Provides residential living in apartments, town houses, or private homes that have access to central health care services such as an infirmary, a clinic, a nursing home, residential physicians, and limited service hospitals.
Skilled nursing facility (SNF)	Provides an intensive, organized program of restorative services of nursing care. Length of stay could be brief for the provision of recuperation or could be life long if custodial care is required.		
Nursing facility (NF)	Provides assistance with activities of daily living, and routine skilled nursing care is available if needed.	Hospice	Provides care for terminally ill. Hospice services are also provided on an outpatient basis under the Medicare hospice benefit. Outpatient hospice care includes palliative services of home health agencies, respite care, services of volunteers, and bereavement care.
Alternate housing (provides self-care focus)			
Group home	Allows patients with severe disability to remain in the community with assistance of personal care attendants who provide assistance with activities of daily living.	Adult day care (medical or social)	Provides care 5 to 12 hr a day for 5 days a week, which provides relief for primary caregivers, particularly those who are employed. Services provided include health maintenance and education, nursing care, restorative therapies, nutrition, personal care, and associate activities and social services.
Foster home	Older client receives care from a family and is able to enjoy living in a home environment.		

SUMMARY

Nurses play a critical role in discharge planning, for they are intimately involved with the patient and his or her family. Nurses are in an ideal position to identify patients who will need continuing care, and their prompt referral of such patients to the discharge planning program will ensure that they receive the mix of services to which they are legally and ethically entitled. For most patients, effective discharge planning will mean a return home or to community-based living.

REFERENCES

American Association of Retired Persons and Administration on Aging (1990). A profile of older Americans, Washington, DC, US Department of Health and Human Services.

Corkery E (1989). Discharge planning and home health care: What every staff nurse should know, Orthop Nurs 8(6):18-27.

Department of Health and Human Services: Health Care Financing Administration (1989). Medicare: Home health agency manual (HCFA Publication 11). Washington, DC, US Government Printing Office.

Folden SL (1990). On the inside looking out: Perceptions of the homebound, J Gerontol Nurs 16(1):9-14.

Gillies DA (1986). Patients suffering from memory loss can be taught self-care, Geriatr Nurs 7(5):357-361.

Johnson J (1989). Where's discharge planning on your list? Geriatr Nurs 10(3):14.

Kim K (1989). Patient education. In Burggraf V and Stanley M, editors: Nursing the elderly: A care plan approach, Philadelphia, JB Lippincott Co, pp 36-47.

Naylor M (1990). Comprehensive discharge planning for hospitalized elderly: A pilot study, Nurs Res 39(3):156-161.

Rorden J and Taft E (1990). Discharge planning for nurses, Philadelphia, WB Saunders Co.

Weinrich SP, Boyd M, and Nussbaum J (1989). Adapting strategies to teach the elderly, J Gerontol Nurs 15(11):17-20.

Zarle N (1987). Continuing care: The process and practice of discharge planning, Rockville, Md, Aspen.

GENERAL BIBLIOGRAPHY

American Association of Retired Persons (1990). A profile of older Americans, PF3049 (1290) D996, Washington, DC, The Association.

Atchley RC (1991). Social forces and aging, ed 6, Belmont, Calif, Wadsworth Publishing Co.

Burggraf V and Stanley M (1989). Nursing the elderly: A care plan approach, Philadelphia, JB Lippincott Co.

Burnside I (1988). Nursing and the aged, ed 3, New York, McGraw-Hill.

Dellasega C (1989). Health in the sandwich generation, Geriatr Nurs 10(5):242-243.

Ebersole P and Hess P (1990). Toward healthy aging, ed 3, St Louis, The CV Mosby Co.

Eliopoulos C (1990). Caring for the elderly in diverse care settings, Philadelphia, JB Lippincott Co.

Eliopoulos C (1990). Health assessment of the older adult, Redwood City, Calif, Addison-Wesley Nursing.

Feil N (1982). Validation, Cleveland, Edward Feil Productions.

Garner BC (1989). Guide to changing lab values in elders, Geriatr Nurs 10(3):144-145.

Gioiella EC and Bevil CW (1985). Nursing care of the aging client. Norwalk, Conn, Appleton-Century-Crofts.

Gress LD and Bahr RT (1984). The aging person, St Louis, The CV Mosby Co.

Hazzard WR (1985). Atherogenesis: Why women live longer than men, Geriatrics 40(1):42-54.

Hogstel MO (1985). Older widowers, Geriatr Nurs 6(1):24-26.

Hogstel MO, editor (1985). Home nursing care for the elderly, Bowie, Md, Brady.

Hogstel MO, editor (1988). Nursing care of the older adult, ed 2, New York, John Wiley & Sons, Inc.

Hogstel MO, editor (1990). Geropsychiatric nursing, St Louis, The CV Mosby Co.

Hooyman NR and Kiyak HA (1990). Social gerontology: A multi-disciplinary perspective, New York: Simon & Schuster.

Institute of Lifetime Learning, American Association of Retired Persons (1983). The best time to grow old: Introduction to gerontology, a lifetime learning mini course study booklet, Washington, DC, The Association.

Johnson L and Keller KL (1989). Staging Alzheimer's disease. Geriatr Nurs 10(4):196-197.

Kane RA and Kane RL (1981). Assessing the elderly, Lexington, Mass, Lexington Books.

Katzen L (1990). Chronic illness and sexuality, Am J Nurs 90(2):56-60.

Kneeshaw MF and Lunney M (1989). Nursing diagnosis: Not for individuals only, Geriatr Nurs 10(5):246-247.

Lueckenotte AG (1990). Pocket guide to gerontologic assessment, St Louis, The CV Mosby Co.

Mace NL and Rabins PV (1981). The 36-hour day, Baltimore, The Johns Hopkins University Press.

Matteson MA and McConnell ES (1988). Gerontological nursing, Philadelphia, WB Saunders Co.

Moore P (1985). Disguised, Waco, Tex, Word Books.

Mowbray CA (1989). Shedding light on elder abuse, J Gerontol Nurs 15(10):20-24.

Newman J et al (1984). Evaluation of a health program, Geriatr Nurs 5(6):234-238.

Osborn CL (1989). Reminiscence: When the past eases the present, J Gerontol Nurs 15(10):6-12.

Resource Directory for Older People (1989). Washington, DC, National Institute on Aging.

Steel K (1984). Geriatric medicine is coming of age, The Gerontologist 24(4):367-372.

Wolfe SM, Fugate L, Hulstrand EP, and Kamimoto LE (1988). Worst pills, best pills, Washington, DC, Public Citizen Health Research Group.

Yurick AG, Spier BE, Robb SS, and Ebert NJ (1989). The aged person and the nursing process, ed 3, Norwalk, Conn, Appleton & Lange.

Zins S (1987). Aging in America: An introduction to gerontology, Albany, NY, Delmar.

APPENDIX A

Standards of Gerontological Nursing Practice*

STANDARD I. Organization of Gerontological Nursing Services

All gerontological nursing services are planned, organized, and directed by a nurse executive. The nurse executive has baccalaureate or master's preparation and has experience in gerontological nursing and administration of long-term care services or acute care services for older clients.

Rationale

The nurse executive uses administrative knowledge to plan and direct nursing services delivered in an environment where nursing is an integral component of the gerontological interdisciplinary team and services. In smaller settings the nurse executive may also serve in a clinical role and coordinate the plan and services to meet the diverse and complex needs of the older client and family. (In this document, the term family refers to family members and significant others.)

In all gerontological settings (day care, home care, ambulatory care, retirement homes and communities, adult homes, health-related facilities, intermediate care and extended care facilities, skilled care nursing homes, and community-based social programs), the nurse executive assures appropriate services, adequately coordinated to meet the multiplicity of conditions and needs of the older population.

STANDARD II. Theory

The nurse participates in the generation and testing of theory as a basis for clinical decisions. The nurse uses theoretical concepts to guide the effective practice of gerontological nursing.

* Reprinted with permission from *Standards and Scope of Gerontological Nursing Practice*, Kansas City, Mo, American Nurses' Association, © 1987.

Rationale

Theoretical concepts from nursing and other disciplines are an essential source of knowledge for professional nursing practice. Theories help organize and interpret isolated information obtained from clients and their families. Theoretical concepts provide a framework for assessing, intervening, and evaluating care to clients, as well as providing the rationale for nursing care to other health professionals. Furthermore, the testing of theory in practice settings is essential for the development of the discipline of nursing.

STANDARD III. Data Collection

The health status of the older person is regularly assessed in a comprehensive, accurate, and systematic manner. The information obtained during the health assessment is accessible to and shared with appropriate members of the interdisciplinary health care team, including the older person and the family.

Rationale

The information obtained from the older person, the family, and the interdisciplinary team, in addition to nursing judgments based on knowledge of gerontological nursing, is used to develop a comprehensive plan of care. This plan incorporates the older person's perceived needs and goals.

STANDARD IV. Nursing Diagnosis

The nurse uses health assessment data to determine nursing diagnoses.

Rationale

Nursing diagnosis is an integral part of the assessment process. Each older person, having a unique perception of health and well-being, responds to aging in a unique way. The basis for nursing intervention rests on the identification of those diagnoses that flow from gerontological nursing theory and scientific knowledge.

STANDARD V. Planning and Continuity of Care

The nurse develops the plan of care in conjunction with the older person and appropriate others. Mutual goals, priorities, nursing approaches, and measures in the care plan address the therapeutic, preventive, restorative, and rehabilitative needs of the older person. The care plan helps the older person attain and maintain the highest level of health, well-being, and quality of life achievable, as well as a peaceful death. The plan of care facilitates continuity of care over time as the client moves to various care settings, and is revised as necessary.

Rationale

Planning guides nursing interventions and facilitates the achievement of desired outcomes. Plans are based on nursing diagnoses and contain goals and interventions with specific time frames for accomplishment.

Goals are a determination of the results to be achieved and are derived from the nursing diagnoses. Goals are directed toward maximizing the older person's state of well-being, health, and achievable independence in all activities of daily living. Goals are based on knowledge of the client's status, the desired outcomes, and current research findings to increase the probability of helping the client achieve maximum well-being.

STANDARD VI. Intervention

The nurse, guided by the plan of care, intervenes to provide care to restore the older person's functional capabilities and to prevent complications and excess disability. Nursing interventions are derived from nursing diagnoses and are based on gerontological nursing theory.

Rationale

The nurse implements a plan of care in collaboration with the client, the family, and the interdisciplinary team. The nurse provides direct and indirect care, using the concepts of health promotion, maintenance, and rehabilitation or restoration. The nurse educates and counsels the family to facilitate their provision of care to the older person. The nurse teaches, supervises, and evaluates care givers outside the health professions and assures that their care is supportive and ethical and demonstrates respect for the client's dignity.

STANDARD VII. Evaluation

The nurse continually evaluates the client's and family's responses to interventions in order to determine progress toward goal attainment and to revise the data base, nursing diagnoses, and plan of care.

Rationale

Nursing practice is a dynamic process that responds to alterations in data, diagnoses, or care plans. Evaluation of the quality of care is an essential component. The effectiveness of nursing care depends on the continuing reassessment of the client's and family's health needs and appropriate revision of the plan of care.

STANDARD VIII. Interdisciplinary Collaboration

The nurse collaborates with other members of the health care team in the various settings in which care is given to the older person. The team meets regularly to evaluate the effectiveness of the care plan for the client and family and to adjust the plan of care to accommodate changing needs.

Rationale

The complex nature of comprehensive care to elderly clients and their family members requires expertise from a number of different health care professions. A multidisciplinary approach is optimal for planning, carrying out, and evaluating care of older adults and their families.

STANDARD IX. Research

The nurse participates in research designed to generate an organized body of gerontological nursing knowledge, disseminates research findings, and uses them in practice.

Rationale

The improvement of the practice of gerontological nursing and the future of health care for older persons depend on the availability and utilization of an adequate knowledge base for gerontological nursing practice.

STANDARD X. Ethics

The nurse uses the Code for Nurses established by the American Nurses' Association as a guide for ethical decision making and practice.

Rationale

The nurse is responsible for providing health care to individuals in settings where decisions about health care are jointly made with client, family, and physician when appropriate. The nurse determines with the client and family the appropriate setting for care during acute and chronic illnesses. Nurses and other care providers are prepared by education and experience to provide the care needed by the older person.

The Code for Nurses provides the parameters within which the nurse makes ethical decisions. Special ethical concerns in gerontological nursing care include informed consent; admission to a health care facility, with collaboration of the client, family, nurse, and physician; emergency interventions; nutrition and hydration; pain management; the need for self-determination by the client; treatment termination; quality-of-life issues; confidentiality; surrogate decision making; nontraditional treatment modalities; fair distribution of scarce resources; and economic decision making.

STANDARD XI. Professional Development

The nurse assumes responsibility for professional development and contributes to the professional growth of in-terdisciplinary team members. The nurse participates in peer review and other means of evaluation to assure the quality of nursing practice.

Rationale

Scientific, cultural, societal, and political changes require a commitment from the nurse to the continuing pursuit of knowledge to enhance professional growth. Peer evaluation of nursing practice, professional education, and participation in collaborative educational programs serve as mechanisms to ensure quality care.

Sample Nursing History Form

Date _____ Name _____

Room _____ Sex: M F Address _____

Private home _____ Apartment _____ Retirement center _____ Nursing home _____

Date of birth _____ Age _____ Date of admission _____ Date of surgery _____

Marital status: M W S D Occupation _____ Retired _____

  If widowed, how long? _____

Religious preference _____

Reason for seeking care (chief complaint) _____

_____

History of present illness/condition/surgery

_____

_____

_____

  Patient's understanding of current condition _____

_____

  Current diet _____

  Medications currently prescribed _____

_____

Past health/medical history

_____

_____

_____

Adapted from Nursing History Form 584, Harris College of Nursing, Texas Christian University, Fort Worth. Used with permission.

Allergies (food, medicines, environmental) _____

_____

Medications and treatments at home _____

_____

Chemical use

Number of cigarettes per day _____   Amount of coffee/tea/carbonated beverages per day _____

Other tobacco per day _____   Amount of alcoholic drinks per day _____

Number of years smoked _____   Type _____

Use of other substances _____

Rest and sleep patterns

Hours worked per day _____   Rest periods or naps (when, number, length) _____

Hours of sleep per night _____   _____

Medications used to aid sleep _____

Other measures to aid sleep _____

Sleep problems _____

Mobility and exercise patterns

Type of activity/exercise _____

Amount (times per week; minutes per day) _____

Restrictions/mechanical aids/prostheses/wheelchair/walker/bedrails

_____

Diet	Breakfast	Lunch	Dinner	Snacks
Typical meal plan at home				

Usual time of meals at home

Ability to feed self _____   Dentures _____

Dietary restrictions/dislikes/difficulty _____

Fluid intake per day (type and amount) _____

Elimination (routines, frequency, problems, aids)

Bowel _____

_____

Urinary _____

_____

Communication

Ability to understand English _____ Language spoken _____

Hearing _____ Sight _____ Aids _____

Educational level _____

Ability to speak _____

Orientation: Person _____ Time _____ Place _____

Present emotional state _____

Activities

Hobbies _____

Part-time employment _____

Volunteer work _____

Other _____

Family history

Composition

Number in household

Roles

Primary support system

History of family health/illness

Other pertinent data

SYSTEM	HISTORY Review of Systems	NOT ASKED
General overview		
Skin, hair, nails		
Head and neck		
Eyes		
Ears		
Nose/sinus		
Mouth/throat		
Respiratory		
Cardiovascular		
Gastrointestinal		
Breasts/axillae		
Genitourinary		
Musculoskeletal		

Neurological

Other pertinent data:

Sample Physical Assessment Form

Name _____ Date _____

Age _____ Height _____ Weight _____

Vital Signs: T _____ P _____ R _____ B/P: Sitting _____ Standing _____ Lying _____

EXAMINATION	DESCRIPTION	NOT EXAMINED
Overall appearance*		
Skin		
Head		
Eyes		
Ears		
Nose and sinuses		
Mouth and pharynx		
Neck		

* See Appendix D for suggested descriptive terms.

Adapted from Physical Assessment Form 584, Harris College of Nursing, Texas Christian University, Fort Worth. Used with permission.

Thorax and lungs

Breasts and axillae

Heart and peripheral vascular

Abdomen

Musculoskeletal

Genitourinary and rectum

Neurological

Mental status

Laboratory and other pertinent data:

APPENDIX D

Sample Physical Assessment Guide

GENERAL INSTRUCTIONS

Use this guide for suggested descriptive terminology for completion of the physical assessment form in Appendix C.

Be specific, descriptive, and objective. Avoid such terms as normal, within normal limits, good, fair, OK, etc. Describe what you see rather than making inferences or judgments.

OVERALL APPEARANCE   Inspection

Sex: Male/female

General Grooming: Clean? Hair combed? Make-up?

Position/Posturing: Supine? Prone? Rigid? Opisthotonos? Erect? Slumped?

Body Size: Thin? Fat? Obese? Emaciated? Flabby? Weight proportionate to height? Mesomorph? Endomorph?

Facial Expressions: Smiling? Frowning? Blank? Apathetic?

Body Language: Eye contact? No eye contact? Arms folded over chest?

Other Observations: Restless? Fidgeting? Lying quietly? Listless? Trembling? Tense?

SKIN   Inspection and palpation

Color and Vascularity: Pink? Tan? Brown? Dark brown? Grayish? Pasty? Yellowish? Flushed? Jaundiced?

Turgor and Mobility: Elastic/nonelastic? Tenting? Wrinkled? Edematous? Tight?

Adapted from Physical Assessment Guide, 1987, Harris College of Nursing, Texas Christian University, Fort Worth. Used with permission.

Temperature and Moisture: Cold? Cool? Warm? Hot? Feverish? Moist? Dry? Clammy? Oily? Sweating? Diaphoresis?

Texture: Smooth? Rough? Fine? Thick? Coarse? Scaly? Puffy?

Nails: Clean? Manicured? Smooth? Rough? Dry? Hard? Brittle? Splitting? Cracking? Angle of nail bed? Clubbing? Curved? Flat? Thick? Yellowing? Paronychia? Nail beds and lunula—Pale? Pink? Cyanotic? Red? Shape of lunula? Blanching? Spooning?

Body Hair Growth: Color? Thick/thin? Coarse/fine? Location and distribution on body? Hirsutism?

Skin Integrity: Intact/not intact? Lesions, birthmarks, moles, scars, and rashes (describe shape, size, and locations)? Nevi? Fissures? Macules? Papules? Pustules? Nodules? Bullae? Cysts? Carbuncle? Wheals? Erythema? Excoriation? Desquamation? Abrasions? Cherry angioma? Senile lentigines? Senile purpura? Senile keratoses? Seborrheic keratoses? Bruises? Insect bites? Crusts? Warts? Pimples? Blackheads? Bleeding? Drainage? Lacerations? Scaly? Ulcers? Lichenification?

HEAD   Inspection and palpation

Shape: Round? Oval? Square? Pointed? Normocephalic?

Face: Shape—Oval? Heart shaped? Pear? Long? Square? Round? Thin? High cheekbones? Symmetrical?

Sensation (Trigeminal Nerve, CN V): Sensation on three branches? Clenched teeth?

Facial Nerve (CN VII): Facial expressions? Smiles?

Hair: Color and growth—Coarse? Fine? Thick? Thin? Sparse? Alopecia? Long? Short? Curly? Straight? Permed? Glossy? Shiny? Greasy? Dry? Brittle? Stringy? Frizzy?

Condition of scalp: Clean? Scaly? Dandruff? Rashes? Sores? Drainage? Masses and lumps (describe location and shape; measure size)?

EYES   Inspection and palpation

Eyebrows: Color and shape? Alignment? Straight? Curved? Thick? Thin? Sparse? Plucked? Scaly?

Eyelashes: Long? Short? Curved? None? Artificial?

Eyelids: Dark? Swollen? Inflamed? Red? Stye? Infected? Open and close simultaneously? Ptosis? Entropion? Ectropion? Lid lag? Xanthomas?

Shape and Appearance of Eyes: Almond? Rounded? Squinty? Prominent? Exophthalmic? Sunken? Symmetrical? Bright? Clear? Dull? Tearing? Discharge? (Serous? Purulent?) Exotropia? Esotropia? Nystigmus? Strabismus?

Sclera: White? Cream? Yellowish? Jaundiced? Injected? Pterygium?

Conjunctiva: Pale pink? Pink? Red? Inflamed? Nodules? Swelling?

Iris: Color and shape—Round? Not round? Coloboma? Arcus senilis?

Cornea: Clear? Milky? Opaque? Cloudy?

Pupils (Oculomotor Nerve, CN III) (pupils equal, round, react to light and accommodation [PERRLA]): Size (measure in mm) and shape—Round? Not round (describe)? Equality—Symmetrical? Anisocoria? Right larger than left? Left larger than right? Convergence? Reaction to light and accommodation? Consensual reaction?
Extraocular movements (Oculomotor, Trochlear, Aducens Nerves, CN III, IV, VI): Intact?

Lacrimal Glands: Tender? Nontender? Inflamed? Swollen? Tearing?

Aids: Glasses? Contact lenses? Prosthesis?

Visual Fields (Optic Nerve, CN II): Intact?

Vision (Optic Nerve, CN II): Reads newsprint? Reports objects across room?

EARS   Inspection and palpation

Pinnae: Size and shape—Large? Small? In proportion to face? Protruding? Oval? Large lobes? Small lobes? Symmetrical? Right larger than left? Left larger than right? Pinnae irregular? Color? Skin intact? Redness? Swelling? Tophi? Cauliflower ear? Furuncles? Darwin's tubercle?

Level in Relation to Eyes: Top of pinnae level with outer cantus of eyes? Top of pinnae lower than outer canthus of eyes? Top of pinnae higher than outer canthus of eyes?

Canal: Clean? Discharge? (Serous? Bloody? Purulent?) Nodules? Inflammation? Redness? Foreign object? Cilia—Present/absent? Cerumen—Present/absent? Color? Consistency?

Tympanic Membrane: Color? Pearly white? Infected? Red? Inflamed? Discharge? Cone of light? Landmarks? Scarring? Bubbles? Fluid level?

Hearing (Auditory Nerve, CN VII): Right—present/absent? Left—present/absent? Hears watch tick? Hears whisper? Responds readily when spoken to? Weber—Lateralizes equally? To left/right side? Rinne—Air conduction > bone conduction 2 : 1? Hearing aid—Right/left?

NOSE AND SINUSES   Inspection and palpation

Size and Shape: Long? Short? Large? Small? In proportion to face? Flat? Broad? Broad based? Thick? Thin? Enlarged? Nares symmetrical/asymmetrical? Pointed? Pug? Swollen? Bulbous? Flaring of nostrils?

Septum: Midline? Deviated right/left? Perforated?

Nasal Mucosa and Turbinates: Pink? Pale? Bluish? Red? Dry? Moist? Discharge? (Purulent? Clear? Watery? Mucus?) Cilia present/absent? Rhinitis? Epistaxis? Polyps?

Patency of Nares: (Close each side and ask client to breathe.)   Right—Patent/partial   obstruction/obstructed?   Left—patent/partial   obstruction/obstructed?

Olfactory Nerve (CN I): Correctly identifies odors?

Sinuses: Tender? Nontender? Transillumination?

MOUTH AND PHARYNX   Inspection

Lips: Color—Pink? Red? Tan? Pale? Cyanotic? Shape—Thin? Thick? Enlarged? Swollen? Symmetrical/asymmetrical? Drooping left side? Drooping right side? Condition—Soft? Smooth? Dry? Cracked? Fissured? Blisters? Lesions (describe)?

Teeth: Color and condition—White? Yellow? Grayish? Spotted? Stained? Darkened? Pitting? Straight? Crooked, protruding? Separated? Crowded? Irregular? Broken? Notching? Peglike? Loose? Dull? Bright? Edentulous? Malocclusion? Caries and fillings—Number and location? Dental hygiene—Clean/not clean?

Breath Odor: Sweet? Odorless? Halitosis? Musty? Acetone? Foul? Fetid? Odor of drugs or food? Hot? Sour? Alcohol?

Gums: Pink? Firm? Swollen? Bleeding? Sensitive? Gingivitis? Hypertrophy? Nodules? Irritated? Receding? Moist? Ulcerated? Dry? Shrunken? Blistered? Spongy?

Facial and Glossopharyngeal Nerves (CN VII and IX): Identifies taste?

Tongue: Macroglossia? Microglossia? Glossitis? Geographic? Red? Pink? Pale? Bluish? Brownish? Swollen? Clean? Thin? Thick? Fissured? Raw? Coated? Moist? Dry? Cracked? Glistening? Papillae?

Hypoglossal Nerve (CN XII)—Tongue
Movement: Symmetry? Lateral? Fasciculation?

Mucosa: Color? Leukoplakia? Dry? Moist? Intact? Not intact? Masses (describe size, shape, and location)? Chancre?

Palate: Moist? Dry? Color? Intact? Not intact?

Uvula: Color? Midline? Remains at midline when saying "ah"? Gag reflex present?

Pharynx: Color? Petechia? Infected? Beefy? Dysphagia?

Tonsils: Present/absent? Cryptic? Beefy? Size 1+ to 4+?

Temporomandibular Joint: Fully mobile? Symmetrical? Tenderness? Crepitus?

NECK   Inspection and palpation

Appearance: Long? Short? Thick? Thin? Masses (describe size and shape)? Symmetrical? Not symmetrical?

Thyroid: Palpable? Nodules? Tender?

Trachea: Midline? Deviated to right/left?

Lymph Nodes (occipital, preauricular, postauricular, submental, submaxillary, tonsilar, anterior cervical, posterior cervical, superficial cervical, deep cervical, supraclavicular): Nonpalpable? Tender? Lymphadenopathy? Shotty? Hard? Firm?

THORAX AND LUNGS   Inspection, palpation, percussion, and ausculation

Respirations: Rate? Tachypnea, eupnea, bradypnea? Apnea? Orthopnea? Labored? Stertorous? Rhythm regular/irregular? Inspiration time greater than expiration time? Expiration time greater than inspiration time? Spasmodic? Gasping? Orthopneic? Deep? Eupneic? Shallow? Flairing of nostrils with respirations? Symmetrical/asymmetrical? Right thorax greater than left? Left thorax greater than right? Ratio of anteroposterior diameter to lateral diameter between 1:2 and 5:7? Ribs sloped downward at 45 degree angle? Well-defined costal space? Accessory muscles used? Pigeon chest? Funnel chest? Barrel chest? Abdominal or chest breather? Skin intact? Lesions? Color? Thin? Muscular? Flabby?

Posterior Thorax: Tenderness? Masses? Respiratory excursion symmetrical/asymmetrical? No respiratory movements on right/left? Subcutaneous emphysema? Crepitus? Fremitus? Estimation of level of diaphragm? Spine alignment? Tenderness? Costovertebral angle tenderness? Resonance? Dull? Hyperresonance? Diaphragmatic excursion 3-5 cm? Comparison of one side to the other? Suprasternal notch located? Costochondral junctions tender? Chest wall stable? Vocal fremitus?

Lung Auscultation: Vesicular? Bronchovesicular? Bronchial? Whispered Pectroliloquy? Adventitious sounds? Rales? Rhonchi? Wheezes? Crackles? Rub? Bronchophony? Egophony?

BREASTS AND AXILLAE   Inspection and palpation

Breasts: Male? Female? Present/absent? Color? Large? Small? Well-developed? Firm? Pendulous? Flat? Flabby? Symmetrical/asymmetrical? Dimpling? Thickening? Smooth? Retraction? Peau d'orange? Venous pattern? Tenderness? Masses (describe)? Gynecomastia?

Nipples: Present/absent? Circular? Symmetrical/asymmetrical? Inverted? Everted? Pale? Brown? Rose? Extra nipples? Discharge? Deviation? Supranumerary?

Axilla: Shaved/unshaved? Odor? Masses or lumps (describe size and shape)?

Lymph Nodes (lateral, central, subscapular, pectoral, epitrochlear): Palpable? Tender? Shotty?

HEART AND PERIPHERAL VASCULAR   Inspection, percussion, auscultation, and palpation

Precordial bulge? Abnormal palpations? Point of maximal impulse? Thrills? Heave or lift with pulsation? S_1 loudest at apex? S_2 loudest at base? S_3? S_4? Splits? Clicks? Snap? Rub? Gallop? Murmurs—Systolic? Diastolic? Holosystolic? Harsh? Soft? Blowing? Rumbling? Grading 1 through 6? High pitch? Medium pitch? Low pitch? Radiating?

Carotid Pulse: *Note: do not check both right and left carotid pulses simultaneously.* Volume—Bounding? Forceful? Strong? Full? Weak? Feeble? Thready? Symmetrical? Right less than left? Left less than right? Rhythm—Regular? Irregular? Symmetrical? Asymmetrical? Bruits present/absent?

Apical Pulse: Record rate. Tachycardia? Bradycardia? Pounding? Forceful? Weak? Moderate? Regular/irregular?

Peripheral Pulses: (Do not count rate of these pulses except radial.) Record character, volume, rhythm, and symmetry of brachial, radial, femoral, popliteal, dorsalis pedis, and posterior tibial pulses. Volume—Full? Strong? Forceful? Bounding? Perceptible? Imperceptible? Weak? Thready? Symmetrical/asymmetrical? Right greater than left? Left greater than right? Rhythm—Regular? Irregular? Symmetrical? Asymmetrical? Symmetry—Record as symmetrical, right greater than left, or left greater than right. Pulse deficit, pulse pressure, blood pressure in both arms, blood pressure lying, sitting, and standing if applicable. Jugular venous distension (record centimeters above level of sternal angle).

ABDOMEN   Inspection, auscultation, percussion, and palpation

Contour: Irregular? Protruding? Enlarged? Distended? Scaphoid? Concave? Sunken? Flabby? Firm? Flat? Flaccid?

Skin: Color? Intact? Not intact? Shiny? Smooth? Scars? Lesions (describe size, shape, and type)? Striae? Umbilicus?

Bowel Sounds: Present? Absent? Hyperactive? High-pitched tinkling? Gurgles? Borborygmus? Percussion—Tympanic? Dull? Flat (describe where)? Liver size 6-12 cm? Splenic dullness sixth to tenth rib? Ascites? Palpation—Splenomegaly? Hepatomegaly? Organomegaly? Masses? Aortic pulse? Diastasis recti? Tenderness? Bulges? Lower pole of kidneys palpable? Inguinal or femoral hernia? Inguinal nodes (describe)?

MUSCULOSKELETAL   Inspection and palpation

Back: Shoulders level? Right shoulder higher than left? Left shoulder higher than right? Alignment? Lordosis? Scoliosis? Kyphosis? Ankylosis?

Vertebral Column Alignment: Straight? Lordosis? Scoliosis? Kyphosis?

Joints: Redness? Swelling? Deformity (describe)? Crepitation? Size? Symmetry? Subluxation? Separation? Bogginess? Tenderness? Pain? Thickening? Nodules? Fluid? Bulging?

Range of Motion: Describe as full, limited, or fixed; estimate degree of limitation. Assess range of motion of neck, shoulders, elbows, wrists, fingers, back, hips, knees, ankles, toes.

Extremities: Compare extremities to each other; describe color and symmetry. Temperature—Hot, warm, cool, cold, moist, clammy, dry? Muscle tone—Firm, muscular, flabby, flaccid, atrophied? Fasciculation? Tremor?

Lower Extremities: Symmetry (describe any variations from normal)? Abrasions? Bruises? Swollen? Edema? Rashes/lesions (describe)? Prosthesis? Varicose veins?

GENITOURINARY AND RECTUM   Inspection

Rectum: Hemorrhoids? Inflammation? Lesions? Skin tags? Fissures? Excoriation? Swelling? Mucosal bulging? Retrocele?

Female Genitalia: Pubic hair distribution and color? Nits? Pediculosis? Lesions? Nodules? Inflammation? Swelling? Pigmentation? Dry? Moist? Shriveled, atrophy, or full labia? Discharge (describe)? Odor? Asymmetry? Varicosities? Uterine prolapse? Smegma? Rash?

Male Genitalia: Pubic hair distribution and color? Nits? Pediculosis? Circumcised/uncircumcised? Phimosis? Epispadias? Hypospadias? Smegma? Priapism? Varicocele? Cryptorchism? Hydrocele? Swelling? Redness? Chancre? Crusting? Rash? Discharge (describe)? Edema? Scrotal sack rugated? Atrophy?

NEUROLOGICAL

Describe tics, twitches, paresthesia, paralysis, coordination.

Gait: Balanced? Shuffling? Unsteady? Ataxic? Parkinsonian? Swaying? Scissor? Spastic? Waddling? Staggering? Faltering? Swaying? Slow? Difficult? Tottering? Propulsive?

Accessory Nerve (CN XI): Shrugs shoulder? Symmetry?

Reflexes: Report as present or absent.

Coordination: Report as to test done.

Cranial Nerves: May be reported here.

MENTAL STATUS

Level of Alertness: Alert? Stuporous? Semicomatose? Comatose?

Orientation: Oriented to time, place, and person? Confused? Disoriented? If confused, check orientation as follows:
Time—Ask client year, month, day, date.
Place—Ask client's residence address, where she/he is now.
Person—Ask client's name, birthday.

Memory: Recent memory—Give client short series of numbers and ask client to repeat those numbers at a later time. Long-term memory—Ask client to recall some event that happened several years ago.

Language and Speech: Language spoken? Speech slurred? Speech slow/rapid? Difficulty forming words? Aphasia?

Responsiveness: Responds appropriately to verbal stimuli? Responds readily? Slow to respond?

Sample Mental Status Assessment Form

Date _____ Room number _____ Date of admission _____

Patient name _____ Date of birth _____ Age _____

Social Security number _____ Marital status: M W S D

Medicaid number _____ Other insurance _____

Primary physician _____ Phone _____

Name of facility _____ Phone _____

Family/relative _____ Phone _____

_____ Phone _____

Medical diagnoses _____

_____

Current behavior requiring evaluation:

ASSESSMENT DATA:
Pertinent medical data from: Medical record _____ Family _____ Self _____ Other _____

Medications/other substances:

Pertinent data from: Staff _____ Family _____

Current physical status

   Mobility:

Adapted from Hogstel MO (1990). Geropsychiatric nursing, St Louis, The CV Mosby Co.

Elimination:

Dietary:

Sleep patterns:

Major physical problems:

Psychosocial assessment

Current stressors:

Coping skills:

Psychiatric history (self and/or family):

Assets:

Patient's view of current problem:

Mental status assessment

Appearance/dress:

Orientation: Person _____   Place _____   Date/time _____

Short portable mental status questionnaire (SPMSQ) _____   Mental status questionnaire (MSQ) _____

Speech:

Eye contact: Good _____   Poor _____

Affect:

Mood:

Memory: Immediate

Recent

Remote

Intelligence: Vocabulary

Calculations

Abstract thinking: Judgment

Proverbs

Analogies

Attention span:

Thought content:

Cognitive impairment ____ yes ____ no

Depressive ____ yes ____ no   Suicidal ____ yes ____ no How? _____

Paranoid beliefs ____ yes ____ no   Type _____

Phobias ____ yes ____ no   Delusions ____ yes ____ no

Hallucinations ____ yes ____ no   ____ Auditory ____ Visual

Other _____

Thought process:

Insight:

Activity level: Appropriate _____ Restless _____ Lethargic _____

Attitude:

Other behavior/observations:

Summary/impressions/recommendations:

Reported to _____

Date _____ Signature _____

Agencies and Organizations Providing Resources and Information for and about Older Adults

Administration on Aging
330 Independence Avenue, SW
Washington, DC 20201
(202) 245-0641

Alzheimer's Disease and Related Disorders Association, Inc.
70 East Lake Street
Chicago, IL 60601
(800) 621-0379

American Association for Geriatric Psychiatry
PO Box 376-A
Greenbelt, MD 20770
(301) 220-0952

American Association of Homes for the Aging
1129 20th Street, NW, Suite 400
Washington, DC 20036-3489
(202) 296-5960

American Association of Retired Persons
601 East Street NW
Washington, DC 20049
(202) 434-2277

American Association of Retired Persons Andrus Foundation
601 East Street, NW
Washington, DC 20049

American Cancer Society
1599 Clifton Road NE
Atlanta, GA 30329
(404) 320-3333

American College of Nursing Home Administrators
4650 East-West Freeway
Washington, DC 20014

American Diabetes Association
1660 Duke Street
Alexandria, VA 22314
(703) 549-1500

American Geriatrics Society
770 Lexington Avenue, Suite 400
New York, NY 10021
(212) 308-1414

American Health Care Association
1200 L Street, NW
Washington, DC 20005
(202) 842-4444

**American Nurses' Association
Council on Gerontological Nursing Practice**
2420 Pershing Road
Kansas City, MO 64108
(816) 474-5720

American Psychiatric Association
1400 K Street, NW
Washington, DC 20005
(202) 682-6239

American Society on Aging
833 Market Street, Suite 516
San Francisco, CA 94103
(415) 543-2617

Arthritis Foundation
1314 Spring Street, NW
Atlanta, GA 30309
(404) 872-7100

Association for Gerontology in Higher Education
600 Maryland Avenue, SW, WW 204
Washington, DC 20024

Children of Aging Parents
1609 Woodbourne Road 302-A
Box KC-791
Levittown, PA 19057

Elder Abuse Hot Line
1-800-252-5400

Federal Council on Aging
330 Independence Avenue, SW, Room 4280 HHS-N
Washington, DC 20201
(202) 245-2451

Gerontological Society of America
1275 K Street, NW, Suite 350
Washington, DC 20005-4006
(202) 842-1275

Gray Panthers
311 South Juniper Street, Suite 601
Philadelphia, PA 19107
(215) 545-6555

National Association for Home Care
519 C Street, NE
Washington, DC 20002
(202) 547-7424

National Association of Area Agencies on Aging
600 Maryland Avenue, SW, Suite 208 W
Washington, DC 20024
(202) 484-7520

National Caucus and Center on the Black Aged, Inc
1424 K Street, NW, Suite 500
Washington, DC 20005
(202) 637-8400

National Council of Senior Citizens
925 15th Street, NW
Washington, DC 20005
(202) 347-8800

National Council on the Aging
600 Maryland Avenue SW, West Wing 100
Washington, DC 20024
(202) 479-1200

National Geriatrics Society
212 West Wisconsin Avenue
Milwaukee, WI 53203

National Institute on Aging
Public Information Office
Federal Building, Room 6C12
9000 Rockville Pike
Bethesda, MD 20892
(301) 496-1752

National League for Nursing
10 Columbus Circle
New York, NY 10019-1350
(212) 582-1022

National Retired Teachers' Association
601 East Street, NW
Washington, DC 20049
(202) 434-2277

Older Women's League
730 Eleventh Street, NW, Suite 300
Washington, DC 20001
(202) 783-6686

Social Security Administration
Office of Public Inquiries
6401 Security Boulevard
Baltimore, MD 21235
(800) 234-5772

Veterans Administration
Office of Public Affairs
810 Vermont Avenue NW
Washington, DC 20420
(202) 233-4000

Journals and Other Publications Related to Gerontology and Gerontological Nursing

Write to the addresses listed for subscription prices and frequency of publication.

AARP Bulletin
3200 E. Carson St.
Lakewood, Calif 90712

Age Page
National Institute on Aging
U.S. Department of Health and Human Services
U.S. Government Printing Office
Washington, DC 20402

Aging
Office of Human Development Services
U.S. Department of Health and Human Services
200 Independence Avenue, SW
Washington, DC 20201

Changes—Research on Aging and the Aged
Superintendent of Documents
U.S. Government Printing Office
Washington, DC 20402

Generations
833 Market Street, Room 516
San Francisco, CA 94103

Geriatric Nursing
Mosby Year-Book
11830 Westline Industrial Drive
St. Louis, MO 63146

Geriatrics
For the Primary Care Physician
Harcourt Brace Jovanovich Publications
1 East First Street
Duluth, MN 55802

The Gerontologist
1275 K Street, NW, Suite 350
Washington, DC 20005-4006

Gerontology Newsletter
Institute of Human Development and Family Studies
Main Building 2300
University of Texas at Austin
Austin, TX 78712

Home Healthcare Nurse
680 Route 206 North
Bridgewater, NJ 08807

The International Journal of Aging and Human Development
Baywood Publishing Co., Inc.
26 Austin Avenue, PO Box 337
Amityville, NY 11701

Journal of the American Geriatrics Society
30 Rutgers Road
Wellesley, MA 02181

Journal of Geriatric Psychiatry
International Universities Press, Inc.
59 Boston Post Road
PO Box 1524
Madison, CT 06443-1524

Journal of Gerontological Nursing
Slack Incorporated
6900 Grove Road
Thorofare, NJ 08086

Journals of Gerontology
1275 K Street, NW, Suite 350
Washington, DC 20005-4006

Long-Term Care Currents
Ross Laboratories
625 Cleveland Avenue
Columbus, OH 43216

Long-Term Care Quarterly
American Nurses' Association
2420 Pershing Road
Kansas City, MO 64108

Modern Maturity
Publication of the American Association
  of Retired Persons
3200 East Carson Street
Lakewood, CA 90712

National Retired Teachers' Association Journal
601 East Street, NW
Washington, DC 20049

Research on Aging
A Quarterly of Social Gerontology &
  Adult Development
Sage Publications, Inc.
2111 West Hillcrest Drive
Newbury Park, CA 91320

INDEX

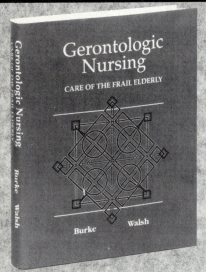
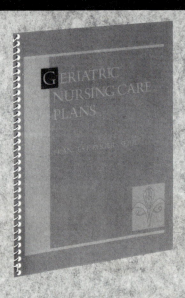
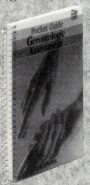
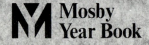